Advances in Veterinary Neurology

Editors

NATASHA J. OLBY
NICHOLAS D. JEFFERY

VETERINARY CLINICS
OF NORTH AMERICA:
SMALL ANIMAL PRACTICE

www.vetsmall.theclinics.com

November 2014 • Volume 44 • Number 6

ELSEVIER

1600 John F. Kennedy Boulevard • Suite 1800 • Philadelphia, Pennsylvania, 19103-2899
http://www.vetsmall.theclinics.com

**VETERINARY CLINICS OF NORTH AMERICA: SMALL ANIMAL PRACTICE Volume 44, Number 6
November 2014 ISSN 0195-5616, ISBN-13: 978-0-323-32690-2**

Editor: Patrick Manley
Developmental Editor: Susan Showalter

Veterinary Clinics of North America: Small Animal Practice (ISSN 0195-5616) is published bimonthly by Elsevier Inc., 360 Park Avenue South, New York, NY 10010-1710. Months of issue are January, March, May, July, September, and November. Business and Editorial Offices: 1600 John F. Kennedy Blvd., Ste. 1800, Philadelphia, PA 19103-2899. Customer Service Office: 3251 Riverport Lane, Maryland Heights, MO 63043. Periodicals postage paid at New York, NY and additional mailing offices. Subscription prices are $310.00 per year (domestic individuals), $500.00 per year (domestic institutions), $150.00 per year (domestic students/residents), $410.00 per year (Canadian individuals), $621.00 per year (Canadian institutions), $455.00 per year (international individuals), $621.00 per year (international institutions), and $220.00 per year (international and Canadian students/residents). To receive student/resident rate, orders must be accompanied by name of affiliated institution, date of term, and the *signature* of program/residency coordinator on institution letterhead. Orders will be billed at individual rate until proof of status is received. Foreign air speed delivery is included in all *Clinics* subscription prices. All prices are subject to change without notice. **POSTMASTER:** Send address changes to *Veterinary Clinics of North America: Small Animal Practice*, Elsevier Health Sciences Division, Subscription Customer Service, 3251 Riverport Lane, Maryland Heights, MO 63043. Customer Service (orders, claims, online, change of address): Elsevier Periodicals Customer Service, Elsevier Health Sciences Division Subscription Customer Service 3251 Riverport Lane Maryland Heights, MO 63043. Tel: 1-800-654-2452 (U.S. and Canada); 314-447-8871 (outside U.S. and Canada). Fax: 314-447-8029. E-mail: journalscustomerservice-usa@elsevier.com (for print support); journalsonlinesupport-usa@elsevier.com (for online support).

Reprints. For copies of 100 or more of articles in this publication, please contact the Commercial Reprints Department, Elsevier Inc., 360 Park Avenue South, New York, NY 10010-1710. Tel.: 212-633-3874; Fax: 212-633-3820; E-mail: reprints@elsevier.com.

Veterinary Clinics of North America: Small Animal Practice is also published in Japanese by Inter Zoo Publishing Co., Ltd., Aoyama Crystal-Bldg 5F, 3-5-12 Kitaaoyama, Minato-ku, Tokyo 107-0061, Japan.

Veterinary Clinics of North America: Small Animal Practice is covered in *Current Contents/Agriculture, Biology and Environmental Sciences, Science Citation Index, ASCA, MEDLINE/PubMed (Index Medicus), Excerpta Medica, and BIOSIS*.

Contributors

EDITORS

NATASHA J. OLBY, VetMB, PhD, MRCVS
Diplomate, American College of Veterinary Internal Medicine (Neurology); Professor of Neurology/Neurosurgery, Department of Clinical Sciences, College of Veterinary Medicine, North Carolina State University, Raleigh, North Carolina

NICHOLAS D. JEFFERY, BVSc, PhD, MSc, FRCVS
Diplomate, European College of Veterinary Neurology; Diplomate, European College of Veterinary Surgeons; Professor of Neurology and Neurosurgery, Department of Veterinary Clinical Sciences, Lloyd Veterinary Medical Center, College of Veterinary Medicine, Iowa State University, Ames, Iowa

AUTHORS

SÒNIA AÑOR, DVM, PhD
Professor and Head of the Neurology-Neurosurgery Service, Facultat de Veterinària, Department of Animal Medicine and Surgery, Veterinary School, Autonomous University of Barcelona, Bellaterra, Barcelona, Spain

DARREN CARWARDINE, BVSc
The School of Veterinary Sciences, University of Bristol, Langford, North Somerset, United Kingdom

JOAN R. COATES, DVM, MS
Diplomate, American College of Veterinary Internal Medicine (Neurology); Professor of Neurology and Neurosurgery, Department of Veterinary Medicine and Surgery, Veterinary Medical Teaching Hospital, College of Veterinary Medicine, University of Missouri, Columbia, Missouri

NICOLAS GRANGER, DVM, PhD, MRCVS
Diplomate, European College of Veterinary Neurology; The School of Veterinary Sciences, University of Bristol, Langford, North Somerset, United Kingdom

ELIZABETH HEAD, MA, PhD
Associate Professor, Department of Pharmacology and Nutritional Sciences, Sanders-Brown Center on Aging, University of Kentucky, Lexington, Kentucky

NICHOLAS D. JEFFERY, BVSc, PhD, MSc, FRCVS
Diplomate, European College of Veterinary Neurology; Diplomate, European College of Veterinary Surgeons; Professor of Neurology and Neurosurgery, Department of Veterinary Clinical Sciences, Lloyd Veterinary Medical Center, College of Veterinary Medicine, Iowa State University, Ames, Iowa

CATHRYN MELLERSH, BSc, PhD
Head of Canine Genetics, Centre for Preventive Medicine, Animal Health Trust, Lanwades Park, Kentford, Newmarket, Suffolk, United Kingdom

HIDETAKA NISHIDA, DVM, PhD
Institute for Regenerative Medicine, Texas A&M Health Science Center, College of Medicine at Scott & White, Temple, Texas

NATASHA J. OLBY, VetMB, PhD, MRCVS
Diplomate, American College of Veterinary Internal Medicine (Neurology); Professor of Neurology/Neurosurgery, Department of Clinical Sciences, College of Veterinary Medicine, North Carolina State University, Raleigh, North Carolina

EDWARD (NED) E. PATTERSON, DVM, PhD
Diplomate, American College of Veterinary Internal Medicine (Small Animal Internal Medicine); Associate Professor, College of Veterinary Medicine, University of Minnesota, St Paul, Minnesota

SIMON PLATT, BVM&S, MRCVS
Diplomate, American College of Veterinary Internal Medicine (Neurology); Diplomate, European College of Veterinary Neurology; Professor Neurology and Neurosurgery Service, Department of Small Animal Medicine and Surgery, College of Veterinary Medicine, University of Georgia, Athens, Georgia

JOHN H. ROSSMEISL, DVM, MS
Diplomate, American College of Veterinary Internal Medicine (Small Animal Internal Medicine and Neurology); Associate Professor, Neurology and Neurosurgery, Department of Small Animal Clinical Sciences, VA-MD Regional College of Veterinary Medicine, Virginia Tech, Blacksburg, Virginia

GANOKON URKASEMSIN, DVM, PhD
Department of Pre-Clinic and Applied Animal Science, Faculty of Veterinary Science, Mahidol University, Salaya, Phuttamonthon, Nakhon Pathom, Thailand

CHARLES H. VITE, DVM, PhD
Diplomate, American College of Veterinary Internal Medicine (Neurology); Associate Professor, School of Veterinary Medicine, Section of Neurology and Neurosurgery, Department of Clinical Studies - Philadelphia, University of Pennsylvania, Philadelphia, Pennsylvania

FRED WININGER, VMD, MS
Diplomate, American College of Veterinary Internal Medicine (Neurology); Department of Neurology/Neurosurgery, Veterinary Specialty Services, Manchester, Missouri; Adjunct Professor-Neurology/Neurosurgery, University of Missouri-College of Veterinary Medicine, Veterinary Medicine and Surgery, Columbia, Missouri

Contents

Preface: Advances in Veterinary Neurology xi

Natasha J. Olby and Nicholas D. Jeffery

New Treatment Modalities for Brain Tumors in Dogs and Cats 1013

John H. Rossmeisl

> Despite advancements in standard therapies, intracranial tumors remain a significant source of morbidity and mortality in veterinary and human medicine. Several newer approaches are gaining more widespread acceptance or are currently being prepared for translation from experimental to routine therapeutic use. Clinical trials in dogs with spontaneous brain tumors have contributed to the development and human translation of several novel therapeutic brain tumor approaches.

Altered States of Consciousness in Small Animals 1039

Simon Platt

> Impaired states of consciousness can be relatively easily identified, although it can occasionally be difficult to assess whether there is a pure disorder of wakefulness or awareness. Regardless, such impairments represent dysfunction of the brainstem and or cerebrum. Acute and severe impairments of consciousness can require immediate assessment, in part currently performed using the modified Glasgow coma scoring system, and emergency stabilization. The prognosis is always guarded and highly sensitive to the underlying etiology.

Corticosteroid Use in Small Animal Neurology 1059

Nicholas D. Jeffery

> Glucocorticoid drugs are frequently used nonspecifically by veterinarians to control clinical signs associated with central nervous system disease. However, this use is infrequently justified and can also be associated with detrimental long-term patient outcomes. First, there are few diseases for which glucocorticoids are the preferred or definitive treatment. Second, their actions may blunt subsequent diagnostic efforts, for instance, by altering MRI appearance or cerebrospinal fluid cell content, or lead owners to abandon pursuit of more appropriate therapies if they perceive the first-line steroid therapy to be a failure.

Canine Hereditary Ataxia 1075

Ganokon Urkasemsin and Natasha J. Olby

> The hereditary ataxias are a group of neurodegenerative diseases that cause a progressive (or episodic) cerebellar ataxia. A large number of different disorders have been described in different breeds of purebred dog, and in some instances, more than one disorder occurs in a single breed, creating a confusing clinical picture. The mutations associated with these disorders are being described at a rapid rate, potentially changing our ability to prevent, diagnose, and treat affected dogs. A breed-related

neurodegenerative process should be suspected in any pure bred dog with slowly progressive, symmetric signs of ataxia.

Canine Paroxysmal Movement Disorders   1091

Ganokon Urkasemsin and Natasha J. Olby

Paroxysmal dyskinesias are episodic movement disorders characterized by muscle hypertonicity that can produce involuntary movements. Signs emanate from the central nervous system; consciousness is not impaired, ictal electroencephalography is normal, and there are no autonomic signs, distinguishing them from seizure disorders. In humans they are classified into 3 groups, each responding to different therapies. A mutation in the gene for brevican (*BCAN*) has been identified as the cause of Episodic Falling in Cavalier King Charles spaniels. Further elucidation of the genetic causes will enhance our ability to identify and treat these canine diseases.

Status Epilepticus and Cluster Seizures   1103

Edward (Ned) E. Patterson

Status epilepticus (SE) is a medical emergency for companion animals, with significant associated morbidity and mortality. Therapy in companion animals and people has been largely with sedatives and anesthetics, many of which have gamma-aminobutyric acid receptor-mediated mechanisms. Early aggressive treatment includes staged first-line therapy with benzodiazepines, and second- and third-line protocols when needed. Recently, intravenous levetiracetam has also been used in for SE in dogs and people, and there are other human intravenous drug preparations that may hold promise for future use in companion animals.

Aging in the Canine and Feline Brain   1113

Charles H. Vite and Elizabeth Head

Aging dogs and cats show neurodegenerative features that are similar to human aging and Alzheimer disease. Neuropathologic changes with age may be linked to signs of cognitive dysfunction both in the laboratory and in a clinic setting. Less is known about cat brain aging and cognition and this represents an area for further study. Neurodegenerative diseases such as lysosomal storage diseases in dogs and cats also show similar features of human aging, suggesting some common underlying pathogenic mechanisms and also suggesting pathways that can be modified to promote healthy brain aging.

Acute Spinal Cord Injury: Tetraplegia and Paraplegia in Small Animals   1131

Nicolas Granger and Darren Carwardine

 Videos of: (1) extension of the digits in response to stimulation of the plantar surface in a dog following severe SCI; (2) 5-year-old male neutered paraplegic Dachshund showing evidence of neuropathic pain around the lesion site; (3) and 8-year-old female neutered Jack Russell terrier following a road traffic accident and complete luxation of the C5-C6 vertebrae accompany this article

Spinal cord injury (SCI) is a common problem in animals for which definitive treatment is lacking, and information gained from its study has benefit for both companion animals and humans in developing new therapeutic approaches. This review provides an overview of the main concepts that are useful for clinicians in assessing companion animals with severe acute SCI. Current available advanced ancillary tests and those in development are reviewed. In addition, the current standard of care for companion animals following SCI and recent advances in the development of new therapies are presented, and new predictors of recovery discussed.

Perspectives on Meningoencephalomyelitis of Unknown Origin   1157

Joan R. Coates and Nicholas D. Jeffery

Meningoencephalomyelitis of unknown origin (MUO) is a heterogeneous group of overlapping central nervous system inflammatory diseases of unknown cause. This article highlights the current understanding of MUO and its phenotypic variants encountered in clinical practice. Diagnostic evaluation of presumptive MUO includes lesion distribution on magnetic resonance imaging and ruling out other acquired diseases. Recent evidence provides further knowledge of immune-mediated processes that underlie the pathogenesis of MUO. Current empiric treatment options include corticosteroids and other adjunctive immunomodulating therapies. As the understanding of neuroimmunology and genetic influences on these disorders evolves, a more targeted treatment approach is becoming attainable.

Biomarkers for Neural Injury and Infection in Small Animals   1187

Hidetaka Nishida

Cross-sectional imaging techniques have facilitated diagnosis of central nervous system (CNS) diseases. However, there is still frequently a lack of definition of the cause of neurologic lesions, because tissue sampling from the pathologic site is often difficult and there are few clinical diagnostic tools to assist diagnosis. Biomarkers can assist in understanding the cause, diagnosis, severity, and prognosis for neural injury. Integration of conventional testing and new diagnostic techniques will overcome shortcomings in understanding infectious diseases of the CNS. Diagnostic tests may be limited by poor positive and negative predictive values, which must be recognized when interpreting test results.

Acute Lower Motor Neuron Tetraparesis   1201

Sònia Añor

Flaccid nonambulatory tetraparesis or tetraplegia is an infrequent neurologic presentation; it is characteristic of neuromuscular disease (lower motor neuron [LMN] disease) rather than spinal cord disease. Paresis beginning in the pelvic limbs and progressing to the thoracic limbs resulting in flaccid tetraparesis or tetraplegia within 24 to 72 hours is a common presentation of peripheral nerve or neuromuscular junction disease. Complete body flaccidity develops with severe decrease or complete loss of spinal reflexes in pelvic and thoracic limbs. Animals with acute generalized LMN tetraparesis commonly show severe motor dysfunction in all limbs and severe generalized weakness in all muscles.

Inherited Neurologic Disorders in the Dog: The Science Behind the Solutions   1223

Cathryn Mellersh

> Canine inherited neurologic diseases are clinically varied and can be congenital, neonatal, or late onset as well as progressive or stationary. Modern genetic technologies are revolutionizing the speed and efficiency with which mutations responsible for inherited neurologic disease are being identified. Clinically similar disorders can be caused by different mutations, even within a single breed, and are thus genetically distinct. DNA tests can be used by dog breeders to reduce the prevalence of inherited neurologic disorders in specific breeds and help the veterinarian diagnose disease.

Neuronavigation in Small Animals: Development, Techniques, and Applications   1235

Fred Wininger

> A persistent obstacle to accurate diagnosis and treatment of brain disease has been the difficulties in safely obtaining representative biopsy material in a live patient. Major problems are the variability in the anatomy between individuals and the inability to reliably locate deep structures through reliance on surface anatomic features. Although stereotaxic devices have been available for many years, they have now been supplanted by frameless systems, which are more accurate and less cumbersome and allow good surgical access and provision of intraoperative feedback of instrument location.

Index   1249

VETERINARY CLINICS OF NORTH AMERICA: SMALL ANIMAL PRACTICE

FORTHCOMING ISSUES

January 2015
Rehabilitation and Physical Therapy
Denis J. Marcellin-Little, David Levine, and Darryl L. Millis, *Editors*

March 2015
Infection Control
Jason Stull and Scott Weese, *Editors*

May 2015
Soft Tissue Surgery
Lisa M. Howe and Harry W. Boothe Jr, *Editors*

RECENT ISSUES

September 2014
Advances in Oncology
Annette N. Smith, *Editor*

July 2014
Clinical Nutrition
Dottie P. Laflamme and Debra L. Zoran, *Editors*

May 2014
Behavior: A Guide for Practitioners
Gary M. Landsberg and Valarie V. Tynes, *Editors*

RELATED INTEREST

Veterinary Clinics of North America: Equine Practice
December 2011, Volume 27, Issue 3
Clinical Neurology
Thomas J. Divers and Amy L. Johnson, *Editors*

THE CLINICS ARE NOW AVAILABLE ONLINE!
Access your subscription at:
www.theclinics.com

Preface

Advances in Veterinary Neurology

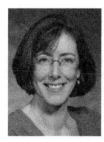 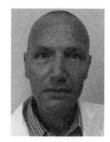

Natasha J. Olby, VetMB, PhD,
MRCVSb

Nicholas D. Jeffery, BVSc,
PhD, MSc, FRCVS

Editors

This issue of *Veterinary Clinics of North America: Small Animal Practice* is focused on "Advances in Veterinary Neurology." This is an easy title to give, because there will always be advances, but we feel it is particularly appropriate now, with veterinary neurology experiencing a dramatic and exciting expansion phase. MRI is now a routine diagnostic modality for veterinary neurologists, and our comfort with advanced imaging modalities is being coupled with advances in computer technology to provide additional diagnostic and therapeutic power. In addition, the revolution in genetic techniques has led to an explosion of knowledge of the genetic cause underpinning hereditary neurologic disorders, providing diagnostic tests, and potentially leading to therapeutic interventions for previously untreatable diseases.

The first section of this issue covers neurologic emergencies; as anyone working in small animal practice knows, diseases of the nervous system frequently present on an emergency basis and require accurate assessment and prompt initiation of the appropriate treatment. In four articles, spanning altered mental status, seizures and status epilepticus, spinal cord disease, and neuromuscular disease, logical approaches to these cases are described, and therapeutic algorithms are discussed. The authors have presented up-to-date information on how to assess the patients and highlighted the most recent advances in treatment.

The second section highlights significant novel advances in veterinary neurology; the application of computer technology to medicine continues unabated. There are two examples in this section: the development of new therapies for brain tumors and precise neuronavigation within the CNS. These both rely on the ability to translate computerized images from one "platform" to another and to use computer analysis to provide feedback on the efficacy of various approaches during the period in which treatment is administered. While these techniques are likely to remain the preserve of specialist facilities, they are both likely to become more widely available and pave the way for

http://dx.doi.org/10.1016/j.cvsm.2014.08.001

vetsmall.theclinics.com

an increase in tertiary referral centers. This section also reviews extremely relevant issues for general practitioners, including the use of corticosteroids in neurology; this article was triggered simply from the numerous questions that continue to arise regarding this subject. The final section covers neurogenetics and neurodegenerative diseases, providing a clear summary of how genetic diseases are mapped and how to use genetic testing, in addition to updates on brain aging, and classification and understanding of a variety of different movement disorders.

We asked each author to approach their subjects from a novel standpoint, with the aim that new information and new approaches will be conveyed and therefore lead to different ways of understanding and responding to diseased animals. Many of these advances have been driven by clinical need or the need for new tools to form the basis of research into possible treatments. This insight provides a window into the thinking behind new therapies in veterinary neurology. We hope that veterinarians will find the new information presented both interesting and useful on a daily basis in the clinic.

We would like to thank John Vassallo for inviting us to edit this issue and for providing us with the freedom to cover really novel topics. We are extremely grateful to the authors who generated cutting-edge articles and suffered our questions with grace and good humor. Finally, we are grateful to our families, Unity Jeffery, and Erik and Izzy Jackson, who have tolerated our lapses in attention and failure to provide dinner at a reasonable time.

Natasha J. Olby, VetMB, PhD, MRCVS
Department of Clinical Sciences
College of Veterinary Medicine
North Carolina State University
Raleigh, NC, USA

Nicholas D. Jeffery, BVSc, PhD, MSc, FRCVS
Department of Veterinary Clinical Sciences
Lloyd Veterinary Medical Center
College of Veterinary Medicine
Iowa State University
Ames, IA, USA

E-mail addresses:
njolby@ncsu.edu (N.J. Olby)
njeffery@iastate.edu (N.D. Jeffery)

New Treatment Modalities for Brain Tumors in Dogs and Cats

John H. Rossmeisl, DVM, MS

KEYWORDS

- Canine • Central nervous system • Convection-enhanced delivery • Feline • Glioma
- Immunotherapy • Oncology • Radiotherapy

KEY POINTS

- Advancements in magnetic resonance (MRI) and functional neuroimaging will continue to improve the clinical management of brain tumors.
- Stereotactic radiosurgery (SRS) is emerging as a viable treatment of many canine and feline brain tumors and can be performed with minimal toxicity using dedicated radiosurgical units or contemporary linear accelerators.
- Convention-enhanced delivery (CED) is a promising therapeutic platform that bypasses the blood-brain barrier (BBB), allowing for direct administration of macromolecular antineoplastic agents to brain tumors.
- CED is used to treat dogs with spontaneous brain tumors but consistent and accurate delivery of drugs remains a challenge to mainstream clinical adoption of this technique.
- Advancements in neuroimmunology and tumor biology have led to the development and clinical translation of several novel immunotherapies with therapeutic potential in canine and human brain tumors.

INTRODUCTION

Transformative advances in MRI over the past 3 decades allow for the detailed neuro-anatomic characterization and presumptive antemortem diagnosis of many canine and feline brain tumors.[1–4] MRI has also served as a fundamental platform for the development of technologies and procedures that have contributed to improvements in the management of brain tumors, including image-guided neuronavigation, functional neuroimaging, surgical and radiotherapeutic planning, and objective therapeutic response assessment.[5–9] Despite this progress, definitive antemortem diagnosis of brain tumors in animals remains uncommon, and few data exist in veterinary medicine

Neurology and Neurosurgery, Department of Small Animal Clinical Sciences, VA-MD Regional College of Veterinary Medicine, Virginia Tech, 215 Duckpond Drive, Mail Code 0442, Blacksburg, VA 24061, USA
E-mail address: jrossmei@vt.edu

Vet Clin Small Anim 44 (2014) 1013–1038
http://dx.doi.org/10.1016/j.cvsm.2014.07.003
0195-5616/14/$ – see front matter Published by Elsevier Inc.
vetsmall.theclinics.com

regarding the influence of treatment on clinical outcomes of animals with brain tumors. Primary brain tumors, in particular the malignant variants, remain a source of significant morbidity and mortality in small animals and humans.[10,11]

Current Therapeutic Options

The prognosis for dogs with palliatively-treated brain tumors is poor. In one study of dogs with brain tumors definitively diagnosed at necropsy, the reported overall median survival was approximately 2 months after diagnosis via brain imaging.[10] Surgical resection and fractionated radiotherapy are currently the principal methods used to treat canine and feline brain tumors, and these therapies are capable of improving both the quality and quantity of life in small animals. However, both surgery and radiotherapy can be associated with treatment-associated morbidity, and local treatment failures after these therapies remain a common cause of death or euthanasia.[12–17] Surgical treatment has been best described for forebrain meningiomas, which is the most common primary brain tumor type in both dogs and cats.[8,12–15] In dogs with meningiomas, the reported median survival after traditional surgical resection is approximately 7 months.[12] In cats, the median survival after surgical resection of forebrain meningiomas is 24 months [13,14] Neurosurgical treatment that incorporates devices that improve intraoperative visualization, such as intracranial endoscopy, or facilitate tumor extirpation have been associated with median survivals ranging from 42 to 70 months.[8,15] Transsphenoidal hypophysectomy has been demonstrated to be an effective surgical technique in dogs and cats with nonenlarged to moderately enlarged pituitary adenomas, with a reported 4-year survival rate of 68% in dogs.[16] Currently available surgical techniques often preclude safe resection of intraparenchymal tumors that are infiltrating the surrounding brain or intimately associated with critical neuroanatomic structures. There is little information available regarding the efficacy of or indications for surgery in canine and feline brain tumors other than meningiomas and pituitary tumors.

Fractionated radiotherapy is beneficial in the treatment of brain tumors as a sole therapeutic modality or as an adjuvant after surgery.[12–18] Studies investigating treatment of a variety of presumptively diagnosed brain tumors in dogs with fractionated radiotherapy reported median survivals that range from approximately 300 to 700 days.[17,18] Dogs with meningiomas treated with 3-D conformal radiation therapy had an overall median survival of 577 days, and the median survival increased to nearly 30 months (ie, approximately 900 days) when dogs dying of causes other than meningioma were excluded.[19] Systemically administered cytotoxic chemotherapeutics, including those agents capable of penetrating BBB, are largely ineffective as sole agents for the treatment of brain tumors. A recent study failed to demonstrate any difference in survival between dogs with brain tumors treated symptomatically with prednisone and anticonvulsant drugs compared with those that received symptomatic therapy and lomustine.[20]

There is increasing recognition of the epidemiologic, neuropathologic, molecular, and genetic homologies between canine and human brain tumors, which has driven the use of dogs with spontaneous brain tumors as a translational disease model.[21–23] This review introduces contemporary therapeutic advancements for brain tumors and illustrates the role that tumor-bearing dogs have made to progressing the field of translational neuro-oncology. Because an exhaustive survey of brain tumor treatment is beyond the scope of this article, it focuses on SRS, CED, and immunotherapy (IT). These therapies hold great promise for the treatment of brain tumors and are being used clinically in dogs and cats.[23–25] Reviews of boron neutron capture therapy, brachytherapy, high-intensity focused ultrasound (HiFU), gene therapy, laser interstitial thermal therapy, proton beam radiotherapy, oncolytic viruses, and pulsed electric fields are available elsewhere.[7,26–34]

These therapeutic approaches are not mutually exclusive. For example, because many molecularly targeted chemotherapeutics, gene-bearing vectors, and boron delivery agents are high-molecular-weight structures that cannot penetrate the BBB when administered systemically, they require delivery by a method that bypasses or disrupts the BBB, such as CED or HiFU.[23,26,30] Distinct advantages are also realized when biologically directed treatments, primarily in the form of target-specific monoclonal antibodies, are conjugated to chemotherapeutics in efforts to sensitize tumors to external beam radiotherapy or radionuclides to allow for more selective tumor irradiation.[35,36]

STEREOTACTIC RADIOSURGERY
Introduction and History

Stereotactic radiation therapy (SRT) broadly encompasses treatments that involve the delivery of high doses of ionizing radiation to a defined anatomic target in a limited number (typically 1–5) of therapeutic sessions. SRS is a subtype of SRT that consists of the treatment delivered as a single fraction.[37] Of the therapies reviewed in this article, only SRT and SRS are currently routinely used in veterinary clinical oncology practice for the treatment of brain tumors.

SRS represents a marriage of stereotactic and radiotherapeutic methods. The origins of the stereotactic method are attributed to Drs Robert Clarke, a surgeon and engineer, and neurosurgeon Victor Horsley, who in 1906 first used a stereotactic frame to lesion the brain of experimental animals.[38] It was not until 40 years later that stereotaxis was used in humans by Speigel and colleagues.[39] Their stereotactic device was based on the Cartesian coordinate system and modeled after the Clarke-Horsley instrument. Speigel and colleagues launched a revolution in stereotaxy that culminated in numerous apparatus, including those of Leksell,[40] Talairach and colleagues,[41] Narabayashi,[42] Riechert and Mundinger,[43] and Todd and Wells,[44] providing the foundations for contemporary stereotactic neurosurgery and SRS.

The concept of using intersecting charged particle beams to ablate intracranial structures can be attributed to Lawrence and colleagues in the late 1940s.[45] However, shortly after introducing his "arc-quadrant" stereotactic frame in 1949, which allowed for greater flexibility for instrument entry and trajectory selection, neurosurgeon Lars Leksell[46] developed and coined the term, SRS. Leksell attached an orthovoltage x-ray unit to his stereotactic frame to produce converging beams, which would intersect at the treatment target. Leksell's prototype device evolved into the Gamma Knife (Elekta AB, Stockholm, Sweden).

Technical Aspects of Stereotactic Radiosurgery

SRS is a noninvasive technique for the precision delivery of highly focused ionizing radiation that is an established therapy for several intracranial disorders in humans, including brain tumors. SRS commonly uses gamma radiation or photons, although it can also be accomplished using protons and other particles.[37] Irrespective of the hardware, software, and radiation source used, SRS includes the delivery of a high dose of radiation in a single treatment, the use of a steep dose gradient with minimal dose delivered to the surrounding brain, stereotactic localization of the target, computerized dosimetry planning, and a highly accurate radiation delivery system.[37] There are numerous radiotherapy devices and software systems capable of SRS, each associated with its own technical nuances, but only Gamma Knife,

CyberKnife (Accuray, Santa Clara, California), and linear accelerator–based SRS are discussed.

Treatment planning is the process of creating a radiation dose distribution that conformally treats the intended target. SRS is usually done using forward planning methods, but some systems allow for inverse planning.[47] Forward planning relies on the expertise of the planner to identify the target and adjacent critical structures as well as for manual trial and error simulations to determine the weights, beam orientation, and use of wedges or collimators to achieve the desired dose distribution. For inverse plans, the planner provides the target dose and dose limits and then a computer algorithm using an objective dose-based or radiobiological model to optimize the plan to closely approximate the input data.[47] Brain tumor treatment plans often involve both CT and MRI sets in planning software for optimal target definition (**Fig. 1**). Reviews of SRS treatment planning are available elsewhere.[48–50]

Stringent quality assurance beginning with patient positioning is essential to successful therapeutic planning and delivery to avoid exposure of normal tissues to high radiation doses. Numerous immobilization devices have been developed to facilitate patient positioning and treatment reproducibility, and it is recommended that patients are imaged in immediate proximity to therapy to confirm positioning (**Fig. 2**) and that therapeutic plans evaluated on phantoms prior to treatment.[25,51,52]

Linear accelerator stereotactic radiosurgery

Standard linear accelerators outfitted with a micromultileaf collimator or stereotactic cones for field shaping represent the most common, economical, and flexible therapeutic platforms currently available to deliver SRS or SRT in both human and veterinary medicine.[51–55] Linear accelerator radiosurgery systems focus a collimated x-ray beam on a stereotactically identified target. The gantry rotates over the patient, producing a target-focused radiation arc. The patient couch also rotates in the horizontal plane, and another arc is generated. Using this method, multiple noncoplanar intersecting arcs of radiation are produced.

Gamma Knife stereotactic radiosurgery

The Gamma Knife is the oldest and best-described dedicated SRS instrument and has been used to treat veterinary patients with intracranial tumors since 2009 (see **Figs. 1–3**).[37,40] Key to the precision and accuracy of the Gamma Knife is the

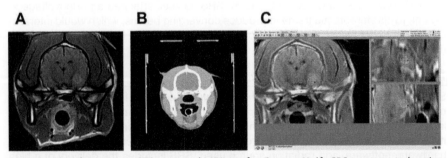

A   **B**   **C**

Fig. 1. Fusion of transverse CT image and MRI sets for Gamma Knife SRS treatment planning in a dog with biopsy confirmed grade II astrocytoma in the left temporal-piriform region. (*A*) Diagnostic, postcontrast T1-weighted MRI. (*B*) Postcontrast fiducial CT image obtained with the patient immobilized in the stereotactic head frame. (*C*) The CT and MRI data sets are imported into Leksell GammaPlan (Elekta AB, Stockholm, Sweden) software and fused for planning purposes.

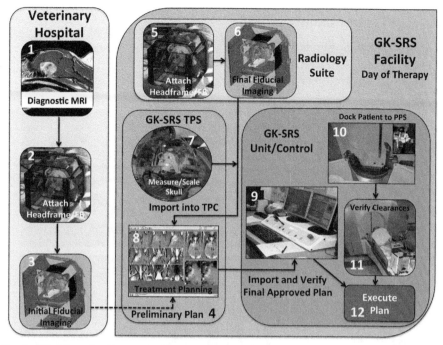

Fig. 2. Workflow for Gamma Knife stereotactic radiosurgical treatment (GK-SRS). Fiducial imaging is typically performed using CT. FB, fiducial box; PPS, patient positioning system; TPC, treatment planning computer; TPS, treatment planning suite.

proprietary rigid head frame that can be docked directly to the patient positioning system, which immobilizes the patient and creates a correspondence between the stereotactic coordinate system defined by the external head frame and the internal coordinate system within the radiotherapy unit (see **Fig. 2**).[56] The current version of the Gamma Knife, Perfexion (Elekta AB, Stockholm, Sweden), contains a hemispheric array of 192 individual cobalt-60 sources aligned with a collimation system. Collimation directs individual gamma radiation beams to a precise focal point. Although individual beams each impart a relatively low radiation dose, which causes minimal biological effect, the superposition of multiple cross-firing beams at the focal point allows precision delivery of high doses in a single therapeutic session.[57]

Cyberknife stereotactic radiosurgery
The CyberKnife system was developed in 1989 by Dr John Adler. It is a frameless, robotic, image-guided SRS system that manipulates a compact linear accelerator.[57] The robotic arm has 6° of freedom and can move in virtually all directions. The treatment suite is equipped with an x-ray stereophotogrammetric guidance system, which uses a patient's axial skeletal structures or implanted radio-opaque markers as stereotactic points of reference. The CyberKnife determines the dose range and quantity by integrating data from the robot and image guidance software, along with inputs from treatment planners, based on imaging studies. The system is capable of modifying the beam in relation to target motion in real-time during treatment. These features allow for frameless therapy, increasing fractionation flexibility, and the treatment of extracranial targets (stereotactic body radiation therapy).[57] The CyberKnife is currently in

Pretreatment

6 Months Post-Treatment

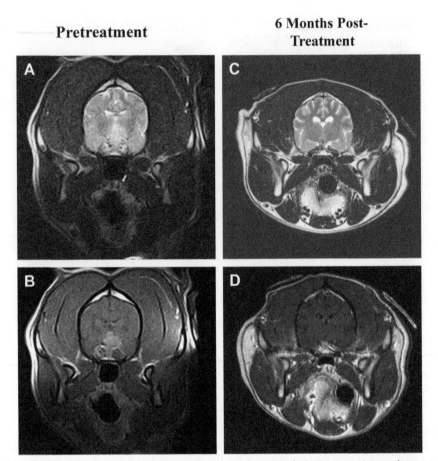

Fig. 3. Objective therapeutic response of a canine functional pituitary corticotroph macro-tumor to SRS. Pretreatment T2-weighted (A) and postcontrast T1-weighted (B) MRI illustrating the macrotumor. At the 6-month post-treatment recheck, the tumor demonstrated a partial response (C, D) and clinical signs of intracranial disease had resolved, but trilostane therapy was required to maintain endocrinologic remission.

clinical use at 2 veterinary referral centers in the United States: one in San Diego, California, and the other in Yonkers, New York.

Radiobiological Considerations

Fractionated radiotherapy relies on the differential susceptibility between normal and tumor tissue to achieve its therapeutic effects. With SRS, however, it is the precision dose delivery and steep peripheral dose gradient (dose avoidance) that provides for tumor control and tissue sparing.[58]

Besides patient and owner convenience associated with single-session therapy, there are several additional proven and potential radiobiological advantages of SRS. Studies have demonstrated that single-session high-dose (>10 Gy) radiotherapy protocols result in significant vascular damage, creating a hypoxic intratumoral microenvironment.[59] The radioprotective effects of hypoxia can be overcome with high-dose fractions, because tumor death occurs through both induction of DNA damage within tumor cells and microvascular dysfunction, resulting from vasculitis and apoptosis via the sphingomyelin pathway.[60,61] Cell cycle redistribution is also affected by high-dose radiation exposure. Single fractions in excess of 15 Gy result in indefinite arrest of the cells in the phases of the cell cycle in which they were irradiated, with arrested cells undergoing interphase death.[62] In the course of a conventional fractionated radiotherapy protocol, tumor cells surviving the radiation exposure proliferate, which increases the number of cells that must be killed during the course of therapy. Cellular repopulation of tumor cells typically occurs 3 to 4 weeks after initiation of radiotherapy. Considering the very short courses of SRS and SRT, compensatory repopulation should be negligible during treatment.[58] SRS therapy can also be repeated or administered after traditional fractionated radiotherapy for rescue treatment of recurrent brain tumors when the risk of adverse events associated with a course of fractionated therapy is considered unacceptable.

SRS has several limitations.[57,58] The extent of repair of sublethal damage in irradiated cells significantly influences their fate, and the repair rate of radiation damage is dependent on dose per fraction, dose rate, and inherent characteristics of irradiated cells. Below dose rates of approximately 1 Gy per minute, cells can repair sublethal damage more quickly than it is generated, which leads to increased survival for a given dose compared with higher dose rates. In fractionated irradiation, delivery of 1 to 2 Gy can be completed in minutes, which minimizes the repair of sublethal damage during the radiation exposure. It has been suggested that the treatment time for SRS may be important, especially for methods, such as Gamma Knife, in which therapeutic durations for delivery of commonly used 15- to 18-Gy single fractions can take an hour or more.[58]

In humans, tumor size is a major limitation of SRS, with masses greater than 3 cm in diameter considered poor candidates for treatment. The geometry of larger tumors lends itself to dose spillover outside the target volume, which increases the risk for symptomatic mass effect and normal tissue damage.[58,63] Although the maximal tumor sizes amenable to SRS in dogs and cats are unknown, it is likely that they are smaller than humans. Finally, despite adverse events associated with SRS uncommonly reported in humans and animals, radiation dose-response relationships in animals are likely different from those in humans and high dose-per-fraction prescriptions may influence the incidence of observed toxicity.[54,64]

Stereotactic Radiosurgery for Canine and Feline Brain Tumors

There are few published reports in the veterinary literature providing clinical data on SRS for the treatment of brain tumors, but SRS and SRT are rapidly evolving fields. Existing reports are promising, however, with regard to both the safety and the efficacy of SRS for canine and feline brain tumors.[25,52–55,65] It is also difficult to extract specific treatment guidelines and efficacy data from the literature for certain tumor types, given the small numbers and lack of histopathologic diagnosis in many canine and feline brain masses treated with SRS.[25,52–55] Despite these limitations, the clinical experience to date indicates SRS is feasible in dogs and cats, can result in comparable clinical outcomes to treatment with conventional fractionated radiotherapy protocols, and that significant toxicities associated with SRS seem uncommon.[25,52–55,65]

Meningiomas have been the most commonly reported intracranial tumor treated with SRS, and available data suggest that the median survival of dogs with meningiomas treated with SRS ranges from 1 to 2 years.[25,53,55,65] Mariani and colleagues[53] treated 38 dogs with presumed or confirmed intracranial meningiomas using a frameless linear accelerator SRS system to a deliver median dose of 15 Gy. In 6 of 9 of these dogs, post-treatment imaging demonstrated objective partial responses or stable disease. The median overall survival for dogs with meningiomas was 399 days.

Preliminary evidence from several other investigators also indicates SRS treatment of canine and feline meningiomas with CyberKnife or linear accelerators is well tolerated and associated with favorable and durable clinical responses.[11,55,65]

SRS and SRT are being investigated at several institutions for the treatment of pituitary tumors (see **Fig. 3**).[52–55] Results of linear accelerator SRS were reported in 11 cats with functional (growth hormone–secreting) pituitary tumors, which resulted in improvement in clinical signs in 7 of 11 (63%) cats, including a reduction in the insulin requirements of 5 of 9 cats with poorly regulated diabetes mellitus and improvement in intracranial neurologic dysfunction in 2 of 2 cats.[54] All cats were initially treated with 15 Gy, and 3 of 11 cats were retreated with SRS after tumor progression. No confirmed acute or late radiation toxicities were observed, and the overall median survival in this cohort of cats was 25 months.[54] In one case series, 4 dogs with pituitary tumors were treated with SRS, with a median reported survival of 118 days.[53]

SRS has been used to treat other brain tumors, including gliomas, choroid plexus tumors, histiocytic sarcomas, and intracranial nerve sheath tumors, but the numbers of cases reported for each of these tumor types are sufficiently small, and objective efficacy measures sufficiently sparse to preclude analyses other than reporting of survival data.[25,53,54] A study by Mariani and colleagues[53] reported median overall survivals of 881 days in 4 dogs with trigeminal sheath tumors and 437 days in 3 dogs with gliomas. Results of a preliminary study investigating CyberKnife SRS suggested a poorer prognosis associated with irradiation of gliomas compared with other tumor types.[65]

SRS is currently used at multiple veterinary referral centers, and the number of facilities capable of performing SRS in dogs and cats has been growing in the past few years. This will provide the means for generation of additional data regarding the efficacy, limitations, dose selection and fractionation, and toxicities of SRS necessary to determine the specific indications in which SRS may offer a survival or other clinical benefit over conventional fractionated radiotherapeutic protocols to dogs and cats with brain tumors. The initial success of SRS for the treatment of canine and feline brain tumors, however, reinforces the fundamental importance of radiotherapy as a primary or adjuvant treatment modality in neurooncology.

CONVECTION-ENHANCED DELIVERY

The BBB has long been recognized as an obstacle to the entry of systemically administered therapeutics into the brain. Tight junctional complexes, active efflux pumps, ion channels, solute carriers, and vesicular transcytosis systems all contribute to the selective and limited permeability of the BBB.[66]

To overcome drug delivery limitations imposed by the BBB, direct infusion of high-molecular-weight substances into the brain parenchyma through small diameter cannulae was developed in 1994.[67,68] This technique was coined CED after showing that positive pressure gradients during infusions into the brain enhanced bulk fluid flow (fluid convection).[68] This landmark study launched the modern field of CED, whose potential for efficient drug delivery is evident by its applications in neoplastic, neurodegenerative, and psychiatric brain disorders.[69]

In neurooncology, CED has been primarily investigated and advocated for use in the treatment of malignant intraparenchymal neoplasms, such as anaplastic astrocytoma or glioblastoma multiforme, that are inherently refractory to other treatments.[69]

Despite significant advancements in CED in the past decade, the technique remains primarily an investigational drug delivery method largely because of its technical challenges and demands. In veterinary medicine, additional practical considerations may result in CED remaining limited to academic institutions treating and assessing the therapy in specific subsets of patients with intra-axial brain tumors.

The Convection-enhanced Delivery Procedure

CED involves creation of a minimally invasive craniectomy to facilitate catheter introduction, stereotactic placement of the catheter(s) into the target, and drug delivery using a microinfusion pump to maintain the positive pressure gradient at the catheter tip, which drives the infusate as an advancing front away from the catheter (**Figs. 4 and 5**).[70,71] CED can be performed safely throughout the central nervous system, including the prosencephalon, brainstem, and spinal cord.[23,69,72]

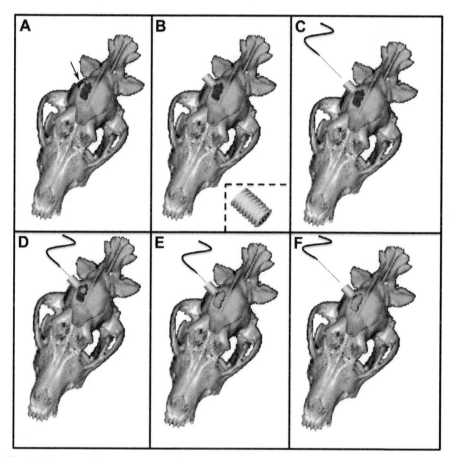

Fig. 4. Schema of CED treatment of canine forebrain glioma. (*A*) Preoperative stereotactic planning determines the location of the minimally invasive craniectomy (*arrow*) required to approach the tumor (*red*). (*B*) A catheter guide pedestal (*inset*) is implanted into the craniectomy defect in a manner that will reproduce the planned catheter trajectory and secure the catheter(s) during intraoperative imaging. (*C*) The catheter is inserted through the catheter guide pedestal to the desired location within the tumor. (*D, E*) Infusate delivery (*yellow*) is monitored with real-time intraoperative imaging and is continued until the target volume of distribution is achieved or a complication, such as reflux, develops. (*F*) The catheter is removed after completion of the infusion.

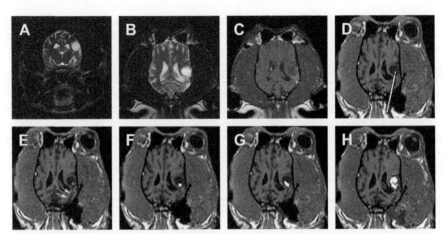

Fig. 5. Treatment of a canine intracranial astrocytoma with CED incorporating intraoperative MRI monitoring of infusate distribution. On pretreatment MRI (*A–D*), the tumor is visible as an ovoid T2-hyperintense (*A, B*) and T1-hypointense, peripherally contrast-enhancing (*C*) mass in the left parietotemporal region. (*D*) Representation of catheter (not to scale) placement into the tumor. Serial, T1-weighted intraoperative images (*E–H*) demonstrating progressive distribution of the gadolinium labeled infusate (T1 hyperintensity) within the tumor over the course of the 2-hour infusion. The arrows (*E*) delineate the CED catheter trajectory traversing the occipital lobe en route to the tumor. (*D–G*) The signal void external to the skull in the left occipital region represents the surgical exposure necessary to implant the catheter guide pedestal through with CED catheters are passed.

The principle advantages of CED are that it allows for direct regional distribution of high concentrations of macromolecular drugs to the brain that are otherwise incapable of penetrating the BBB and relatively safe administration of drugs that have narrow therapeutic indices when administered systemically.[67–69] Although other methods of direct drug delivery to the brain exist, such as implantable biodegradable polymers and catheter-reservoir devices, these techniques are diffusion dependent. Limitations of diffusion include unpredictable distribution volumes that are constrained to the tissue immediately surrounding the drug source.[73] CED has been shown to increase the volume of drug distribution in the brain by at least an order of magnitude relative to simple diffusion.[74] The potential to safely saturate large volumes of brain tissue with high concentrations of antineoplastic drugs has been the primary motivation for use of CED in treatment of malignant gliomas, whose phenotypes are characterized by extensive microscopic invasion of neoplastic cells into brain parenchyma.[23,68,75]

Technical Factors Governing Infusate Distributions in the Brain

Extensive clinical experience with CED has indicated that there are many interdependent factors at all steps of the procedure that ultimately influence the volume of drug distribution (see **Figs. 4–8**) and thus the therapeutic outcome.[70,71,75–87] Identifying, modeling, and optimizing these potential confounders have been a focus of CED research, and a significant amount of this work has been performed in animals with gliomas.[23,69–79]

The numerous catheters for CED (see **Figs. 6 and 7**) reflect the absence of an ideal design.[80–84] Backflow and reflux of the infusate along the insertion track or leakage into nontargeted regions are common problems and have been reported in up to 25% of all CED infusions.[70] Once reflux occurs, there is negligible further distribution of the infusate into the targeted region (see **Figs. 7 and 8**).[70,75,76] Catheters less than

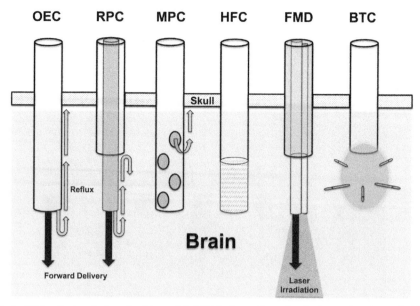

Fig. 6. CED catheter designs (not to scale). BTC, balloon-tipped catheter variant intended for infusion into resection cavities; FMD, fiberoptic microneedle device capable of photothermochemotherapy; HFC, hollow fiber catheter; MPC, multiport, single-lumen catheters, notorious for infusate efflux from most proximal port only; OEC, open-ended catheter; RPC, reflux-preventing catheter with a step-down at distal tip.

27 gauge (0.4 mm) in diameter afford greater resistance to reflux.[82] Reflux-preventing catheter designs consist of a single-end port coupled with step-down design at the distal tip (see **Figs. 5–8**) and are the most commonly used catheters for clinical CED infusions.[80,82]

Even in the normal brain, where the interstitial fluid pressure ranges from 1 to 3 mm Hg, heterogeneous tissue conditions contribute to nonuniform spatial infusate dispersion.[75] White matter tracts and perivascular spaces provide routes of lower resistance to interstitially delivered fluids, and pial surfaces along the cerebral convexities provide barriers to drug distribution.[71,75] Tissue heterogeneity is considerably greater in the peritumoral microenvironment. The intratumoral interstitial fluid pressure is typically high and regionally variable, which limits infusate entry into high-pressure zones. Peritumoral white matter edema is exquisitely permeable to fluid, and resection and cystic cavities represent low-pressure foci that can complicate infusion (see **Fig. 8**). The CED infusion itself also dynamically alters the poroelastic properties of the brain.[75]

Given the contributions of boundary conditions and tissue heterogeneity to infusate distribution, catheter placement is a huge consideration in CED. Ideally, infusates would be contained within a predetermined target volume (ie, tumor [see **Figs. 4 and 5**]). Early CED efforts relied on the experience of neurosurgeons to define the catheter trajectory and termination point. Extensive modeling of CED has led to numeric solutions and shape-fitting algorithms that allow pretreatment simulation of CED from diagnostic MRI studies.[75,76,88,89] Currently, neurosurgical software platforms that can account for the numerous technical factors affecting infusate distribution are used to plan CED procedures and optimize catheter placement.[75,76,88,89]

Catheter placement technique is also paramount to efficient function. Excessive tissue trauma during insertion can result in an insertion track defect larger than the outer

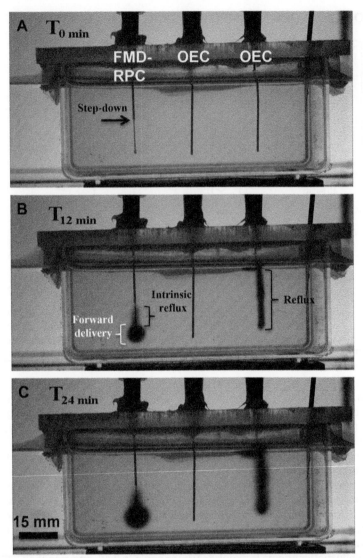

Fig. 7. Time-lapsed in vitro CED simulations in agarose brain phantoms, comparing a fiber-optic microneedle device with reflux prevention feature (FMD-RPC) (*A, left*) to open-ended catheters (OEC) (*A, middle and right*). Infusion of Evans blue albumin conjugate was performed at a rate of 2 μL/min through the left and right catheters. Reflux occurs with both catheters but is mitigated by the step-down feature on the FMD-RPC catheter (*B*), which permits continual forward delivery of the infusate over time. Once the infusate refluxes up the shaft of the OEC, virtually no forward distribution occurs (*B, C*).

diameter of the cannula, which greatly favors reflux. Catheter motion after placement can also disrupt seal formation at the catheter-tissue interface.

Convection-enhanced Delivery Infusion Techniques

Currently in veterinary medicine, 2 CED infusion techniques are being investigated. The first incorporates real-time imaging confirmation of the volume of distribution of

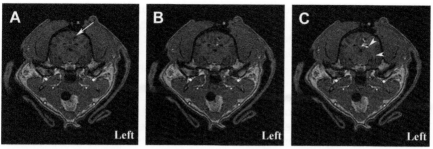

Fig. 8. Serial, intraoperative T1-weighted transverse MRIs of CED treatment of a canine astrocytoma in the left frontoparietal lobes demonstrating unintended infusate penetration into the ventricular system. (A) On the preinfusion image, the caudal aspect of the tumor is visible as a hypointense region (*arrow*). The implanted catheter guide pedestal (*asterisk*) is visible in all panels. (B) Image obtained 119 minutes into the infusion. The infusate, labeled with a liposomal gadoteridol tracer, can be seen as hyperintensity within the cystic portion of the tumor as well as extending into the periventricular white matter. (C) Penetration of the infusate into lateral ventricle (*arrowheads*) is evident on MRIs obtained 137 minutes into the infusion, at which point the CED procedure was terminated.

infusates into the procedure (see **Figs. 4, 5,** and **8**).[23,70,79,89] MRI, single-photon emission tomography, and positron emission tomography can be used for monitoring.[23,70,75] This technique is performed with an anesthetized patient immobilized in the MRI gantry to allow for repeated imaging of the brain during the infusion. Seminal work by Dickinson and colleagues[23] in dogs with spontaneous gliomas has illustrated the feasibility and importance of real-time imaging monitoring of CED for confirmation of catheter placement and target coverage as well as providing an opportunity to detect and remedy any local adverse effects of treatment, such as infusate reflux or brain hemorrhage and edema (see **Figs. 5 and 8**).[70] Numerous, paramagnetic MRI contrast agents, including free gadolinium, have been evaluated as surrogates of the infusate distribution and can be delivered as co-infusions with or conjugated to therapeutic agents.[79,83] The necessity for real-time monitoring of CED was further realized when a retrospective analysis of a trial in human glioblastoma incriminated suboptimal drug distribution as a potential contributor to therapeutic failure.[71]

The real-time monitoring of CED presents several practical challenges. This technique requires prolonged periods of anesthesia, because durations of infusions can range from 1 to 6 hours, and accessibility to patients for anesthetic monitoring is limited while they are in the MRI. Depending on the size of an individual patient and technical specifications of the MRI scanner, physical constraints of the MRI bore or coil configurations can potentially limit approach angles and catheter trajectories to the tumor. The procedure also requires use of specialized and expensive MRI compatible head frames, catheter assemblies, and microinfusion pumps.[23]

The second CED technique that has been investigated in dogs is referred to as ambulatory CED,[90] in which pretreatment images are used to plan placement of the CED catheter(s). During surgery, the catheter is placed into the target and secured, and then the patient is recovered from anesthesia. The actual CED infusion takes place in a conscious patient while under observation in the ICU. Infusions using this technique typically last 12 to 72 hours and are delivered with an external, programmable reservoir pump attached to the patient.[90] Compared with CED monitored with real-time MRI, ambulatory CED is not constrained by the need for extensive MRI compatible instrumentation and offers the additional advantage of reduced anesthetic duration. Limitations of ambulatory CED include the largely blind manner in which infusates are delivered to the target and the potential for the catheter movement or dislodgement during the infusion.[71,90]

Ultimately, infusion parameters will depend on the pharmacologic properties of the therapeutic agent, nuances of the delivery technique, and the number of catheters required to provide coverage of the target volume. Increasing the flow rate will facilitate convective flow and theoretically result in larger total volumes of distribution. The risk of tissue damage and reflux also increases, however, with higher flow rates. In clinical applications, infusions are initiated at low flow rates (0.5–1 µL/min) and escalated up to a ceiling of 5 µL/min. This range of infusion rates represents a reasonable balance between desired drug distribution and risk of adverse events.[29,45] In canine studies, total CED infusion volumes have ranged from approximately 50 to 2000 µL.[23,79,90]

Convection-enhanced Delivery for Treatment of Canine Brain Tumors

The optimum time to perform CED in relation to other therapies in canine and feline patients with brain tumors is currently unknown. In dogs with gliomas, CED has been performed as a single therapeutic modality as well as prior to and immediately after surgical resection.[23,90] CED delivery of infusate is facilitated if a mass has been resected, but resection can also limit distribution of the infusate beyond the local low-pressure region that is created. Finally, depending on the mechanism of action and pharmacokinetics of the infused therapeutic agent, multiple CED infusions may be necessary to achieve durable tumor responses.[23]

Several clinical trials are currently using CED for the treatment of canine intracranial gliomas. In the most advanced trial reported to date, Dickinson and colleagues[23] evaluated CED of the topoisomerase-1 inhibitor, irinotecan in 9 dogs with forebrain gliomas. This study demonstrated the feasibility and safety of CED with irinotecan and the clinical utility of a reflux-preventing catheter and reaffirmed the necessity for intraoperative MRI of CED in the clinical setting.[23,78] Although the study was not designed to evaluate therapeutic efficacy, data supporting efficacy were presented. The median survival for all dogs was 190 days.[23]

Two additional clinical trials at University of Georgia and Virginia Tech are using CED to treat canine gliomas. The therapeutic rationale of these trials is discussed later, because both use monoclonal antibodies for therapeutic targeting.[90–93] The Virginia Tech trial is modeled after the work performed by Dickinson and colleagues,[79] in which CED is performed as a sole therapy in dogs with forebrain gliomas over a several-hour period using stereotactically placed reflux-preventing catheters, and infusions are monitored with real-time MRI and gadolinium-based imaging tracer (see **Fig. 5**).[91,92] The University of Georgia trial is investigating ambulatory CED in the postresection setting using a commercial cerebrospinal fluid drainage catheter and a superparamagnetic iron-oxide nanoparticle imaging agent.[90,93]

IMMUNOTHERAPY

Immense progress has been made in cancer biology and neuroimmunology over the past 2 decades.[94–97] The brain is no longer considered an immune-privileged organ unfavorable to IT interventions and instead there is increasing elucidation and exploitation of the unique mechanisms that characterize immunocompetency and tumor-host interactions within the brain.[94,97] Cancer IT consists of diverse strategies whose unifying goal is to use an immune response in the host to kill the tumor.[96]

History of and Rationale for Brain Tumor Immunotherapy

It has been long observed that changes in immune function are common in cancer patients and intimately related to survival. The benefits of immune activation were first documented more than a century ago when Dr William Coley reported that the development of postoperative infection in cancer patients improved outcomes.[98] Similar survival advantages were observed in humans with glioblastoma multiforme who developed perioperative infections compared with those who did not, as well as in those persons whose tumors were infiltrated by cytotoxic T cells.[99] The potential of IT to specifically recognize and kill tumor cells is particularly attractive for malignant brain tumors given their inherent chemo- and radioresistance and ability to induce a state of systemic cell-mediated immunosuppression in the host. The potential to preserve normal tissue function in the sensitive biological environment of the brain through the selective killing of neoplastic cells is also important.[97,100,101]

Basic Immunotherapeutic Strategies

Passive and active approaches represent the 2 fundamental arms of IT.[96,101] Passive IT does not activate a patient's immune system. Instead, a specific immune component is administered to the patient. Passive IT can be subdivided into 3 strategies: cytokine immunomodulation, monoclonal antibodies, and adoptive (cell-based) IT. In contrast, active IT stimulates an inherent immune response by exposing patients to antigens and is commonly referred to as tumor vaccination.

Passive immunotherapy: cytokine immunomodulation
Cytokine immunomodulation attempts to enhance the immune response by administration of cytokines, such as interferons or interleukin (IL)-2, that have antitumor effects, or via agents inhibiting endogenous immunosuppressive cytokines or tumor growth promoters, such as transforming growth factor β. There has been some success using interferon-alpha in the treatment of human malignant or unresectable meningiomas, but cytokine immunomodulation has been ineffective for the treatment of gliomas.[102,103]

Passive immunotherapy: monoclonal antibodies
Another passive IT approach involves administration of monoclonal antibodies capable of interaction with tumor-associated or -specific antigens, often referred to as *targeted therapy*. Monoclonal antibodies can be delivered naked or used as delivery vehicles for conjugated radioisotopes, drugs, or biological toxins to tumor cells.[53,58] Although naked monoclonal antibodies have revolutionized IT in human malignancies, as indicated by the success of trastuzumab in breast cancer and rituximab in lymphoma, none of them is able to effect a cure for cancer as a single agents.[104] Naked monoclonal antibodies can induce tumor responses through inhibition of DNA synthesis and cellular proliferation as well as through complement-mediated and antibody-dependent cell-mediated cytotoxicity.[96] Both beneficial and detrimental off-target biological responses may be observed when using monoclonal antibodies. The human experience has highlighted the limitations of naked monoclonal antibodies, including redundancy of signaling pathways leading to cancer cell survival, inefficient effector cell interaction due to Fc receptor polymorphism, up-regulation of inhibitory receptors, and competition with circulating immunoglobulins.[104,105]

Bevacizumab, the most extensively studied monoclonal antibody in human brain tumors, binds and neutralizes vascular endothelial growth factor (VEGF) ligand.[101,106] VEGF is a tumor-associated protein crucial for angiogenesis in solid cancers, and patterns of VEGF and VEGF receptor expression are similar in human and canine brain tumors.[107,108] Bevacizumab's mechanism of action is antagonism of the ligand that activates VEGF receptors on tumor vasculature, thus inhibiting angiogenesis and tumor growth as well as mitigating vasogenic edema formation.[108] Bevacizumab may also be synergistic with chemotherapeutics and radiotherapy by concentrating drugs within the tumor through modulation of vascular tone and improving tumor oxygenation.[108] Bevacizumab has improved the radiologic response rate, progression-free survival, and quality of life in humans with malignant gliomas but has had questionable impact on overall survival.[108]

A mutation of the epidermal growth factor receptor (EGFR) gene, EGFRvIII, results in a constitutively activated tyrosine kinase not found in normal tissues but frequently expressed in malignant gliomas and other cancers.[108–110] Because it is tumor specific, EGFRvIII represents an ideal IT target. Although human glioma trials investigating systemic administration of naked monoclonal antibody targeting EGFRvIII have been disappointing, therapeutic success has been observed in a rodent glioma model in which cetuximab, an EGFRvIII inhibitor, has been delivered with CED.[110,111] The University of Georgia canine clinical trial seeks to exploit EGFR overexpression in canine gliomas, which occurs in 28% to 57% of astrocytomas and correlates with tumor grade, as well as in a minority of high-grade oligodendrogliomas.[108,109] In this canine trial, cetuximab conjugated to an iron-oxide magnetic nanoparticle is delivered with CED after surgical resection of the glioma. The superparamagnetic nanoparticle allows for visualization of the MRI distribution of cetuximab in the brain.[93] The feasibility and safety of the cetuximab-nanoparticle conjugate for CED have been demonstrated in dogs and encouraging preliminary results from the trial have been reported.[90,112]

Conjugated monoclonal antibodies, composed of a targeting ligand and a radioisotope, drug, or bacterial cytotoxin effectors, are being investigated in brain tumors. My colleagues and I demonstrated the validity of targeting the receptors IL-13 alpha 2 (IL-13Rα2) and ephrin receptor A2 (EphA2) in canine high-grade gliomas, because these tumor-associated receptors are expressed at high levels in most gliomas and are virtually absent in normal brain (**Fig. 9**).[91,113] IL-13Rα2 is a cancer/testis-like tumor antigen representing a downstream gene target after activation of EGFRvIII.[114,115] We have designed canine monoclonal antibodies generated against IL-13Rα2 demonstrating cross-reactivity with human and canine receptors, and a conjugate containing this canine monoclonal antibody and a *Pseudomonas* exotoxin A derivative is capable of specific and efficient killing of glioma cells in vitro.[91] These developments form the therapeutic rationale for the Virginia Tech canine glioma clinical trial, which is currently recruiting patients.[92] Our work also illustrated the presence of IL-13Rα2 on canine meningiomas and choroid plexus tumors, identifying them as candidates for IL-13Rα2–targeted therapies (see **Fig. 9**).[91]

Passive immunotherapy: adoptive immunotherapy

Adoptive IT involves harvesting a patient's immune effector cells, either lymphocyte-activated killer cells or cytotoxic T lymphocytes; activating and expanding them ex vivo; and then administrating them back to the patient systemically or intratumorally. Although activated lymphocyte-activated killer cells are capable of providing a robust cytotoxic immune response, it is not necessarily tumor specific. A majority of brain tumor studies have investigated lymphocyte-activated killer cells for adoptive IT in human malignant glioma and have not identified any significant impact on survival.[116,117]

Because evidence exists that T cells are the major effectors in antitumor immunity, cytotoxic T lymphocyte adoptive IT is a promising approach. Cytotoxic T lymphocytes are obtained by collecting peripheral blood mononuclear cells or tumor-infiltrating

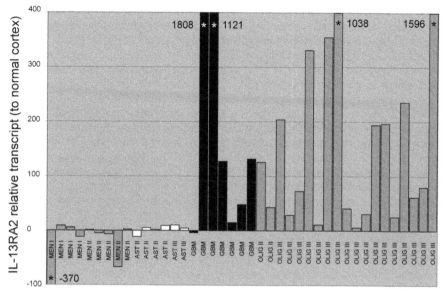

Fig. 9. Quantitative TaqMan real-time polymerase chain reaction comparing expression of IL-13Rα2 in canine primary brain tumors. Elevated expression, relative to normal canine brain cortex, is seen predominantly in high-grade glial tumors, essentially mirroring protein expression determined by Western blotting. Off-scale values are marked with an asterisk and value. AST, astrocytoma; GBM, glioblastoma multiforme; MEN, meningioma; OLIG, oligodendroglioma. (*From* Debinski W, Dickinson P, Rossmeisl JH, et al. New agents for targeting of IL-13RA2 expressed in primary human and canine brain tumors. PLoS One 2013;8(10):e77719.)

lymphocytes and then antigenically stimulating or genetically manipulating them ex vivo.[118] Autologous tumor cells are often used for antigen stimulation, which yields cytotoxic T lymphocytes with tumor specificity. Although this technique has shown potential for the treatment of human brain tumors, it has not been attempted in veterinary medicine, likely because the methodology is labor intensive, often requires host immunodepletion, and genetic engineering of cytotoxic T lymphocytes is complicated by the need for viral transduction.[119–123]

Active immunotherapy

Active IT, or tumor vaccination, enhances a patient's immune response by priming it through antigen exposure. Active immunization can occur using peptide- and cell-based therapies.[124] Peptides selected for tumor vaccines are usually able to bind to major histocompatibility complex class I molecules, which subsequently activate cytotoxic T lymphocytes.[101,118] Cell-based active IT uses activated antigen-presenting cells to prime the immune system in lieu of the native antigen.[101,124] Dendritic cells, given their capacity as professional antigen-presenting cells, have been the most widely studied for cell-based active IT.[119,124] Dendritic cells are usually prepared from autologous peripheral blood mononuclear cells cultured in the presence of growth factors or cytokines. Mature dendritic cells are then activated by antigens obtained from whole tumor cells, tumor lysates, peptides eluted or mRNA derived from activated tumor cells, or viral-derived antigens.[123,124] Activated dendritic cells are then returned to the patient by intradermal, subcutaneous, intranodal, or intratumoral injection.

As active IT has evolved, brain tumor trials have moved away from single peptide or autologous dendritic cell vaccines to use approaches in which patients are treated with some combination of tumor antigens or antigen-presenting cells with a stimulatory agent, such as a cytokine or immunoadjuvant, and often in conjunction with another synergistic therapy.[24,124–129] Combination IT approaches have been used in dogs with spontaneous brain tumors.[24,127–130] Culture-free dendritic cell vaccination of glioma-bearing dogs with tumor cell lysates containing a Toll-like receptor ligand adjuvant in combination with in situ adenoviral interferon gamma gene transfer demonstrated sufficient safety and promise to result in rapid translation of this immunogenetic therapy to a human glioblastoma clinical trial.[24,130] In dogs with intracranial meningiomas, vaccination with an autologous tumor cell lysate combined with synthetic Toll-like receptor ligands after cytoreductive surgery increased survival (median 645 days) compared with surgically treated historic controls (median 222 days).[127] In these studies, it was demonstrated that vaccines induced systemic or local tumor-reactive antibodies.[24,127]

Future Directions of Immunotherapy

IT has just begun the journey toward achieving robust, specific, durable, and clinically beneficial antitumor immune responses in cancer patients. Although brain tumor IT has yielded promising results in both humans and dogs, current trials are limited by small numbers of patients as well as study design complexity implicit to IT in which efficacy and toxicity are not clearly dose related, and dose limitation is often defined

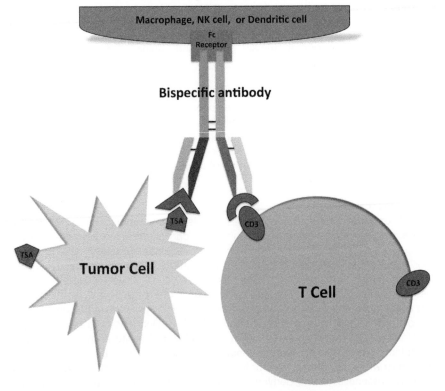

Fig. 10. Schematic of bispecific antibodies of the T-cell engager class. NK, natural killer; TSA, tumor-specific antigen.

by the availability of cells and not the appearance of adverse effects.[131] The data indicate, however, that CED can feasibly deliver IT, and brain tumor IT is generally safe and capable of inducing tumor-specific immune responses in the host. There remains a need for the incorporation of validated endpoints that assess the immune response into clinical trials and investigation of fundamental subjects, such as the optimal route and frequency of administration of tumor vaccines.[24,117–127]

Current and future IT efforts seek to enhance antigen presentation, circumvent tumor-induced immunotolerance, optimize activation of antitumor effectors, and improve the production efficiency and standardization of cell-based therapies. The fabrication of bispecific antibodies of the T-cell engager class (**Fig. 10**) represents a unique method for redirecting cytotoxic activity from circulating T cells. These bispecific antibodies consist of 2 different variable region fragments, one that binds tumor-specific antigen and the other directed against the T-cell ligand CD3. The net effect is a direct connection between one or more immunocytes and tumor cells, which greatly enhances specificity and cytotoxicity (see **Fig. 10**). A bispecific antibody approach targeting EGFRvIII in human glioblastoma is under investigation.[132]

REFERENCES

1. Whelan HT, Clanton JA, Wilson RE, et al. Comparison of CT and MRI brain tumor imaging using a canine glioma model. Pediatr Neurol 1988;4:279–83.
2. Wisner ER, Dickinson PJ, Higgins RJ. Magnetic resonance imaging features of canine intracranial neoplasia. Vet Radiol Ultrasound 2011;52:S52–61.
3. Cherubini GB, Mantis P, Martinez TA, et al. Utility of magnetic resonance imaging for distinguishing neoplastic from non-neoplastic brain lesions in dogs and cats. Vet Radiol Ultrasound 2005;46:384–7.
4. Troxel MT, Vite CH, Massicotte C, et al. Magnetic resonance imaging features of feline intracranial neoplasia: retrospective analysis of 46 cats. J Vet Intern Med 2004;18:176–89.
5. Chen AV, Wininger FA, Frey S, et al. Description and validation of a magnetic resonance imaging-guided stereotactic brain biopsy device in the dog. Vet Radiol Ultrasound 2011;53:150–6.
6. Zhao Q, Lee S, Kent M, et al. Dynamic-contrast enhanced magnetic resonance imaging of canine brain tumors. Vet Radiol Ultrasound 2010;51:122–9.
7. Garcia PA, Pancotto TE, Rossmeisl JH, et al. Non-thermal irreversible electroporation (N-TIRE) and adjuvant fractionated radiotherapeutic multimodal therapy for intracranial malignant glioma in a canine patient. Technol Cancer Res Treat 2011;10:73–83.
8. Klopp LS, Rao S. Endoscipic-assisted intracranial tumor removal in dogs and cats: long-term outcome of 39 cases. J Vet Intern Med 2009;23:108–15.
9. Rossmeisl JH Jr, Garcia PA, Daniel GB, et al. Invited review- Neuroimaging response assessment criteria for brain tumors in veterinary patients. Vet Radiol Ultrasound 2014;55:115–32. http://dx.doi.org/10.1111/vru.12118.
10. Rossmeisl JH, Jones JC, Zimmerman KL, et al. Survival time following hospital discharge in dogs with palliatively treated brain tumors. J Am Vet Med Assoc 2013;242:193–8.
11. Huse JT, Holland EC. Targeting brain cancer: advances in the molecular pathology of malignant glioma and medulloblastoma. Nat Rev Cancer 2010;10:319–31.
12. Axlund TW, McGlasson ML, Smith AN. Surgery alone or in combination with radiation therapy for treatment of intracranial meningiomas in dogs: 31 cases 1989-2002. J Am Vet Med Assoc 2002;221(11):1597–600.

13. Gordon LE, Thacher C, Matthiesen DT, et al. Results of craniotomy for the treatment of cerebral meningioma in 42 cat. Vet Surg 1994;23:94–100.

14. Gallagher JG, Berg J, Knowles KE, et al. Prognosis after surgical excision of cerebral meningiomas in cats: 17 cases (1986-1992). J Am Vet Med Assoc 1993; 10:1437–40.

15. Greco JJ, Aiken SA, Berg JM, et al. Evaluation of intracranial meningioma resection with a surgical aspirator in dogs: 17 cases (1996-2004). J Am Vet Med Assoc 2006;229:394–400.

16. Hanson JM, van t'Hoofd MM, Voorhout G, et al. Efficacy of transsphenoidal hypohysectomy in dogs with pituitary-dependent hyperadrenocorticism. J Vet Intern Med 2005;19:687–94.

17. Bley CR, Sumova A, Roos M, et al. Irradiation of brain tumors in dogs with neurologic disease. J Vet Intern Med 2008;19:849–54.

18. Brearley MJ, Jeffrey ND, Phillips SM, et al. Hypofractionated radiation therapy of brain masses in dogs: a retrospective analysis of survival of 83 cases (1991–1996). J Vet Intern Med 1999;13:408–12.

19. Keyerleber MA, McEntee MC, Farrely J, et al. Three-dimensional conformal radiation therapy alone or in combination with surgery for treatment of canine intracranial meningiomas. Vet Comp Oncol 2013. http://dx.doi.org/10.1111/vco.12054.

20. Van Meervenne S, Verhoeven PS, de Vos J, et al. Comparison between symptomatic treatment and lomustine supplementation in 71 dogs with intracranial, space-occupying lesions. Vet Comp Oncol 2014;12:67–77.

21. Kimmelman J, Nalbantoglu J. Faithful companions: a proposal for neurooncology trials in pet dogs. Cancer Res 2007;67:4541–4.

22. Thomas R, Duke SE, Wang HJ, et al. Putting our heads together: insights into genomic conservation between human and canine intracranial tumors. J Neurooncol 2009;94:333–49.

23. Dickinson PJ, LeCouteur RA, Higgins RJ, et al. Canine spontaneous glioma: a translational model system for convection-enhanced delivery. Neuro Oncol 2010;12:928–40.

24. Pluhar GE, Grogan PT, Seiler C, et al. Anti-tumor immune-response correlates with neurological symptoms in a dog with spontaneous astrocytoma treated by gene and vaccine therapy. Vaccine 2010;28:3371–8.

25. Lester NV, Hopkins AL, Bova FJ, et al. Radiosurgery using a stereotactic headframe for irradiation of brain tumors in dogs. J Am Vet Med Assoc 2001;219:1562–7.

26. Barth RF, Vicente MF, Harling OK, et al. Current status of boron neutron capture therapy of high grade gliomas and recurrent head and neck cancer. Radiat Oncol 2012;7:146.

27. Gavin PR, Kraft SL, Swartz CD, et al. Boron neutron capture therapy of spontaneous intracranial tumors in dogs. In: Mishima Y, editor. Cancer neutron capture therapy. New York: Springer; 1996. p. 763–8.

28. Schwarz EB, Thon N, Nikolajek K, et al. Iodine-125 brachytherapy for brain tumors: a review. Radiat Oncol 2012;7:30.

29. Murphy AM, Rabkin SD. Current status of gene therapy for brain tumors. Transl Res 2013;161:339–54.

30. Al-Bataineh O, Jenne J, Huber P. Clinical and future applications of high intensity focused ultrasound in cancer. Cancer Treat Rev 2012;38:346–53.

31. Sloan AE, Ahluwalia MS, Valerio-Pascua J, et al. Results of the neuroblate system first-in-humans phase I clinical trial for recurrent glioblastoma. J Neurosurg 2013;118:1202–19.

32. Gridley DS, Grover RS, Lordeo LN, et al. Proton-beam therapy for tumors of the CNS. Expert Rev Neurother 2010;10:319–30.
33. Kirson ED, Dbaly V, Frantisek T, et al. Alternating electric fields arrest cell proliferation in animal tumor models and human brain tumors. Proc Natl Acad Sci U S A 2007;24:10152–7.
34. Garcia PA, Rossmeisl JH Jr, Neal RE, et al. Intracranial nonthermal irreversible electroporation: in vivo analysis. J Membr Biol 2010;236:127–36.
35. Chang JE, Khuntia D, Robins HI, et al. Radiotherapy and radiosensitizers in the treatment of glioblastoma multiforme. Clin Adv Hematol Oncol 2007;5(11): 894–902.
36. Tomblyn MB, Katin MJ, Wallner PE. The new golden era for radioimmunotherapy: not just for lymphomas anymore. Cancer Control 2013;20:60–71.
37. Kondziolka D, Lunsford LD, Loeffler JS, et al. Radiosurgery and radiotherapy: observations and clarifications. J Neurosurg 2004;101:585–9.
38. Clarke RH, Horsley VA. On a method of investigating the deep ganglia and tracts of the central nervous system (cerebellum). Br Med J 1906;2:1799–800.
39. Speigel EA, Wycis HT, Marks M, et al. Stereotaxic apparatus for operations on the human brain. Science 1947;106:349–50.
40. Leksell L. A stereotactic apparatus for intracerebral surgery. Acta Chir Scand 1949;99:229–33.
41. Talairach J, He'caen M, David M, et al. Recherches sur la coagulation therapeutique des structures sous-corticales chez l'homme. Rev Neurol 1949;81:4–24.
42. Narabayashi H. Stereotaxic instrument for operation on the human basal ganglia. Psychiatr Neurol Jpn 1952;54:669–71.
43. Riechert T, Mundinger F. Beschreibung und Anwendung eines Zielgerates fur stereotaktische Hirnoperationen (II. Modell). Acta Neurochir Suppl 1955;3:308–37.
44. Nadelhaft I, Morgan C, Herbert DL. Stereotactic brain surgery: a method for rapid and precise positioning of a target in the Todd-Wells stereotactic instrument. Appl Neurophysiol 1977–1978;40:13–25.
45. Lawrence JH, Tobias CA, Born JL, et al. Heavy-particle irradiation in neoplastic and neurologic disease. J Neurosurg 1962;19:717–22.
46. Leksell L. The stereotaxic method and radiosurgery of the brain. Acta Chir Scand 1951;102:316–9.
47. Hacker F. Compared with inverse-planning, forward planning is preferred for IMRT stereotactic radiosurgery. For the proposition. Med Phys 2003;30:731–2.
48. Rowshanfarzad P, Sabet M, O'Connor DJ, et al. Isocenter verification for linac-based stereotactic radiosurgery: review of principles and techniques. J Appl Clin Med Phys 2011;12:3645.
49. Zamecnik P, Essig M. Perspectives of 3T magnetic resonance imaging in radiosurgical treatment planning. Acta Neurochir Suppl 2013;116:187–91.
50. Flickinger JC, Kano H, Niranjan A, et al. Dose selection in stereotactic radiosurgery. Prog Neurol Surg 2013;27:49–57.
51. Harmon J, Van UD, LaRue S. Assessment of a radiotherapy patient cranial immobilization device using daily on-board kilovoltage imaging. Vet Radiol Ultrasound 2009;50:230–4.
52. Kent MS. Stereotactic radiosurgery for brain tumors: clinical trial update [PFN01]. In: Proceedings of the American College of Veterinary Internal Medicine Forum. Red Hook, NY: Curran Associates; 2012. p. 25–6.
53. Mariani CL, Schubert TA, House RA, et al. Frameless stereotactic radiosurgery for the treatment of primary intracranial tumours in dogs. Vet Comp Oncol 2013. http://dx.doi.org/10.1111/vco.12056.

54. Sellon RK, Fidel J, Houston R, et al. Linear-accelerator-based modified radiosurgical treatment of pituitary tumors in cats: 11 cases (1997-2008). J Vet Intern Med 2009;23:1038–44.
55. LaRue SM. Advances in radiotherapy treatment of neurological tumors [S171]. In: Proceedings of the American College of Veterinary Internal Medicine Forum. Red Hook, NY: Curran Associates; 2013. p. 426–7.
56. Leksell L, Lindquist C, Adler JR, et al. A new fixation device for the Leksell stereotaxic system. Technical note. J Neurosurg 1987;66:626–9.
57. Levivier M, Gevaert T, Negretti L, et al. Gamma knife, cyberknife, tomotherapy: gadgets or useful tools? Curr Opin Neurol 2011;24:616–25.
58. Hall EJ, Brenner DJ. The radiobiology of radiosurgery: rationale for different treatment regimes for AVMs and malignancies. Int J Radiat Oncol Biol Phys 1993;25:381–5.
59. Vaupel P, Kallinowski F, Okunieff P. Blood flow, oxygenation and nutrient supply, and metabolic microenvironment of human tumors: a review. Cancer Res 1989; 49:6449–65.
60. Ch'ang HJ, Maj JG, Paris F, et al. ATM regulates target switching to escalating doses of radiation in the intestines. Nat Med 2005;11:484–90.
61. Sharp CD, Jawahar A, Warren AC, et al. Gamma knife irradiation increases cerebral endothelial expression of intercellular adhesion molecule 1 and E-selectin. Neurosurgery 2003;53:154–60.
62. Park H, Lyon JC, Griffin RJ, et al. Apoptosis and cell cycle progression in an acidic environment after irradiation. Radiat Res 2000;153:295–304.
63. Luxton G, Petrovich Z, Jozsef G, et al. Stereotactic radiosurgery: principles and comparison of treatment methods. Neurosurgery 1993;32:241–59.
64. Lawrence JA, Forrest LJ, Turek MM, et al. Proof of principle of ocular sparing in dogs with sinonsal tumors with intensity-modulated radiation therapy. Vet Radiol Ultrasound 2010;51:561–70.
65. Charney SC, Witten MR, Berg JM, et al. Cyberknife radiosurgery for irradiation of brain tumors in dogs and cats. [abstract]. In: Proceedings of the American College of Veterinary Internal Medicine Forum. Red Hook, NY: Curran Associates; 2010.
66. Abbott NJ, Patabendige AA, Dolman DE, et al. Structure and function of the blood-brain barrier. Neurobiol Dis 2010;37:13–25.
67. Morrison PF, Laske DH, Bobo H, et al. High-flow microinfusion: tissue penetration and pharmoacodynamics. Am J Physiol 1994;266:R292–305.
68. Bobo RH, Laske DW, Akbasak A, et al. Convection-enhanced delivery of macromolecules in the brain. Proc Natl Acad Sci U S A 1994;91:2076–80.
69. Vogelbaum MA. Convection-enhanced delivery for treating brain tumors and selected neurological disorders: a review. J Neurooncol 2007;83:97–109.
70. Varenika V, Dickinson PJ, Bringas J, et al. Detection of infusate leakage in the brain using real-time imaging of convection-enhanced delivery. J Neurosurg 2008;109:874–80.
71. Sampson JH, Archer G, Pedain C, et al. Poor drug distribution as a possible explanation for the results of the PRECISE trial. J Neurosurg 2010;113:301–9.
72. Murad GJ, Walbridge S, Morrison PF, et al. Image-guided convection-enhanced delivery of gemcitabine to the brainstem. J Neurosurg 2007;106:351–6.
73. Gallia GL, Brem S, Brem H. Local treatment of malignant brain tumors using implantable chemotherapeutic polymers. J Natl Compr Canc Netw 2005;3:721–8.
74. Lieberman DM, Laske DW, Morrison PF, et al. Convection-enhanced distribution of large molecules in gray matter during interstitial drug infusion. J Neurosurg 1995;82:1021–9.

75. Raghavan R, Brady ML, Rodriguez-Ponce MI, et al. Convection-enhanced delivery of therapeutics for brain disease, and its optimization. Neurosurg Focus 2006;20:E12.
76. Raghavan R, Brady M. Predictive models for pressure-driven fluid infusions into brain parenchyma. Phys Med Biol 2011;56:6179.
77. Motion JP, Huynh GH, Szoka FC, et al. Convection and retro-convection enhanced delivery: some theoretical considerations related to drug targeting. Pharm Res 2011;28:472–9.
78. Fiandaca MS, Forsayeth JR, Dickinson PJ, et al. Image-guided convection-enhanced delivery platform in the treatment of neurological diseases. Neurotherapeutics 2008;5:123–7.
79. Dickinson PJ, LeCouteur RA, Higgins RJ, et al. Canine model of convection-enhanced delivery of liposomes containing CPT-11 monitored with real-time magnetic resonance imaging: laboratory investigation. J Neurosurg 2008;108: 989–98.
80. Debinski W, Tatter SB. Convection-enhanced delivery for the treatment of brain tumors. Expert Rev Neurother 2009;9:1519–27.
81. Olson JJ, Zhang Z, Dillehay D, et al. Assessment of a balloon-tipped catheter modified for intracerebral convection enhanced delivery. J Neurooncol 2008; 89:156–68.
82. Krauze MT, Saito R, Noble C, et al. Reflux-free cannula for the convection-enhanced high-speed delivery of therapeutic agents. J Neurosurg 2005;105: 923–9.
83. Hood RL, Andriani RT, Emch S, et al. Fiberoptic microneedle device facilitates volumetric infusate dispersion during convection-enhanced delivery in the brain. Lasers Surg Med 2013;45:418–26.
84. Oh S, Odland R, Wilson SR, et al. Improved distribution of small molecules and viral vectors in the murine brain using a hollow-fiber catheter. J Neurosurg 2007; 107:568–77.
85. Hood RL, Rossmeisl JH Jr, Andriani RT, et al. Intracranial hyperthermia through local photothermal heating with a fiberoptic microneedle device. Lasers Surg Med 2013;45:167–74.
86. Chen MY, Hoffer A, Morrison PF, et al. Surface properties, more than size, limiting convective distribution of virus-sized particles and viruses in the central nervous system. J Neurosurg 2005;103:311–9.
87. Saito R, Krauze MT, Noble CO, et al. Tissue affinity of the infusate affects the distribution volume during convection-enhanced delivery into rodent brains: implications for local drug delivery. J Neurosci Methods 2006;154:225–32.
88. Sampson JH, Raghaven R, Brady ML, et al. Clinical utility of a patient-specific algorithm for simulating intracerebral drug infusions. Neuro Oncol 2007;9: 343–53.
89. Rosenbluth KH, Martin AJ, Mittermeyer S, et al. Rapid inverse planning for pressure-driven drug infusions in the brain. PLoS One 2013;8(2):e56397.
90. Platt S, Nduom E, Kent M, et al. Canine model of convection-enhanced delivery of cetuximab-conjugated iron-oxide nanoparticles monitored with magnetic resonance imaging. Clin Neurosurg 2012;59:107–13.
91. Debinski W, Dickinson P, Rossmeisl JH, et al. New agents for targeting of IL-13RA2 expressed in primary human and canine brain tumors. PLoS One 2013;8(10):e77719.
92. Rossmeisl JH. Molecular combinatorial therapy for canine malignant gliomas. In: Virginia Maryland Regional College of Veterinary Teaching Hospital Current

Clinical Trials Website. 2013. Available at: http://www.vetmed.vt.edu/research/rossmeisl/. Accessed October 23, 2013.

93. Platt SR, Kent MK, Northrup N. The treatment of canine brain tumors with Cetuximab administered using convection enhanced delivery (CED). In: University of Georgia College of Veterinary Medicine Clinical Trials Website. 2013. Available at: http://vet.uga.edu/research/clinical/current. Accessed November 1, 2013.

94. Sehgal A, Berger MS. Basic concepts of immunology and neuroimmunology. Neurosurg Focus 2000;9(6):e1.

95. Rivest S. Regulation of innate immune responses in the brain. Nat Rev Immunol 2009;9:429–39.

96. Rosenberg SA. Progress in human tumour immunology and immunotherapy. Nature 2001;411:380–4.

97. Mitchell DA, Fecci PE, Sampson JH. Immunotherapy of malignant brain tumors. Immunol Rev 2008;222:70–100.

98. Nauts HC, McLaren JR. Coley toxins-the first century. Adv Exp Med Biol 1990; 267:483–500.

99. De Bonis P, Albanese A, Lofrese G, et al. Post-operative infection may influence survival in patients with glioblastoma: simply a myth? Neurosurgery 2011;69:864–9.

100. Dix AR, Brooks WH, Roszman TL, et al. Immune defects observed in patients with primary malignant brain tumors. J Neuroimmunol 1999;100:216–32.

101. Wainwright DA, Nigam P, Thaci B, et al. Recent developments on immunotherapy for brain cancer. Expert Opin Emerg Drugs 2012;17(2):181–202.

102. Sioka C, Kyritsis AP. Chemotherapy, hormonal therapy, and immunotherapy for recurrent meningiomas. J Neurooncol 2009;92:1–6.

103. Dillman RO. Cancer immunotherapy. Cancer Biother Radiopharm 2011;26:1–64.

104. Donaldson JM, Kari C, Fragoso RC, et al. Design and development of masked therapeutic antibodies to limit off-target effects. Cancer Biol Ther 2009;8:2147–52.

105. Harris M. Monoclonal antibodies as therapeutic agents for cancer. Lancet Oncol 2004;5:292–302.

106. Narita Y. Drug review: safety and efficacy of bevacizumab for glioblastoma and other brain tumors. Jpn J Clin Oncol 2013;43:587–95.

107. Rossmeisl JH, Duncan RB, Huckle WR, et al. Expression of vascular endothelial growth factor in tumors and plasma from dogs with primary intracranial neoplasms. Am J Vet Res 2007;68:1239–45.

108. Dickinson PJ, Roberts BN, Higgins RJ, et al. Expression of receptor tyrosine kinases VEGFR-1 (FLT-1), VEGFR-2 (KDR), EGFR-1, PDGFRa and c-Met in canine primary brain tumours. Vet Comp Oncol 2006;4:132–40.

109. Higgins RJ, Dickinson PJ, LeCouteur RA, et al. Spontaneous canine gliomas: overexpression of EGFR, PDGFRalpha and IGFBP2 demonstrated by tissue microarray immunophenotyping. J Neurooncol 2010;98:49–55.

110. Neyns B, Sadones J, Joosens E, et al. Stratified phase II trial of cetuximab in patients with recurrent high-grade glioma. Ann Oncol 2009;20:1596–603.

111. Hadjipanayis CG, Machaidze R, Kaluzova M, et al. EGFRvIII antibody-conjugated iron oxide nanoparticles for magnetic resonance imaging-guided convection enhanced delivery and targeted therapy of glioblastoma. Cancer Res 2010;70:6303–12.

112. Cox Media Group. Killing canine brain tumors. In: WFTV Channel 9 News (www.wftv.com). 2013. Available at: http://www.wftv.com/news/news/local/killing-canine-brain-tumors/nY3zY/. Accessed November 4, 2013.

113. Debinski W, Gibo D, Wykosky J, et al. Canine gliomas over-express IL-13Ralpha2, EphA2, and Fra-1 in common with human high-grade astrocytomas [abstract]. Neuro Oncol 2007;9(4):535–6.
114. Debinski W, Gibo DM. Molecular expression analysis of restrictive receptor for interleukin 13, a brain tumor-associated cancer/testis antigen. Mol Med 2000; 6:440–9.
115. Lal A, Glazer CA, Martinson HM, et al. Mutant epidermal growth factor receptor up-regulates molecular effectors of tumor invasion. Cancer Res 2002;62: 3335–9.
116. Lillehei KO, Mitchell DH, Johnson SD, et al. Long-term follow-up of patients with recurrent malignant gliomas treated with adjuvant adoptive immunotherapy. Neurosurgery 1991;28:16–23.
117. Boiardi A, Silvani A, Ruffini PA, et al. Loco-regional immunotherapy with recombinant interleukin-2 and adherent lymphokine-activated killer cells (A-LAK) in recurrent glioblastoma patients. Cancer Immunol Immunother 1994; 39:193–7.
118. Rosenberg SA, Yang JC, Restifo NP. Cancer immunotherapy: moving beyond current vaccines. Nat Med 2004;10(9):909–15.
119. Vauleon E, Avril T, Collet B, et al. Overview of cellular immunotherapy for patients with glioblastoma. Clin Dev Immunol 2010;2010. http://dx.doi.org/10.1155/2010/689171. pii:689171.
120. Morgan RA, Dudley ME, Wunderlich JR, et al. Cancer regression in patients after transfer of genetically engineered lymphocytes. Science 2006;314: 126–9.
121. Tsuboi K, Saijo K, Ishikawa E, et al. Effects of local injection of ex vivo expanded autologous tumor-specific T lymphocytes in cases with recurrent malignant gliomas. Clin Cancer Res 2003;9:3294–302.
122. Quattrocchi KB, Miller CH, Cush S, et al. Pilot study of local autologous tumor infiltrating lymphocytes for the treatment of recurrent malignant gliomas. J Neurooncol 1999;45:141–57.
123. Wood GW, Holladay FP, Turner T, et al. A pilot study of autologous cancer cell vaccination and cellular immunotherapy using anti-CD3 stimulated lymphocytes in patients with recurrent grade III/IV astrocytoma. J Neurooncol 2000;48: 113–20.
124. Yamanaka R. Cell- and peptide-based immunotherapeutic approaches for glioma. Trends Mol Med 2008;14:228–35.
125. Yamanaka R, Homma J, Yajima N, et al. Clinical evaluation of dendritic cell vaccination for patients with recurrent glioma: results of a clinical phase I/II trial. Clin Cancer Res 2005;11:4160–7.
126. Kikuchi T, Akasaki Y, Abe T, et al. Vaccination of glioma patients with fusions of dendritic and glioma cells and recombinant human interleukin 12. J Immunother 2004;27:452–9.
127. Andersen BM, Pluhar GE, Seiler CE, et al. Vaccination for invasive canine meningioma induces in situ production of antibodies capable of antibody-dependent cell-mediated cytotoxicity. Cancer Res 2013;73:2987–97.
128. Xiong W, Candolfi M, Liu C, et al. Human Flt3L generates dendritic cells from canine peripheral blood precursors: implications for a dog glioma clinical trial. PLoS One 2010;5:e11074.
129. Candolfi M, Pluhar GE, Kroeger K, et al. Optimization of adenoviral vector-mediated transgene expression in the canine brain in vivo, and in canine glioma cells in vitro. Neuro Oncol 2007;9:245–58.

130. CBS Interactive, Inc. Man's best friend: key to brain cancer cure? In: CBS News (www.cbsnews.com). 2011. Available at: http://www.cbsnews.com/video/watch/?id=7390631n&tag=cbsnewsMainColumnArea. Accessed November 8, 2013.

131. Postel-Vinay S, Arkenau HT, Olmos D, et al. Clinical benefit in phase-I trials of novel molecularly targeted agents: does dose matter? Br J Cancer 2009;100: 1373–8.

132. Gedeon PC, Choi BD, Hodges TR, et al. An EGFRvIII-targeted bispecific T-cell engager overcomes limitations of the standard of care for glioblastoma. Expert Rev Clin Pharmacol 2013;6:375–86.

Altered States of Consciousness in Small Animals

Simon Platt, BVM&S, MRCVS

KEYWORDS

- Consciousness • Confusion • Stupor • Coma • Intracranial pressure
- Small animals

KEY POINTS

- Consciousness is best represented by both wakefulness and awareness.
- Abnormalities of consciousness indicate a brainstem and/or forebrain localization.
- Any disease that affects intracranial structures can cause abnormalities of consciousness.
- Severely impaired consciousness can represent a medical emergency.
- Immediate fluid therapy and oxygen therapy are the most successful supportive measures for acute impaired states of consciousness.

INTRODUCTION

The terms consciousness, confusion, stupor, unconsciousness, and coma have been endowed with so many different meanings that it is almost impossible to avoid ambiguity in their usage. The word consciousness is the most difficult of all to define. For practical and didactic purposes, consciousness is often described as having 2 main components: awareness and wakefulness. At present, there is no single marker of awareness, but its presence can be clinically deduced from behavioral signs, such as visual pursuit or responses to command. Wakefulness describes the state of arousal, often apparent by opened eyes.

Abnormalities of consciousness usually indicate diseases or intoxications that result in dysfunction of the brainstem and/or the cerebrum. Clinical abnormalities may be acute or chronic in nature and may vary from subtle to profound dysfunction. Assessment of consciousness is based on an animal's responses, either appropriate or inappropriate, to its environment, and stimuli, both normal and abnormal, within that environment. As such, familiarity with the range of normal responses of cats versus

Department of Small Animal Medicine & Surgery, College of Veterinary Medicine, University of Georgia, 501 DW Brooks Drive, Athens, GA 30602, USA
E-mail address: srplatt@uga.edu

Vet Clin Small Anim 44 (2014) 1039–1058
http://dx.doi.org/10.1016/j.cvsm.2014.07.012   vetsmall.theclinics.com

dogs, young animals versus old animals, and highly active breeds, such as terriers, versus less-active giant breeds is important in the assessment of consciousness.

STATES OF NORMAL AND IMPAIRED CONSCIOUSNESS

The following definitions aim to describe the states of consciousness in terms of awareness and wakefulness so that they can be practically identified and related to underlying disease of the nervous system (**Table 1**):

A. *Normal consciousness.* This is the condition of the normal animal when awake. In this state, the animal is fully responsive.
B. *Confusion.* The term confusion lacks precision but in general it denotes an inability to think with appropriate speed and clarity. This is obviously open to subjective interpretation in veterinary medicine, but it is proposed here as the term that describes an abnormal state of awareness because of its simplicity and its intuitive implication. Assessing an animal to be either normally aware versus confused relies on an interpretation of an animal's behavior, which itself is defined as the observable response of an animal to environmental or specific stimuli (**Fig. 1**). Behavior suggestive of confusion includes getting trapped in corners or under furniture, unprovoked vocalization, staring at the floor or wall for protracted periods of time, and loss of house training. The words delirium and dementia have been inappropriately used in the veterinary literature to describe abnormal states of awareness. In human neurology, delirium describes a mental disturbance denoted by excitement, restlessness, and unprovoked vocalization often associated with hallucinations, whereas dementia is defined as impaired intellectual function involving memory and judgment, as well as changes in personality. Accurate assessment of these states in veterinary medicine is not obviously possible; additionally they

Table 1
States of consciousness in animals

State of Consciousness	Wakefulness	Awareness	Interpretation
Normal consciousness	Preserved	Preserved	No evidence of intracranial disease but it cannot be ruled out.
Drowsy	Reduced	Preserved	Possible primary brainstem or forebrain disease but systemic disease, intoxication, and even pain could be responsible. A drowsy and confused state would isolate the disease to the forebrain.
Confused	Preserved	Reduced	Isolates the disease to the forebrain. A drowsy and confused state also can be possible with this lesion localization.
Stupor	Absent	Absent	This indicates severe disease of the brainstem and/or bilateral cerebral hemispheres. The animal can be aroused with noxious stimulation.
Coma	Absent	Absent	As for stupor, this indicates severe disease of the brainstem and or bilateral cerebral hemispheres. The animal cannot be aroused with noxious stimulation but some cranial nerve reflexes may still be present if the brainstem is not involved.

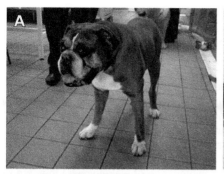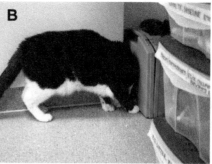

Fig. 1. (A) A 7-year-old boxer demonstrates abnormal consciousness. This could represent a drowsy state and/or a confused state. Without observing environmental interactions and responses, such an assessment could not be made. (B) A 3-year-old domestic short hair cat is "trapped" in a corner, which is one of several behavioral manifestations of a confused state.

do not determine a different or more specific lesion localization or a distinct set of differentials in comparison with the use of the more encompassing term confusion.

C. *Drowsiness.* This term denotes a reduced ability to sustain a normally wakeful state without the application of external stimuli (see **Fig. 1**). Slow arousal is usually elicited by speaking to the animal or applying a tactile stimulus. A state of drowsiness does not necessarily imply primary dysfunction of the central nervous system (CNS), but disorders of the brainstem and occasionally bilateral cerebral hemisphere disease may be responsible. The terms lethargy, obtundation, and depression have synonymously and inappropriately been used in the veterinary literature to describe the state of drowsiness. Lethargy describes a lowered level of consciousness, with drowsiness, listlessness, and apathy; the latter obviously cannot be assessed in dogs and cats. Obtundation is defined as a state of mental blunting with mild to moderate reduction in alertness and a diminished sensation of pain, which cannot be accurately assessed in dogs and cats. Depression represents a mental state of altered mood characterized by feelings of sadness, despair, and discouragement, which obviously cannot be assessed in veterinary medicine.

D. *Stupor.* This term describes an animal that is unconscious, essentially unresponsive to normal environmental stimuli, but is responsive to painful stimuli. Such cases either have a disease of or affecting (ie, toxicity) both cerebral hemispheres and more usually the brainstem.

E. *Coma.* An animal in this state is unconscious and unresponsive to any stimulus, including noxious pain. As for stupor, diseases of or affecting bilateral hemispheres or the brainstem are suggested.

NEURO-ANATOMICAL BASIS OF CONSCIOUSNESS

Clinicopathological correlation and neurophysiological experimentation have shown that coma is caused by diffuse bilateral cerebral hemisphere damage, failure of the ascending reticular activating system, or both.[1,2] The reticular formation is composed of a network of both ascending and descending neuronal communications and forms an extensive component of the neuraxis in all mammals.[2] The ascending component of the reticular system forms a diffuse midline system in the brainstem and spinal cord and receives input from all sensory modalities (except muscle and joint proprioception) and projects this information diffusely to the cerebral cortex via the thalamus. The ascending reticular formation arouses all areas of the cerebral cortex, resulting in a normal level of consciousness. Therefore, the ascending reticular formation is often referred to as the reticular activating system (RAS).

Experimental work in animals suggests that the following structures play key roles in the maintenance and modulation of wakefulness: cholinergic nuclei in the upper brainstem and basal forebrain; noradrenergic nuclei, in particular the locus coeruleus; a histaminergic projection from the hypothalamus; and probably dopaminergic and serotonergic pathways arising from the brainstem.[2] Additionally, hypocretins (orexins) are more recently described hypothalamic neuropeptides thought to have an important role in the regulation of sleep and arousal states.[3] Much of the influence exerted by all of these pathways is mediated by the thalamus, which is regarded as the apex of the RAS, as well as a critical synaptic relay for most sensory pathways.[2] The function of these activating structures is not confined to the maintenance of wakefulness: they are of profound importance to a wide range of interrelated functions, including motivation, attention, learning, and movement.[4] Some specific contributions made by these and other structures to the regulation of conscious states have been defined. For example, the suprachiasmatic nucleus of the hypothalamus provides a timekeeper function.[2] Additionally, transection experiments have established the key importance of cholinergic nuclei at the pontomesencephalic junction, the laterodorsal tegmental and pedunculopontine nuclei, in the reduction of consciousness during sleep.[2] More caudally, the rostral pons and caudal midbrain make a critical contribution to the RAS and are important in mediating the effects of CNS depressants and stimulants.

The true seat of consciousness is the cerebral cortex; however, the RAS is critical for adjusting the level of cerebral activity, and damage to either area or interruption of the communication between the RAS and the cerebrum will result in abnormal levels of wakefulness. Extensive bilateral dysfunction of cerebral hemisphere function is required to produce coma and therefore a unilateral hemisphere lesion will not result in coma unless there is secondary brainstem compression that compromises the ascending reticular activating system. Bilateral thalamic and hypothalamic lesions also cause coma by interrupting activation of the cortex.[1] The speed of onset, site, and size of a brainstem lesion determine whether it results in coma, so brainstem infarction or hemorrhage often cause coma, whereas other brainstem conditions (eg, neoplasia) rarely do so. Drugs and metabolic disease produce coma by depression of both cortex and RAS function.

In the assessment of the poorly responsive animal, it is important to analyze quality of the consciousness (normal vs confused) as well as the quantity. Normal behavior requires the complex interaction of numerous components of the thalamus and cerebral cortex. Of particular interest is the limbic system, which is associated with emotional and behavioral patterns in animals. It functions in the nonolfactory part of the rhinencephalon (the part of the brain once thought to be concerned entirely with olfactory functions). The name limbic (edge or border) is used because the nuclei that primarily comprise the nonolfactory rhinencephalon lie in 2 incomplete rings on the medial aspect of the telencephalon at its border with the diencephalon. The term now includes other anatomically distant nuclei, such as those in the brainstem. The major structures of the limbic system include the amygdaloid, hippocampus, and cingulate gyrus in the telencephalon, the thalamus and hypothalamus in the diencephalon, and the reticular formation of the mesencephalon. The function of the limbic system is to influence visceral motor activity, primarily through its influence on the hypothalamus. Neurons in this system receive projections from the olfactory, optic, auditory, exteroceptive, and interoceptive sensory systems. It is the portion of the brain in humans that is involved in basic drives, sexual activity, emotional experiences, memories, fears, and pleasures.

NEUROLOGIC EVALUATION OF THE ANIMAL WITH IMPAIRED CONSCIOUSNESS

The clinician needs to determine what type of lesion is responsible for the impaired consciousness and its severity. The first component of a complete neurologic examination consists of general observations, including the level of consciousness. If possible, an animal should be allowed to move around freely so that its response to both the local environment and people can be assessed. This may be accomplished while the examiner is obtaining the pertinent history and presenting complaints from the owner.

Using the Modified Glasgow Coma Scoring System

In humans, traumatic brain injury is graded as mild, moderate, or severe on the basis of the level of consciousness or the Glasgow Coma Scale.[5–11] Mild traumatic brain injury in humans is usually the result of concussion, and full neurologic recovery routinely occurs. A patient with moderate traumatic brain injury is drowsy, and a patient with severe injury is stuporous or comatose. Patients with severe traumatic brain injury have a high risk of hypotension, hypoxemia, and brain swelling.[6–11] If these sequelae are not prevented or managed properly, they can exacerbate the brain injury and increase the risk of death. The clinical point at which to initiate therapy for a veterinary patient with head trauma, the extent of appropriate therapy, and the length of time that such treatment is necessary are poorly documented. The effectiveness of specific treatment and the prognosis for any given animal will always be difficult to assess because of the multifactorial nature of the injury.

A modification of the Glasgow Coma Scale used in humans has been proposed for use in veterinary medicine (**Table 2**).[12] This scoring system enables grading of the initial neurologic status and serial monitoring of the patient with impaired consciousness. Although primarily investigated for its prognostic value in head trauma, this modified scale could be used to assess baseline function whatever the underlying cause of cerebral dysfunction, creating a baseline against which the patient can be monitored. Such a system can facilitate the assessment of prognosis, which is crucial information for both the veterinarian and owner. An almost linear correlation between this scoring system and short-term survival of dogs with head trauma has now been demonstrated.[12] It should be noted that long-term survival and functional outcome have not been evaluated using these scales in dogs or cats.

Each of the 3 categories of the examination (ie, level of consciousness, motor activity, brain stem reflexes) is assigned a score from 1 to 6. The level of consciousness provides information about the functional capabilities of the cerebral cortex and the reticular activating system in the brain stem.[13]

Levels of consciousness

The level of consciousness is the most reliable empiric measure of impaired cerebral function after head injury. Impairment of consciousness is stratified in terms of the responses to external stimuli, and serial records of these responses provide an important guide to treatment.

Decreasing levels of consciousness indicate abnormal function of the cerebral cortex or interference with transmission of sensory stimuli by the reticular activating system. Human patients who arrive in a state of coma generally have bilateral or global cerebral abnormalities or severe brain stem injury and have a guarded prognosis.[14]

Limb movements, posture, and reflexes

Spontaneous and evoked limb movements are studied as part of the coma scale examination.[12] It is important for the clinician to determine whether spinal cord injury or severe orthopedic abnormalities are present before extensive manipulation of the patient.

Table 2 Small animal Modified Glasgow Coma Scale (MGCS)	
Assessment Parameter	**Score**
Motor activity	
Normal gait, normal spinal reflexes	6
Hemiparesis, tetraparesis, or decerebrate activity	5
Recumbent, intermittent extensor rigidity	4
Recumbent, constant extensor rigidity	3
Recumbent, constant extensor rigidity with opisthotonus	2
Recumbent, hypotonia of muscles, depressed or absent spinal reflexes	1
Brain stem reflexes	
Normal pupillary light reflexes and oculocephalic reflexes	6
Slow pupillary light reflexes and normal to reduced oculocephalic reflexes	5
Bilateral, unresponsive miosis with normal to reduced oculocephalic reflexes	4
Pinpoint pupils with reduced to absent oculocephalic reflexes	3
Unilateral, unresponsive mydriasis with reduced to absent oculocephalic reflexes	2
Bilateral, unresponsive mydriasis with reduced to absent oculocephalic reflexes	1
Level of consciousness	
Occasional periods of alertness and responsiveness to environment	6
Depression or delirium, capable of responding but response may be inappropriate	5
Semicomatose, responsive to visual stimuli	4
Semicomatose, responsive to auditory stimuli	3
Semicomatose, responsive only to repeated noxious stimuli	2
Comatose, unresponsive to repeated noxious stimuli	1

A score is given to each of 3 categories of the neurologic examination: motor activity, brain stem reflexes, and level of consciousness. Within each category, a score of 1 to 6 exists, representing the most severe to the mildest of clinical pictures. A total score can then be helpful (1) in estimating the severity of the initial condition, which determines the most appropriate level of therapy; (2) assessing the prognosis for survival within the first 72 hours; and (3) assessing the effect of therapy.

From Platt SR, Radaelli ST, McDonnell JJ. The prognostic value of the modified Glasgow Coma Scale in head trauma in dogs. J Vet Intern Med 2001;15:581; with permission.

Motor activity may be affected by the animal's level of consciousness; the best motor response detected is the most important. Animals that are not comatose, but have an altered state of consciousness, usually maintain some voluntary motor activity.

Muscle tone is assessed by putting the limbs through a full range of passive movement, keeping in mind the possibility of a long-bone or joint fracture. The tendon reflexes are elicited; these reflexes have very little value in the diagnosis of acute cerebral injuries, but localized absence of tendon jerks may disclose a nerve injury. Exaggerated reflexes can be seen in all 4 limbs in patients with cerebral injury (or cervical spinal cord trauma), but severely affected comatose animals lose muscle tone and reflex activity.

Opisthotonus with hyperextension of all 4 limbs is suggestive of decerebrate rigidity, which results from a midbrain lesion and is caused because the reticular formation in the brainstem facilitates gamma motor activity and the vestibulospinal system facilitates alpha motor neuron activity. Severe and acute injury rostral to these structures can result in their "release," causing increased extensor tone of all limbs. This posture is occasionally seen in animals recumbent as a result of craniocerebral trauma, and can provide further information about the severity of the brain injury. Variable flexion and extension of the hind limbs is seen in rigidity with cerebellar injury accompanied by a normal level of consciousness; this is termed decerebellate rigidity (**Fig. 2**).[14]

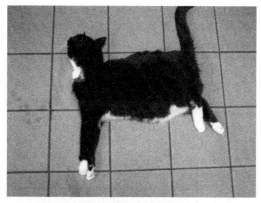

Fig. 2. A 9-year-old cat exhibits decrebellate rigidity. The thoracic limbs demonstrate increased extensor tone and the pelvic limbs demonstrate increased flexor tone, which is most classic for a severe and often acute lesion affecting the cerebellum. The animal's consciousness may be unaffected if a pure cerebellar lesion is responsible.

Neuro-ophthalmologic examination

Pupillary responses Proper assessment of the pupillary responses requires a bright light in a dimmed room. The clinician should be aware that prior and ongoing ophthalmic disease of any nature, concomitant trauma to the eye, and the use of drugs, such as atropine, dopamine, and opioids, can all have effects on pupillary reactions that may be misleading. Pupil size, shape, and reactivity are recorded routinely during the initial examination and should be checked at frequent intervals thereafter (**Table 3**).

Table 3
Anatomic interpretation of pupillary abnormalities

Injury	Ipsilateral Pupil	Associated Findings
Oculomotor nerve	Dilated and fixed to direct light No consensual constriction from contralateral light but normal consensual constriction in contralateral pupil	Ptosis and ventrolateral strabismus
Optic nerve	Fixed to direct light Absent consensual constriction in contralateral pupil Normal consensual constriction from contralateral light	Spontaneous fluctuations in pupil size
Oculomotor and optic nerve	Dilated and fixed to direct light No consensual constriction from contralateral light and no consensual constriction in contralateral pupil	Ptosis and ventrolateral strabismus
Iris or ciliary body	Dilated and fixed to direct light No consensual constriction from contralateral light but normal consensual constriction in contralateral pupil	Often signs of orbital injury No strabismus
Cervical sympathetic pathway	Constricted and fixed or sluggish to direct light and contralateral light but normal consensual constriction in contralateral pupil	Ptosis

The pupillary light reflex (PLR) is tested by shining a bright light into the pupil and assessing for pupillary constriction (direct reflex). The opposite pupil should constrict at the same time (consensual or indirect reflex). A slight dilation usually follows the initial pupillary constriction (pupillary escape) as a consequence of light adaptation of photoreceptors. The PLR involves an afferent arm and an efferent arm. The afferent arm of this reflex shares some common pathways (ipsilateral retina, optic nerve, optic chiasm, and contralateral optic tract) with part of the afferent arm of the menace response and visual placing (**Fig. 3**). These tests use different integration centers within the brain and different efferent pathways. The PLR does not test the animal's vision and the cerebrum is not involved in the PLR pathway. The efferent arm of the PLR reflex is mediated by the parasympathetic portion of cranial nerve III (oculomotor nerve). Although axons involved in vision reach the conscious level after synapse with the lateral geniculate nucleus, the axons involved in the PLR synapse with a third neuron in the pretectal nucleus. Most of the axons arising from this nucleus decussate (cross over) again and synapse in the parasympathetic component of the oculomotor nucleus (ipsilateral to the stimulated eye) in the mesencephalon. There are also neurons that do not decussate and that project to the oculomotor nucleus on the contralateral side of the stimulated eye. The proportion of axons that decussate is higher than the ones that do not decussate, explaining why the direct response (constriction in the eye receiving the light stimulus) is greater than the consensual response (constriction in the eye not receiving the light stimulus). Combining the results of the menace response and PLR testing helps to localize the lesion as being within the common pathways or not.

Pupillary abnormalities may be bilateral or unilateral. Mild size discrepancy between the 2 pupils (<3 mm) has not been significantly associated with patient outcome in humans but has not been assessed in veterinary patients.[15] There are simplistically 3 situations that may be identified in the comatose animal, recognizing that asymmetry of the disease can affect the evaluation.

i. Pupils that are of normal size and are considered to respond normally to stimulation with light. This is compatible with normal structure and function of the visual pathways, which includes the thalamus and brainstem.

ii. Miotic pupils, which remain that way in a dimly lit environment. In the absence of concurrent ocular trauma, miosis may indicate a diencephalic (thalamic) lesion, particularly in the hypothalamus, because this area represents the origin of the sympathetic pathway responsible for pupillary dilation.[14] Bilateral miotic pupils also have been noted in association with more diffuse CNS diseases, such as toxic and metabolic encephalopathies.

iii. Mydriatic and unresponsive pupils (**Fig. 4**). Pupils that are widely dilated at the time of initial examination may indicate an irreparable primary midbrain lesion or advanced caudal transtentorial herniation, although it is important to be aware that profound sympathetic stimulation (as is likely in many injured animals) also can elicit similar findings. Pupils that are initially miotic and then become mydriatic are indicative of a progressive brainstem lesion. If this is the case, severe impairment of consciousness is likely, emphasizing that pupil size and response cannot be interpreted in isolation.

Dazzle reflex This reflex is poorly described in the literature, but is stimulated by a bright light shone in each eye resulting in "squinting" or complete closure of the palpebral fissure. The anatomic pathways involve the retina, optic nerve, and tract to the level of the lateral geniculate nuclei. From the lateral geniculate nuclei, axons project to the rostral colliculi from which tectonuclear pathways stimulate eyelid closure.

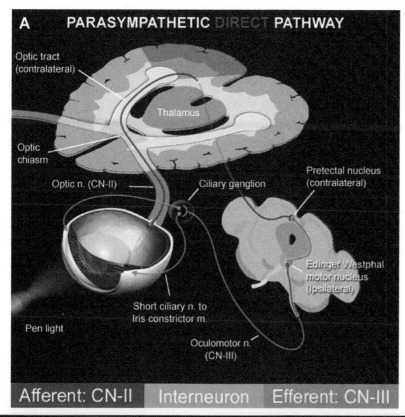

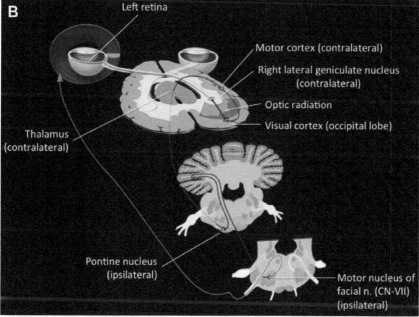

Fig. 3. (*A*) Anatomic pathway responsible for the pupillary light reflex. (*B*) Anatomic pathway responsible for the menace response. (*Courtesy of* Kip Carter, Department of Educational Resources, University of Georgia.)

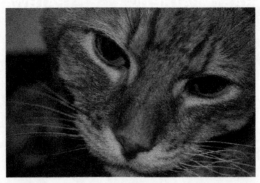

Fig. 4. A domestic short hair cat presents in a profound drowsy state, poorly responsive to external stimuli, and exhibiting mydriasis with reduced response to light stimulation. The mydriasis in combination with the altered consciousness suggest a severe intracranial parenchymal lesion.

As the pathway does not involve the cerebrum, this reflex is maintained despite severe cerebral disease.[16]

Ocular mobility The cranial nerve nuclei (III, IV, and VI) responsible for extraocular muscle innervation are adjacent to the brainstem areas responsible for arousal; thus, evaluation of eye movement is a valuable guide to the presence and level of brainstem disease causing coma. Normal reflex eye movements (physiologic nystagmus) imply that the pontomedullary junction to the level of the oculomotor nucleus in the midbrain is functional. Physiologic (or vestibular) nystagmus is a nystagmus that occurs in normal animals, whereas pathologic nystagmus reflects an underlying vestibular disorder. In both instances, the nystagmus has a slow and fast phase (ie, "jerk" nystagmus). A physiologic nystagmus can be induced in healthy individuals by rotation of the head from side to side (oculovestibular reflex). It is best performed on a cat or a small dog by holding the animal at arm's length, rotating from side to side; it may be seen only at the end of the animal's movement. This physiologic nystagmus functions to stabilize images on the retina during head movement. It is always observed in the plane of rotation of the head and consists of a slow phase in the direction opposite that of the head rotation and a fast phase in the same direction as the head rotation. In the absence of head movement, normal animals do not exhibit nystagmus.

In the unconscious patient, spontaneous ocular movements always should be assessed. If there are none, physiologic nystagmus is tested by rotating the head in vertical and horizontal planes. This should be done only after a cervical spinal injury has been excluded. Physiologic nystagmus may be impaired in animals with brainstem lesions as a result of either involvement of cranial nerve nuclei that innervate the extraocular muscles, the vestibulocochlear nuclei, or the interconnecting ascending medial longitudinal fasciculus within the pons and midbrain.

In addition to their localizing value, eye movements have been considered indices of head injury severity. The ability of the patient to fix its eyes on a target and follow it is a favorable finding, and absence of eye movements is an ominous finding. Absence of eye movements on irrigating the external auditory canal with ice-cold water (oculovestibular reflex) is indicative of profound brain stem failure and is an accepted criteria of brain death in humans. The implications of this finding have not been described in companion animals and this test should not be performed if there is any suspicion of a cranioaural fistula or a skull base fracture. Between the presence and absence of inducible eye movements, there are many ill-defined disturbances with unknown diagnostic and prognostic implications.

DIAGNOSTIC APPROACH TO THE ANIMAL WITH IMPAIRED CONSCIOUSNESS

Coma is an acute, life-threatening situation. In this emergency, the approach is to stabilize (airway, breathing, circulation [ABCs]), to diagnose, to manage, and to critically assess information one step at a time,[17] while urgent steps are taken to minimize further neurologic damage.[18] Assessment should initially comprise a thorough history, a general physical examination, and a neurologic assessment, as described previously.[1]

Systemic and metabolic diseases are a major cause of decreased levels of consciousness in many animals (**Table 4**). Before pursuing specific neurodiagnostic procedures, it is essential to evaluate hematology, serum chemistry, urinalysis, and, probably, thoracic radiographs (in case of trauma or suspected metastatic lesions).

The choice of specific neurodiagnostic techniques depends on the most likely underlying cause and location of the lesion. Although some diagnostic techniques, such as computed tomography (CT) or magnetic resonance imaging (MRI), may be indicated to investigate potential intracranial disease, the overall medical condition of the patient must be assessed and the risks and benefits calculated, particularly when general anesthesia is required (eg, patients with head trauma). Advanced imaging and other diagnostic procedures may be possible in the unanesthetized animal if the animal is already stuporous or comatose.

Laboratory and Ancillary Investigations

Hematology and serum chemistry evaluation play a prominent role in the assessment of an acute unresponsive patient and can often lead to rapid diagnosis. More specific testing should be tailored to the clinical history, physical examination, and imaging findings; for instance, urine and blood screens should be obtained if toxicity is suspected and a specific test is available. In animals presenting with fever and/or an elevated white blood cell count, blood cultures are a necessity. Analysis of serum troponin levels could be considered if there is any suspicion of an acute cardiac lesion.[19] It is important to also consider the anion and osmolar gaps, as these can aid in diagnosis of an acute intoxication. The anion gap can increase in the presence of unmeasured anions, such as ethanol and salicylate intoxications. A difference between the calculated and measured osmolality can indicate intoxication with atypical alcohols, such as ethylene glycol.

Although more invasive, a cerebrospinal fluid (CSF) tap and analysis can be considered in all unresponsive animals with the suspicion of CNS infection or inflammation, or when advanced imaging tests are normal and no explanation exists for the decreased responsiveness. Disease targets that might be identified through this means include viral, bacterial, fungal, rickettsial, and protozoal infections or evidence for noninfectious inflammatory brain disease. However, CSF sampling can be hazardous if there is an increase in intracranial pressure and so a CT or MRI scan would ideally precede a CSF tap to exclude cases at high risk of parenchymal shift associated with a mass lesion.

Neuroimaging

Unfortunately, many unresponsive or comatose animals lack true localizing features on examination and may not have abnormal laboratory findings. In such instances, neuroimaging may help in determining the underlying etiology. Even in an animal

Table 4
Differential diagnosis of altered states of consciousness

Disease Mechanisms (Vitamin D)	Specific Disease
Vascular	Brain infarct Brain hemorrhage Hypertension
Inflammatory/Infectious	Infectious encephalitis (distemper, rabies, toxoplasma, neospora, fungal, bacterial, rickettsial, feline infectious peritonitis) Meningo-encephalitis of unknown etiology (GME, necrotizing, idiopathic)
Trauma	Head trauma 2° Herniation
Toxic	Anticoagulants (2° hemorrhage) Avermectins and milbemycins Hexachlorophene Barbiturates Ethylene glycol Lead Metaldehyde Theobromine (chocolate) Opioids Phenothiazine tranquilizers Recreational drugs Anticonvulsants
Anomalous	Hydrocephalus
Metabolic	Hypoxia/ischemia Syncope (transient) Excitotoxicity (Postictal) Hepatic encephalopathy Uremia Hyperthermia Osmotic abnormalities (Na^+ imbalance) Hypoglycemia Ketoacidosis Hypoadrenocortical crisis Hypothyroidism
Idiopathic	Narcolepsy
Neoplastic	Primary or metastatic brain tumor
Nutritional	Thiamine deficiency

Abbreviation: GME, granulomatous meningoencephalitis.

whose examination allows the clinician to localize the lesion, imaging and laboratory investigation continue to play key roles. For instance, the examination may suggest a lesion involving the midbrain, but the lesion may be an infarct or neoplasia (among other diagnoses), with widely differing prognoses. In the evaluation of an unresponsive patient, CT scans can be excellent at detecting hydrocephalus or intracranial hemorrhage.[20,21] CT scans also are useful in the detection of edema, although the underlying cause of the edema may be elusive.[22] CT is particularly useful for investigation of head trauma if calvarial fractures are suspected. Limitations of CT include poor detail of the caudal fossa secondary to "beam-hardening artifact," especially in cats, as well as reduced anatomic differentiation in comparison with MRI, which may not allow precise etiologic determination.

MRI scans allow greater definition of cortical and subcortical structures and may show cortical injury, laminar necrosis, or white matter disease that is not so apparent on a CT scan (**Fig. 5**).[23–25] The major drawbacks of MRI include accessibility, cost, and time necessary to complete the scan; however, recent work suggests that it can be a valuable prognostic tool, at least in dogs with head trauma.[26]

Advances in task-based functional MRI (fMRI), resting-state fMRI (rs-fMRI), and arterial spin labeling (ASL) perfusion MRI have occurred at a rapid pace in recent years in humans.[27] These techniques for measuring brain function have great potential to improve the accuracy of prognostication for patients with traumatic coma. In addition, fMRI, rs-fMRI, and ASL perfusion MRI have provided novel insights into the pathophysiology of traumatic disorders of consciousness, as well as the mechanisms of recovery from coma.[27] At this time, there is no information on and limited potential for the use of fMRI in veterinary patients to assess traumatic coma.

Electrodiagnostic Evaluation

- *Brainstem auditory evoked response (BAER).* Assessment of the central auditory pathway allows indirect assessment of overall brainstem function.[28] Complete loss of BAER is a poor prognostic indicator in comatose animals (assuming peripheral hair cells are functional). Middle latency auditory evoked responses recorded from the cortex may be used to assess cortical function in addition to brainstem function. However, cortical function will be difficult to evaluate if there is also severe brainstem disease.
- *Electroencephalography (EEG).* EEG allows for assessment of cortical function.[24] Low amplitude or flat trace (0.5 μV) following auditory and painful stimuli carries a poor prognosis in comatose animals. The role of an urgent EEG in an unresponsive patient is somewhat limited, with the exception of nonconvulsive status epilepticus.[29,30] Nonconvulsive status epilepticus should be suspected in any patient with a history of seizures that becomes acutely unresponsive, but also can be considered in otherwise unexplained cases of acute unresponsiveness.[17,29]

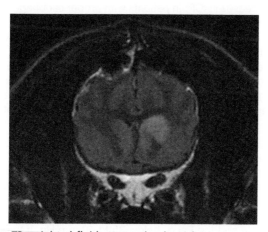

Fig. 5. A transverse T2-weighted fluid attenuation inversion recovery magnetic resonance image of a 6-year-old poodle with an acute-onset altered consciousness. A reasonably well-defined hyperintense lesion can be identified associated with caudate nucleus and causing no adjacent mass effect. This lesion was most compatible with an ischemic infarction based on further imaging sequences and was not visible on CT imaging.

- *Somatosensory evoked potentials.* Recording of potentials from the head following stimulation of sensory nerves in a limb may be used to assess conduction of information to the cortex through the brainstem.[31]

IMMEDIATE EMERGENCY THERAPY OF IMPAIRED CONSCIOUSNESS
General Care

Assessment and stabilization of systemic vital parameters are the first priorities when dealing with an animal presenting in a coma (**Fig. 6**). The underlying cause may not be apparent and so a general approach is necessary, making an assumption that the animal may have elevated intracranial pressure (ICP) and the potential for brain herniation. Until the underlying cause is known, an accurate treatment regimen will not be possible.

A patent airway and normal ventilation, normovolemia, and normotension should be the initial treatment goals to optimize cerebral oxygenation and cerebral perfusion pressure (**Fig. 7**). Secondary goals include intervening for emergent neurologic complications, which include related seizure disorders, clinical neurologic deterioration secondary to uncompensated intracranial hypertension, or metabolic derangements. For animals with metabolic derangements, parenteral fluid therapy and medications should be administered as indicated. Once the patient is systemically stabilized, advanced neuroimaging studies are performed to prioritize the differential diagnoses and identify appropriate ancillary diagnostic and therapeutic plans.

Urinary catheters can be considered to aid in bladder management in recumbent patients and to monitor urinary output. Adequate urine output is between 1 and 2 mL/kg per hour, but should match the volume of fluid given to the patient. Adequate nutrition is critical to the recovery of patients after brain injury[32]; however, hyperglycemia should be avoided because it increases cerebral metabolic rate and promotes anaerobic metabolism, leading to cerebral acidosis. Initially, nutrition may be supplemented through naso-esophageal feeding tubes. Placement may be contraindicated in patients with elevated ICP, because placement can stimulate sneezing, which causes transient increases in ICP. In patients with proper esophageal function, esophagostomy tubes allow medium-term to long-term management of feeding. Gastrostomy tubes offer nutritional support in patients with poor esophageal function and allow long-term nutritional support.

Recumbent patients require proper bedding and monitoring to prevent the development of decubital ulcers. Bedding should be well padded and evaluated frequently to maintain a clean and dry surface. Patients require alternation of recumbency every 4 to 6 hours and frequent evaluation of pressure points for development of decubital ulcers.

Specific Care

Management of oxygen and carbon dioxide
Oxygen supplementation should be considered in all patients presenting in a coma. Control of the partial pressure of oxygen in the arterial blood supply (Pao$_2$) and Paco$_2$ is mandatory and will affect both cerebral hemodynamics and ICP. The goal of oxygen therapy and management of ventilation is to maintain Pao$_2$ greater than or equal to 90 mm Hg and the Paco$_2$ below 35 to 40 mm Hg. If the patient is able to ventilate spontaneously and effectively, supplemental oxygen should be delivered via "flow-by"; confinement within an oxygen cage prevents frequent monitoring. Face masks and nasal catheters should be avoided if possible, as they can cause anxiety, which may contribute to elevations of ICP. Permissive hypercapnea should be

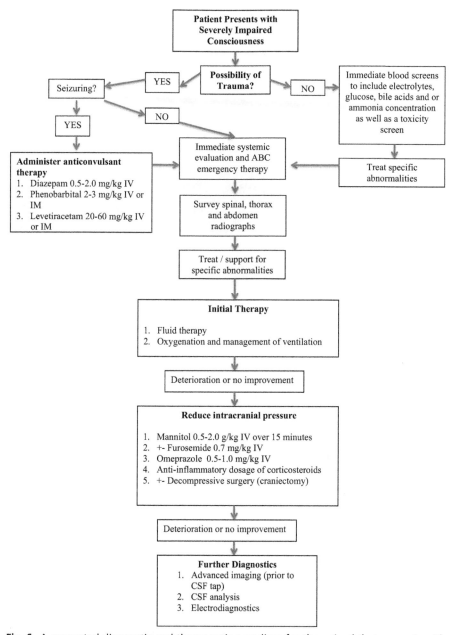

Fig. 6. A suggested diagnostic and therapeutic paradigm for the animal that presents with severely impaired consciousness. IV, intravenous.

avoided because of its cerebral vasodilatory effect, which increases ICP. Excessive hypocapnea can produce cerebral vasoconstriction through serum and CSF alkalosis, although moderate hypocapnea (30–35 mm Hg) can be helpful in reducing ICP. Reduction in cerebral blood flow and ICP is almost immediate, although peak ICP reduction may take up to 30 minutes after P_{CO_2} has been changed.[33]

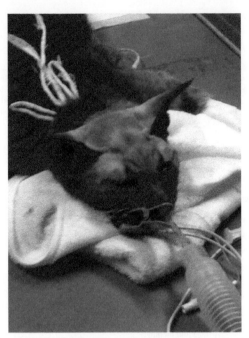

Fig. 7. A 3-year-old cat presenting for an acute loss of consciousness is supportively and symptomatically managed with fluids and intubation to ensure appropriate oxygenation is achieved in the face of a poor ventilatory status.

The amount of oxygen within the blood can be assessed by pulse oximeter (Spo_2), or measuring the Pao_2 with blood gas analysis in conjunction with measurement of circulating hemoglobin concentration. Calculation of oxygen delivery to the tissues requires measurement of both arterial oxygen content and cardiac output. Measurement of mixed venous oxygen can provide an indirect measure of adequacy of oxygen supply to the tissues. The amount of CO_2 within the blood can be assessed by arterial blood gas analysis or by capnography, which provides breath-by-breath assessment of adequacy of ventilation assuming normal cardiovascular function. This technique measures CO_2 in the expired patient gases ($P'ETCO_2$), which approximates to Pco_2 in the alveoli. As alveolar gases should be in equilibrium with arterial blood, $P'ETCO_2$ can be used to approximate $Paco_2$ unless severe pulmonary dysfunction is present.

Fluid therapy
The goal of fluid therapy in a patient with impaired consciousness is to ensure a normovolemic state. It is deleterious to dehydrate an animal in an attempt to reduce cerebral edema. Aggressive fluid therapy and systemic monitoring are required to ensure normovolemia to maintain adequate cerebral perfusion pressure.

Crystalloid and hypertonic fluids should be given concurrently to help restore and maintain blood volume following trauma. Crystalloids are usually given initially for the treatment of systemic shock if necessary. These balanced electrolyte solutions may be given at shock doses (90 mL/kg for dogs, 60 mL/kg for cats). Typically, it is recommended that the shock dose be given in fractions, starting with one-third to one-fourth of the calculated volume, frequently reassessing the patient for normalization of mean arterial blood pressure, mentation, and central venous pressure, if monitored, and giving additional fractions if needed. Unfortunately, crystalloid solutions will extravasate into the interstitium within 1 hour of administration, requiring additional fluid resuscitation.

Hypertonic saline improves cerebral perfusion pressure and blood flow by rapidly restoring intravascular blood volume. Additionally, the high sodium content of hypertonic saline draws water from the interstitial and intracellular spaces, subsequently reducing ICP. Contraindications to administration of hypertonic saline include systemic dehydration and hypernatremia. Hypertonic saline remains within the vasculature for only approximately 1 hour; therefore, it should be followed by colloids to maximize its effects, although its effects on ICP are apparent for approximately 18 hours. A dose of 5 to 6 mL/kg (dogs) and 2 to 4 mL/kg (cats) of 7.5% NaCl should be given over 5 to 10 minutes.

Colloids (ie, Hetastarch, Dextran-70) allow for low-volume fluid resuscitation, especially if total protein concentrations are below 50 g/L or 5 g/dL. These fluids also draw fluid from the interstitial and intracellular spaces, but have the added benefit of staying within the intravascular space longer than crystalloids. Hetastarch is typically given at boluses of 5 to 6 mL/kg in dogs and 2 to 4 mL/kg in cats over 5 to 10 minutes, with frequent patient reevaluation. A total dose of 20 mL/kg per day may be given, although the undocumented benefits and the potential adverse effects of this fluid type make it a contentious choice in veterinary medicine.

Diuretics ICP can be aggressively addressed with the administration of osmotic diuretics. Osmotic diuretics, such as mannitol, should not be given to any patient without being certain that the patient has been volume resuscitated. If not, their use can precipitate acute renal failure. For this reason, they are reserved as therapy secondary to oxygen and fluids.

Mannitol improves cerebral blood flow and reduces ICP by decreasing edema. After administration, mannitol expands the plasma volume and reduces blood viscosity, which improves cerebral blood flow and delivery of oxygen to the brain. Additionally, mannitol assists in scavenging free radicals, which contribute to secondary injury processes. Vasoconstriction occurs as a sequela to the increased partial pressure of oxygen leading to an immediate decrease in ICP. Additionally, the osmotic effect of mannitol reduces extracellular fluid volume within the brain.

Mannitol (0.5–2.0 g/kg) should be given as a bolus over 15 minutes to optimize the plasma-expanding effect. Continuous infusions of mannitol increase the permeability of the blood brain barrier exacerbating edema. Lower doses of mannitol are as effective at decreasing ICP as higher doses, but may not last as long. Mannitol reduces brain edema over approximately 15 to 30 minutes after administration and has an effect for approximately 2 to 5 hours. Repeated dosing of mannitol can cause diuresis, leading to reduced plasma volume, increased osmolarity, intracellular dehydration, hypotension, and ischemia. Therefore, adequate isotonic crystalloid and colloid therapy are critical to maintain hydration. Additionally, administration of mannitol should be reserved for critical patients (Modified Glasgow Coma Scale [MGCS] of <8), deteriorating patients, or patients failing to respond to other treatment, such as hypertonic saline. Multiple reports exist documenting a potentially more beneficial effect in reducing ICP associated with hypertonic saline as compared with mannitol.[34,35]

Administration of furosemide (0.7 mg/kg) before administration of mannitol has a synergistic effect in lowering ICP. Currently, there is no evidence to support that mannitol is contraindicated in cases of intracranial hemorrhage, as has previously been suggested.

PROGNOSIS

There have been no long-term functional outcome studies in dogs or cats with severely impaired consciousness from any cause. There is an obvious need for an accurate assessment of outcome, because patients surviving head trauma, or other causes of stupor/coma, may be left with multiple neurologic deficits that markedly affect quality of life (or at least the owner's perception of the animal's quality of life). Exceptional owner commitment may enable some very disabled patients to return home, but conversely, minor neurologic deficits may be viewed by some owners as unacceptable.

The Glasgow Outcome Scale used in humans is based on the overall social capability of the patient, which takes into account specific mental and neurologic deficits. It was devised for victims of brain damage in general, because it was required for studies both of head injury and of nontraumatic coma. Four categories of survival are recognized and are listed as good recovery, moderate disability (independent but disabled), severe disability (conscious but dependent), and vegetative state. There is variation within each category, but much of this may not be applicable to veterinary patients because it is based on the ability of the patient to communicate and be self-sufficient. There remains a need, therefore, for the modified Glasgow Coma Scale to be correlated with an outcome scale in veterinary medicine, because this would truly assist with defining a prognosis in small-animal patients. Until this time, coma scales can be used only as a guide of the immediate success of therapy and, more importantly, when to initiate this treatment.

COMA SCALES IN THE FUTURE

The use of coma scales in veterinary medicine is still very crude and potentially subject to much interrater variability. The use of the MGCS in isolation could lead to misinterpretation of the prognosis or potential response to aggressive treatment. Evaluation of concurrent systemic injuries or disease and the results of clinical pathology evaluation and imaging evaluations must also be taken into consideration.

A new coma scale named the Full Outline of UnResponsiveness (FOUR) score has recently been introduced in human medicine.[36–41] The FOUR score is based on the bare minimum of tests necessary for assessing a patient with altered consciousness, but also includes much important information that is not assessed by the human Glasgow Coma Scale, including measurement of brainstem reflexes; determination of eye opening, blinking, and tracking; and abnormal breathing rhythms and respiratory drive.

The FOUR score has 4 components: eye responses, motor responses, brainstem reflexes, and respiratory pattern. Each component has a maximal value of 4. As expected, some of the evaluations that comprise this scoring system are not easily translated into a veterinary scoring system, but because it has been proven to be simpler, more accurate, and more consistent in its use in human medicine,[38–41] it is likely that a similar improved scoring system will be available in veterinary medicine in the near future.

SUMMARY

Impaired states of consciousness can be relatively easily identified, although it can occasionally be difficult to assess whether there is a pure disorder of wakefulness or awareness. Regardless, such impairments represent dysfunction of the brainstem and or cerebrum. Acute and severe impairments of consciousness can require immediate assessment, in part currently performed using the modified Glasgow coma scoring system, and emergency stabilization. The prognosis is always guarded and highly sensitive to the underlying etiology.

REFERENCES

1. Bateman DE. Neurological assessment of coma. J Neurol Neurosurg Psychiatr 2001;71(Suppl 1):i13–7.
2. Zeman A. Consciousness. Brain 2001;124(Pt 7):1263–89.
3. Ebrahim IO, Howard RS, Kopelman MD, et al. The hypocretin/orexin system. J R Soc Med 2002;95(5):227–30.
4. Marrocco RT, Witte EA, Davidson MC. Arousal systems. Curr Opin Neurobiol 1994;4(2):166–70.
5. Ghajar J. Traumatic brain injury. Lancet 2000;356(9233):923–9.
6. Mullie A, Verstringe P, Buylaert W, et al. Predictive value of Glasgow coma score for awakening after out-of-hospital cardiac arrest. Cerebral Resuscitation Study Group of the Belgian Society for Intensive Care. Lancet 1988;1(8578):137–40.
7. Schefold JC, Storm C, Kruger A, et al. The Glasgow Coma Score is a predictor of good outcome in cardiac arrest patients treated with therapeutic hypothermia. Resuscitation 2009;80(6):658–61.
8. Juarez VJ, Lyons M. Interrater reliability of the Glasgow Coma Scale. J Neurosci Nurs 1995;27(5):283–6.
9. Menegazzi JJ, Davis EA, Sucov AN, et al. Reliability of the Glasgow Coma Scale when used by emergency physicians and paramedics. J Trauma 1993;34(1):46–8.
10. Fielding K, Rowley G. Reliability of assessments by skilled observers using the Glasgow Coma Scale. Aust J Adv Nurs 1990;7(4):13–7.
11. Gill MR, Reiley DG, Green SM. Interrater reliability of Glasgow Coma Scale scores in the emergency department. Ann Emerg Med 2004;43(2):215–23.
12. Platt SR, Radaelli ST, McDonnell JJ. The prognostic value of the modified Glasgow Coma Scale in head trauma in dogs. J Vet Intern Med 2001;15(6):581–4.
13. Dewey CW. Emergency management of the head trauma patient. Principles and practice. Vet Clin North Am Small Anim Pract 2000;30(1):207–25, vii–viii.
14. Winter CD, Adamides AA, Lewis PM, et al. A review of the current management of severe traumatic brain injury. Surgeon 2005;3(5):329–37.
15. Chesnut RM, Gautille T, Blunt BA, et al. The localizing value of asymmetry in pupillary size in severe head injury: relation to lesion type and location. Neurosurgery 1994;34(5):840–5 [discussion: 845–6].
16. Gelatt KN. Visual disturbance: where do I look? J Small Anim Pract 1997;38(8):328–35.
17. Moore SA, Wijdicks EF. The acutely comatose patient: clinical approach and diagnosis. Semin Neurol 2013;33(2):110–20.
18. Teasdale G, Jennett B. Assessment of coma and impaired consciousness. A practical scale. Lancet 1974;2(7872):81–4.
19. Boswood A. Biomarkers in cardiovascular disease: beyond natriuretic peptides. J Vet Cardiol 2009;11(Suppl 1):S23–32.
20. Sidman R, Connolly E, Lemke T. Subarachnoid hemorrhage diagnosis: lumbar puncture is still needed when the computed tomography scan is normal. Acad Emerg Med 1996;3(9):827–31.
21. Perry JJ, Stiell IG, Sivilotti ML, et al. Sensitivity of computed tomography performed within six hours of onset of headache for diagnosis of subarachnoid haemorrhage: prospective cohort study. BMJ 2011;343:d4277.

22. Stevens RD, Sutter R. Prognosis in severe brain injury. Crit Care Med 2013;41(4): 1104–23.
23. Samain JL, Haven E, Gille M, et al. Typical CT and MRI features of cortical laminar necrosis. JBR-BTR 2011;94(6):357.
24. Bruno MA, Gosseries O, Ledoux D, et al. Assessment of consciousness with electrophysiological and neurological imaging techniques. Curr Opin Crit Care 2011; 17(2):146–51.
25. Lescot T, Galanaud D, Puybasset L. Exploring altered consciousness states by magnetic resonance imaging in brain injury. Ann N Y Acad Sci 2009;1157:71–80.
26. Beltran E, Platt SR, McConnell JF, et al. Prognostic value of early magnetic resonance imaging in dogs after traumatic brain injury: 50 cases. J Vet Intern Med 2014;28(4):1256–62.
27. Edlow BL, Giacino JT, Wu O. Functional MRI and outcome in traumatic coma. Curr Neurol Neurosci Rep 2013;13(9):375.
28. Higgins MA, Rossmeisl JH Jr, Panciera DL. Hypothyroid-associated central vestibular disease in 10 dogs: 1999-2005. J Vet Intern Med 2006;20(6):1363–9.
29. Lovell B, Lander M, Negus R. Non-convulsive status epilepticus as a cause for prolonged delirium: an under-diagnosed phenomenon? Acute Med 2012;11(4):222–5.
30. Raith K, Steinberg T, Fischer A. Continuous electroencephalographic monitoring of status epilepticus in dogs and cats: 10 patients (2004-2005). J Vet Emerg Crit Care (San Antonio) 2010;20(4):446–55.
31. Koenig MA, Kaplan PW. Clinical neurophysiology in acute coma and disorders of consciousness. Semin Neurol 2013;33(2):121–32.
32. Wang X, Dong Y, Han X, et al. Nutritional support for patients sustaining traumatic brain injury: a systematic review and meta-analysis of prospective studies. PLoS One 2013;8(3):e58838.
33. Yoshihara M, Bandoh K, Marmarou A. Cerebrovascular carbon dioxide reactivity assessed by intracranial pressure dynamics in severely head injured patients. J Neurosurg 1995;82(3):386–93.
34. Wakai A, McCabe A, Roberts I, et al. Mannitol for acute traumatic brain injury. Cochrane Database Syst Rev 2013;(8):CD001049.
35. Dostal P, Dostalova V, Schreiberova J, et al. A Comparison of Equivolume, Equiosmolar Solutions of Hypertonic Saline and Mannitol for Brain Relaxation in Patients Undergoing Elective Intracranial Tumor Surgery: a Randomized Clinical Trial. J Neurosurg Anesthesiol 2014. [Epub ahead of print].
36. Wijdicks EF, Bamlet WR, Maramattom BV, et al. Validation of a new coma scale: the FOUR score. Ann Neurol 2005;58(4):585–93.
37. Fischer M, Ruegg S, Czaplinski A, et al. Inter-rater reliability of the Full Outline of UnResponsiveness score and the Glasgow Coma Scale in critically ill patients: a prospective observational study. Crit Care 2010;14(2):R64.
38. Idrovo L, Fuentes B, Medina J, et al. Validation of the FOUR Score (Spanish Version) in acute stroke: an interobserver variability study. Eur Neurol 2010; 63(6):364–9.
39. Sadaka F, Patel D, Lakshmanan R. The FOUR score predicts outcome in patients after traumatic brain injury. Neurocrit Care 2012;16(1):95–101.
40. Stead LG, Wijdicks EF, Bhagra A, et al. Validation of a new coma scale, the FOUR score, in the emergency department. Neurocrit Care 2009;10(1):50–4.
41. Iyer VN, Mandrekar JN, Danielson RD, et al. Validity of the FOUR score coma scale in the medical intensive care unit. Mayo Clin Proc 2009;84(8):694–701.

Corticosteroid Use in Small Animal Neurology

Nicholas D. Jeffery, BVSc, PhD, MSc, FRCVS

KEYWORDS

- Glucocorticoid • Meningoencephalomyelitis • Inflammation • Immunosuppression
- Dog • Intracranial pressure • Tumor

KEY POINTS

- Glucocorticoids have a multitude of effects on diseases affecting the central nervous system (CNS) but are frequently misused.
- There are few diseases for which glucocorticoids are the preferred or definitive therapy, most of which are immune-mediated conditions, such as meningoencephalomyelitis of unknown origin and steroid-responsive meningitis.
- Glucocorticoid effects can impede and impair subsequent diagnostic workup if they are given at early stages of disease.
- Glucocorticoids may have beneficial effects to reduce edema associated with CNS neoplasia.
- For owners who wish to optimize treatment for their pets, it is almost always preferable to delay treatment with glucocorticoids until a specific diagnosis has been attained.

INTRODUCTION

In many veterinarians' minds, neurology and corticosteroids go together like a horse and carriage. It is therefore surprising to consider that there are only a few neurologic conditions in animals for which corticosteroids are the treatment of choice and many more for which their use is unwarranted or even detrimental. A particular concern is that early initiation of corticosteroid therapy can cause confusion in subsequent attempts to confirm a diagnosis, consequently impeding timely application of definitive effective interventions. In reality, much corticosteroid use for neurologic disease in small animals is a default option chosen because of a lack of clear diagnosis and the perception that there is little other option for treating neurologic disease. This viewpoint is disappointing because owners of affected animals will often appreciate the immediate benefit from the initial use of corticosteroids and may then be less likely to pursue accurate diagnosis afterward, because of the perception that the "first-choice" therapy has failed. In almost all instances, it would be preferable to offer

Department of Veterinary Clinical Science, College of Veterinary Medicine, Iowa State University, 1600 South 16th Street, Ames, IA 50011, USA
E-mail address: njeffery@iastate.edu

Vet Clin Small Anim 44 (2014) 1059–1074
http://dx.doi.org/10.1016/j.cvsm.2014.07.004
0195-5616/14/$ – see front matter
vetsmall.theclinics.com

pursuit of accurate diagnosis and targeted specific treatment before submitting to the (often) temporary and nonspecific "feel-good" effect of corticosteroid therapy.

Somewhat counterintuitively, it could be considered that primary care practice in veterinary medicine demands greater attention to constructing a differential diagnosis list than does working in referral practice. In the neurologic referral practice especially, because of access to high-tech equipment, it commonly is possible to make a precise diagnosis, meaning that treatment plans can be accurately constructed and applied to each individual as required. In contrast, in primary care practice, it is often not possible to make a definitive neurologic diagnosis (because of the precluding cost of appropriate tests), meaning that pragmatic therapy is often required. For optimal application of such pragmatic therapy, it is essential to have a comprehensive differential diagnosis list by which to weigh the potential beneficial and detrimental effects of any specific course of action. When considering corticosteroid therapy, there are many possible detrimental consequences associated with both the known desired effects (eg, immunosuppression) and the side effects (eg, gut ulceration), which, in many instances, may not outweigh the potential benefits. However, of course, there are instances when it is rational to use corticosteroids as a pragmatic treatment. The aim of this article is to provide the background information to aid in deciding when corticosteroid therapy is appropriate for treating neurologic disease in specific small animal patients.

MECHANISMS OF CORTICOSTEROID ACTIVITY

Corticosteroids are lipophilic and can therefore pass freely through cell membranes and have a very wide range of activity mediated via both intranuclear and intracytoplasmic interactions. There are 2 forms of corticosteroid receptor in cells: the mineralocorticoid and glucocorticoid receptors and, although they have relatively high affinities for their respective classes of corticosteroid, they will each interact with the other class. In the brain, glucocorticoids are major ligands for mineralocorticoid receptors, but this effect is ameliorated in many other tissues (such as the kidney) by the enzyme 11β-hydroxysteroid dehydrogenase type II, which metabolizes cortisol to cortisone (which is inactive). This article is concerned only with glucocorticoids (GC).

Immunosuppressive effects of GC result from their effects on pro-inflammatory and anti-inflammatory cytokine production, which culminate in a reduced immune response to stimuli.[1] The effects are most evident on cell-mediated immune responses, although reduction in antibody production also occurs at high dosage.[2]

Activity via Nuclear Effects

GC, of which the most physiologically important is cortisol, bind to the glucocorticoid receptor, which is expressed in almost every cell in the body.[1] GC receptors are inactive in the cytoplasm until they bind their ligand[3]; activated GC receptors then translocate to the cell nucleus, where they have 2 modes of action. First, they can bind to specific DNA base sequences termed the glucocorticoid response element and there act as transcription factors to regulate expression of a variety of genes that regulate metabolism and immune function. Second, the activated receptors can bind to other transcription factors to alter their function. The first process is termed transactivation and is not thought to contribute to the anti-inflammatory effects[4] but has been associated with many of the negative side effects of GC administration.[5] The second process, termed transrepression, is associated with negative modulation of pro-inflammatory cytokines and much effort has been dedicated to emphasizing these effects in developing new synthetic GC drugs.[6]

Overall, the most pronounced effect of GC is to reduce pro-inflammatory cytokine production,[7] which can occur both directly and indirectly. GC receptor interaction with DNA reduces transcription of these cytokines, but GC also increase production of proteins that destabilize cytokine mRNA.[8] GC also increase production of anti-inflammatory cytokines, most notably TGFβ, through both pretranscriptional and posttranscriptional mechanisms.[9] Increased production of lipocortin-1, which then reduces availability of prostaglandins, increases the anti-inflammatory effect.[10]

GC also have direct cellular effects, profoundly depressing the proliferative response of lymphocytes to mitogens[10] and inducing apoptosis in a variety of cell types, including T cells, monocytes, and eosinophils.[1] GC administration decreases interleukin-12 responsiveness through inhibition of a specific phosphorylation reaction, which changes the balance between Th1 and Th2 responses toward a Th2 humoral response phenotype through preferential inhibition of T-helper cells and Th1 cytokines, which reduces the immune and inflammatory response.[11]

Activity via Nongenomic Effects

Although the intranuclear activity of GC is well-known, GC also act through a variety of nongenomic mechanisms, including direct and indirect interactions with cytoplasmic proteins, cell and mitochondrial membranes, and direct effects on neuronal function.[12,13] There are many mechanisms proposed for how intracytoplasmic effects of GC might negatively regulate pro-inflammatory cytokine production.[4] For instance, GC receptor inactivates NF-κB[4] and AP-1[14] through a tethering mechanism, and GC also increase expression of IkB-α, which can sequester NF-κB in the cytoplasm, thereby inhibiting its activity to induce inflammatory cytokine production. GC interact with many categories of protein kinase, through which they can mediate a multitude of effects on both immune cell and neuronal function, for instance, elevating nitric oxide production in specific body locations.[12]

Therapeutic Effects of GC

Corticosteroids have a multitude of physiologic and pharmacologic effects. Their physiologic effects can be appreciated in the clinical signs that are apparent in the deficiency state, hypoadrenocorticism (Addison's disease), in which hypotension and low blood glucose are prominent signs. Although most of the effects of hypoadrenocorticism are the result of mineralocorticoid deficiency, exogenous GC may also be required for maintenance or (especially) management of periods of stress in Addison's disease.

More commonly, GC are used pharmacologically to achieve one or more of the following: (1) immunosuppression; (2) anti-inflammatory effects; (3) anti-edema effects; and, (4) specific cytotoxicity versus neoplastic lymphocytes (ie, as part of a cytotoxic protocol for lymphoma). Each of these effects constitutes a clear rationale for their use in specifically diagnosed conditions (see later discussion).

Metabolic Effects

Gluconeogenic effects

This activity is mediated through the liver, in which there is increased synthesis of glucose from nonsaccharide substrates, including amino acids and glycerol. There is also inhibition of glucose uptake into the liver and adipose tissue from the blood. The metabolic effects of GC are occasionally valuable in clinical medicine, for instance, maintaining blood glucose levels in animals with (metastatic or nonoperated cases of) insulinoma[15]; it has been estimated that methylprednisolone will increase activity of the glucose-6-P cycle by 15-fold.[16]

Effects on blood pressure

GC have several effects in regulation of vascular tone. First, they appear to sensitize blood vessels to the effects of epinephrine,[17] and a lack of GC, as observed in hypo-adrenocorticism, is associated with a dramatic loss of blood pressure and collapse. GC inhibit nitric oxide release from endothelial cells, thereby inhibiting its potent vaso-dilating effect.[18] GC also act at mineralocorticoid receptors and therefore have some direct effect through aldosterone signaling pathways; in fact, the MR has the same affinity for GC as for aldosterone, although GC action at this receptor is limited by its inactivation by a specific dehydrogenase found in the endoplasmic reticulum.[19]

Reduction in cerebrospinal fluid production

Several experiments have demonstrated that exogenous GC can reduce cerebrospinal fluid (CSF) production and intraventricular pressure. Betamethasone (investigated in the cited study and similar in effect to dexamethasone) is estimated to reduce production of CSF by about 50%.[20] Sato and colleagues[21] state that this effect occurs within an hour of dexamethasone injection, but there is uncertainty about how quickly the clinical effect can be observed.[22] There is also evidence that GC can increase the rate of absorption of CSF.[23]

Effects on the Immune System

Immunosuppression, anti-inflammatory effect, and cytotoxicity versus lymphocytes

The immunosuppressive and anti-inflammatory effects of GC are well-established and have been extensively reviewed elsewhere; here follows an introduction to the mechanisms of action as it pertains to the nervous system specifically. Pro-apoptotic factors are up-regulated by GC and this mechanism of glucocorticoid-induced inflammatory cell death is widely thought to be responsible for beneficial effects in laboratory animal models of central nervous system (CNS) inflammatory disease.[24] GC-mediated restoration of the blood-brain barrier provides another avenue for effect, because it impedes entry of inflammatory cells into the brain, and the required receptors for adhesion on T cells are down-regulated after methylprednisolone administration.[25] This effect is combined with the reduced expression and secretion of pro-inflammatory cytokines (as described above). Pro-inflammatory cytokines, such as interferon-γ, tumor necrosis factor-α, and nitric oxide, all have direct effects on neural function, sometimes directly blocking axonal conduction.[26] There is also evidence that both endogenous and exogenous GC can directly affect neuronal function in various regions of the brain through nongenomic mechanisms.[27]

Reduction of CNS edema in association with tumors

Although GC have no effect to reduce the edema that accompanies acute trauma (see later discussion), they have long been used to shrink the zone of edema that surrounds brain tumors.[28] It is thought that vascular endothelial growth factor (VEGF), which is highly expressed by CNS tumors, and is responsible for the proliferation of blood vessels and increased permeability of the blood-brain barrier, mediates much of the edema formation associated with brain tumors. Clinical signs can be improved within 24 hours of administration of GC, although it may take 2 days to significantly reduce intracranial pressure.[29] This reduction in intracranial pressure occurs through many mechanisms, but the end result is to decrease the permeability of the blood-brain barrier. In vitro experiments demonstrate that the effect of GC is to increase levels of ANG-1 (which reduces blood vessel permeability) and reduce levels of VEGF in astrocytes, pericytes, and endothelial cells in the brain.[30] It would seem that these effects are mediated via GC receptors, but it is not clear whether changes in gene transcription are required. Endothelial effects include alteration of the tight junctions to make them less permeable[31] and NF-κB-mediated effects also restore blood-brain barrier function, thereby preventing leukocyte recruitment into the parenchyma.[32]

In contrast, GC do not reduce CNS edema resulting from cytotoxic lesions, in which a lack of energy supply (through lack of blood, oxygen, glucose, or other metabolic disturbances), for instance, that occur following trauma to the CNS, impairs ion channel and exchanger mechanisms. Cytotoxic edema is a consequence of loss of function in the sodium-potassium exchanger, leading to accumulation of sodium (and therefore water) within the cells and eventual loss of membrane integrity. Because GC cannot restore the function of the sodium-potassium exchanger (because it is lost as a consequence of impaired energy supply), they have no effect on this disorder; this largely explains why GC are not useful for reduction of edema that follows traumatic injury to the CNS.

Direct effect of GC on tumors
GC have a well-recognized effect on hematologic tumors[33] but may also have effects on other tumors too (see Ref.[28]). For instance, high-dose dexamethasone is thought to have a direct antitumor effect on (experimental) glioma cells,[34] although it also may interfere with the cytotoxic effects of other chemotherapeutics, such as temozolomide[35] and cisplatin.[36]

ROLE OF GLUCOCORTICOID TREATMENT OF SPECIFIC CONDITIONS
Conditions for Which GC Are Definitely Indicated

Immune-mediated disease
There are many neurologic conditions that are known or suspected to have an immune-mediated component and these are clearly targets for treatment with GC. However, the signalment and presentation associated with these types of disease do not aid in suggesting their pathogenesis, meaning that there will be no indication from clinical signs alone that pragmatic use of GC would be indicated. Indeed, many of the differential diagnoses will be infectious diseases, for which GC treatment may well be unhelpful or detrimental.

Therefore, a sufficiently specific working diagnosis is required, which can often be achieved via CSF analysis, often combined with various imaging studies, electrodiagnostics, and blood tests, although histopathologic diagnosis would be ideal.

Corticosteroid-responsive meningitis This condition produces a characteristic clinical syndrome of spinal pain associated with fever and reluctance to move, usually without accompanying neurologic deficits, except in prolonged cases.[37,38] The condition is most commonly diagnosed in large-breed young dogs, and a predisposition has been noted in several breeds (beagle, Bernese mountain dogs, boxers, and Nova Scotia duck tolling retrievers).

Diagnosis is made through ruling out other diagnoses, most commonly bacterial meningitis, through imaging, CSF analysis, culture, and sensitivity testing. The use of GC in this condition, at immunosuppressive doses, is highly efficacious (as would be expected) and the condition generally has an excellent prognosis, although animals that are treated later in the course of the disease seem to require more prolonged periods of therapy.[39] Affected animals may suffer recurrences, which have been suggested to be more common if the initial GC dose is too cautious[37]; relapses sometimes necessitate the use of combinations of GC with other immunosuppressive drugs, such as azathioprine.[38] The prognosis for this condition is excellent, although several cycles of treatment are occasionally required. Various trigger factors for the condition have been suspected but not proven.[40,41]

Meningoencephalomyelitis of unknown origin Meningoencephalomyelitis of unknown origin (MUO) is associated with a great variety of clinical signs, including localized and generalized neurologic deficits and pain syndromes.[42] Typically affected dogs are small, middle-aged, and female, but many types and ages of dog can be affected.[43] This condition is sometimes confused with corticosteroid-responsive meningitis (discussed above), but it is important to make a clear differentiation, because the prognosis for MUO is variable and can be poor, especially for some of the breed-specific variants.[44] Diagnosis depends on imaging and CSF analysis, but it can be difficult to definitively rule out some differential diagnoses without examination of histopathological specimens. Although the underlying triggers for this condition are currently unknown,[45] it has long been suspected to be an immune-mediated condition, and many types of immunosuppressive regime have been shown to be effective in prolonging life expectancy and remitting the clinical signs. Most commonly, GC are used alone; although it has been suggested that procarbazine, cytarabine, or other drugs are more efficacious,[46,47] there is, as yet, no definitive evidence on which to recommend more complicated therapy.[48] The prognosis for MUO is extremely variable, some reported case series suggest a median survival of 10 days for granulomatous meningoencephalomyelitis (GME),[49] but others suggest a much better prognosis; many cases can certainly survive for many years, some even without prolonged therapy.

Immune-mediated myositis Although myositis can have an infectious cause (eg, Protozoal infections[50]), most cases in adult dogs are the result of an immune-mediated disease.[51] Several forms exist: masticatory muscle myositis (in which the masticatory muscles are the only group clinically affected), extraocular myositis (a rare condition causing abnormal eye movements in dogs; see Ref.[52]), dermatomyositis (in which immune-mediated disease of both muscle and skin occur concurrently; most commonly seen in collie dogs), and generalized myositis, which can have an acute, waxing and waning, or chronic course. Although masticatory muscle myositis is easy to recognize during the acute or chronic phases (because of pain and swelling in the former and muscle atrophy in the latter) and dermatomyositis is easy to recognize because of the breeds affected and the concurrent skin lesions, the generalized condition can be difficult to recognize because the clinical signs can be rather nonspecific. Although severely affected animals may walk with a stiff gait, be reluctant to rise from recumbency, or reluctant to walk any distance at all, many other affected cases may exhibit very indistinct signs, such as a general reluctance to exercise or showing nonspecific signs of "depression."

In all myositis conditions, evaluation of CK levels in the blood can be a useful aid to diagnosis, although because of the short half-life of this enzyme,[53] a normal level does not rule out muscle disease. Levels above ~2000 to 3000 IU are generally regarded as abnormal. Further diagnostic evaluation involves electrodiagnostic tests and muscle biopsy, which can reveal inflammatory cell infiltration, usually by lymphocytes or macrophages. Masticatory muscle myositis can be diagnosed by blood samples demonstrating a raised level of the type 2M antibodies that are specific for this condition.[54]

Treatment of all 3 types of immune-mediated muscle disease is generally very gratifying, although cases with severe muscle atrophy may not recover full muscle mass or even full range of motion in affected regions if there has been extensive fibrosis as a secondary consequence of muscle inflammation. GC are well recognized to cause muscle atrophy, especially of the masticatory muscles, and so this can complicate evaluation of response in some cases. Large doses of GC can cause muscle weakness,[55] which, anecdotally at least, seems to be more clinically significant in larger dogs; for long-term treatment, it is often preferable to use other immunosuppressive therapy to avoid these possible complications.

Conditions for Which GC May Be Helpful

CNS neoplasia

The blood-brain barrier is frequently defective in CNS neoplasia, because of VEGF secretion, meaning that edema will develop in the vicinity of the tumor; this effect can greatly enlarge the "effective size" of a tumor within the skull, so that not only the actual tumor region but also a large zone on its periphery will be dysfunctional. GC can be immensely effective in reducing this zone of edema, and clinical signs can dramatically regress following their administration. Although beneficial, if misinterpreted, this effect can deter owners from pursuing definitive diagnosis and therapy, which may be detrimental in the long term. For instance, although the effects may initially be dramatic, it has been estimated that dogs with brain tumors treated with palliative therapy alone (primarily GC) have a median life expectancy of ~2 months.[56] Therefore, it is necessary to counsel owners carefully before embarking on GC therapy in this condition.

A second use of GC in the context of brain tumors is to reduce the swelling of the tumor and its surrounding areas during the course of radiotherapy, which is regarded as fairly routine.[57] The tumor destruction associated with radiotherapy will lead to a zone of edema and inflammation (associated with the response to dead cells) that can be reduced using GC.

Last, GC can be used as a part of the cytotoxic protocol for treating some hematological tumors, notably lymphoma.[58,59] The mechanism of this effect is incompletely understood but may result from activation of death-inducing transcription pathways, but also perhaps by reducing expression of survival genes. It seems that the effects of GC are different from those by which cells can become resistant to other chemotherapeutic agents. However, it has also been shown that GC can induce P-glycoprotein drug transporter expression in dogs,[60] which may increase resistance to chemotherapeutic drugs. Indeed, there is direct evidence that dexamethasone reduces susceptibility to other chemotherapeutic agents,[61] and this may lead to the observation that pretreatment with GC may lead to decreased survival.[62] However, it also would seem that the response to chemotherapy can be predicted by the response to GC monotherapy at induction.[63] Furthermore, there was no detectable effect in a direct test of the hypothesis that cotreatment with GC would reduce response to chemotherapy of lymphoma in dogs.[64]

Conditions for Which GC Have Dubious Value

Polyradiculoneuritis and myasthenia gravis

The most common type of polyradiculoneuritis is the acute form that, in the United States, may be associated with a raccoon bite, although similar syndromes (where raccoons do not exist) are recognized worldwide. It has been established that, although the cause is likely to be immune-mediated, GC therapy does not aid in recovery. In fact, it would seem that GC might be detrimental, probably through increasing the risk of complications and exacerbating muscle loss.[65] Similarly, immune-mediated myasthenia gravis in dogs does not necessarily require treatment with GC, because remission can occur within about 6 months without immunosuppression.[66]

Chronic polyradiculoneuritis is a less common disease that can be difficult to recognize, in which dogs or cats can develop progressive weakness affecting all 4 limbs and sometimes the cranial nerve distribution also.[67] The most common cause of this pattern of clinical signs is a degenerative peripheral neuropathy, as is common in older Labrador retrievers,[68] but occasional cases can be recognized that appear to have a chronic inflammatory cause. Such cases can be diagnosed through careful and in-depth electrodiagnostic tests plus CSF analysis that identifies an inflammatory component through elevated protein or cell content or through nerve biopsy. Such cases can be candidates for immune-suppression using GC alone or in combination with other immunosuppressive agents, although such therapy does not invariably lead to resolution of clinical signs.

Infectious disease

In general, infectious disease is usually assumed to be a contraindication to the use of GC, because of their effects in reducing inflammatory and immune responses to eliminate or repel the infectious process. Although this is generally true with regard to the ability to overcome viral infections, which relies largely on nonspecific inflammation and then generation of an immune response, all of which are detrimentally affected by GC, GC therapy does have some possible benefits in other types of infection, albeit when used in combination with anti-infective drugs.

Most notably, it has been argued that GC use in combination with antibiotics can be helpful in the treatment of acute bacterial meningitis in human patients. Reduced levels of nitric oxide may be a mechanism by which GC exert these beneficial effects.[69] However, the clinical effect remains controversial, with some studies suggesting benefits and some showing detrimental effects, suggesting that the net result may depend on the environmental conditions.[70] In dogs, bacterial meningitis can usually be treated using antibiotics alone and so the need to add GC can be reserved for cases in which there has been a failure to respond adequately.

Low doses of GC are commonly given together with antifungal drugs when treating fungal infections, such as blastomycosis or cryptococcosis in animals.[71] The justification is that the widespread death of fungal organisms creates an inflammatory response that can be damaging in itself and lead to severe detrimental sequelae.[72]

Although in general there are strong reasons to wish to avoid GC in the face of a viral infection, for the reasons described above, there can be specific examples in which GC therapy may be beneficial for the individual. Most notable in neurology is the notion that canine distemper virus leads to "bystander" demyelination caused by the inflammatory reaction to the infection.[73] Use of low doses ($\sim$1 mg/kg/d) of prednisolone can reduce this effect and therefore are often recommended for treatment.[74]

Use for pain control or other nonspecific purposes
Pain

In general practice, there is often a great deal of pressure on veterinarians to administer a treatment that will alleviate the signs of pain to which an owner attributes a pet's abnormal behavior. Although nowadays there are many options for pain relief in small animals, including long-acting opioid therapy (fentanyl patches), nonsteroidal anti-inflammatory drugs (NSAIDs) of many types, and Tramadol, many veterinarians remain more comfortable with using GC as a form of pain relief. Common reasons for this choice include the detrimental effects that have been highlighted in association with the other options, including risk of owner abuse, cost, risk of seizures, and detrimental gastrointestinal effects. Although some of these are well founded, the risks of NSAIDs seem to have been overestimated by many academic veterinarians compared with the actual number of reports of side effects,[75] and therefore, avoidance of this class of drugs may be misplaced. Even so, for treatment of radicular (nerve root) pain, a common source of pain for human "back" patients, a recent *Cochrane Review* suggested that NSAIDs were of no benefit over placebo.[76]

Specifically considering neurologic diseases, intervertebral disc degeneration can lead to pain through many mechanisms, including stretching of the annulus and entrapment of nerve roots (reviewed by Ref.[77]). Although many of these causes can be readily addressed through surgery, there are some instances, for instance, postoperatively, or if owners are reluctant to allow their animals to undergo surgery, in which GC might potentially be thought useful for pain relief. In humans, radicular pain has been shown to be controlled in the short term by using epidural corticosteroid injections,[78] although this advantage is not consistent, nor strong,[79] and disappears over longer periods. On the other hand, it seems that single intravenous doses of methylprednisolone sodium succinate (MPSS), or tapering oral prednisone, are no better than placebo in the treatment of acute back pain in human patients.[80]

In itself, use of GC to pragmatically treat spinal pain is not necessarily problematic, because it may alleviate clinical signs that the owners present for treatment, but problems can arise because of the consequences that follow. For instance, (1) the use of GC may change the clinical signs to such an extent that the owner will assume that the patient has "recovered" even though the condition itself has not been (adequately) treated, or even perhaps not diagnosed, leading to delayed diagnosis, which could be detrimental in itself, but may also mean that subsequent clinical examination does not identify the same signs as were initially apparent, leading to incorrect diagnostic pathways; (2) GC administration will change many blood sample parameters so that it becomes difficult to make a diagnosis, most notable will be changes in alkaline phosphatase and white cell counts, but, for example, urine specific gravity will also be affected. Specific tests such as thyroid function will be impossible to interpret after recent GC administration; (3) until the diagnosis has been made, the use of GC cannot be considered risk-free; it might be that the condition is caused by an infection that could be exacerbated by their use.

Therefore, for most conditions in which there is pain, it is better to wait until a diagnosis of the cause has been attained before resorting to GC.

Nonspecific use
As outlined above, although GC may give many apparent benefits to the animals from the owners' point of view, these are often illusory. For instance, increasing an animal's appetite through GC administration may also reduce glycogen stores, increase muscle catabolism, reduce bone mass, and increase the risk of diabetes mellitus. Infectious diseases may also be potentiated. Again, therefore, the use of GC should be avoided until a diagnosis has been made.

Conditions for Which GC Are Not Indicated

CNS trauma
The use of GC in the treatment of trauma to the CNS is a long-standing source of controversy in both human and veterinary medicine. The theory is that inflammation follows trauma and therefore it would be logical to use GC to ameliorate this consequence. In fact, there is even evidence from experimental laboratory studies that therapy with MPSS, either at the time of injury or immediately afterward, will ameliorate the detrimental structural and functional consequences of spinal cord injury (reviewed by[81]). Despite the positive results of laboratory studies, these beneficial effects have not been replicated in practice in real-life clinical trials. Dexamethasone was long used in human and veterinary medicine for spinal cord injury and has never been shown to be of benefit.[82] More recently, MPSS was used in a series of clinical trials based on the effects that had been detected in laboratory studies. Initially, the response was designated as a positive effect of this GC[83] but subsequent analysis

has suggested that the apparent benefit was a consequence of the manner that the analysis was conducted.[84] Reanalysis of the data has suggested that there was no beneficial effect and, in addition, there has been concern that the detrimental effects of steroids in promoting infections and muscle loss outweigh any possible benefits anyway.[85] In veterinary medicine, there is even less reason to trust that GC have benefits because those that were purported to occur in the human trials depended on the effects on gray matter rather than white, which is often not the prime target in dogs and cats (because of the common sites of spinal cord injury in these species). More pertinently, a specific study on spinal cord injury in dogs did not detect a benefit of MPSS,[86] although that could also be a consequence of low study power.

In human medicine, in which head trauma is a more major problem, GC had long been used as a first-line treatment. However, the CRASH study,[87] which systematically investigated the benefits of GC (MPSS) in head injury, concluded very strongly that they were detrimental, so detrimental that the study was terminated early because of excess deaths in the GC group. No similar trials have been conducted in veterinary medicine, but there is little reason to suppose that the results would be any different. Although the mechanisms that underlie this detrimental effect of GC in head trauma are not fully understood, and may result from more general effects on metabolism and blood pressure, it has been shown that GC exacerbate neuronal death following a wide range of insults to the CNS.[3] The effects of GC on immune cells may also contribute to these detrimental outcomes.

In conclusion, there is no good reason to support the use of GC in CNS trauma.

DETRIMENTAL EFFECTS OF CORTICOSTEROID THERAPY
Immunosuppression

Although immunosuppression can be a desirable effect, it may be detrimental by potentiating infection and, because its cause is the same as that leading to benefits, cannot be eliminated as a "side effect." When considering CNS diseases in dogs, fungi and Protozoal infections are the main pathogens to beware of that could be potentiated.[88]

Gut Ulceration, Vomiting, Diarrhea

These side effects can be fatal if there is severe gut ulceration. In one study on concurrent spinal surgery (after imaging by myelography) and MPSS therapy, there was ~90% incidence of gastrointestinal ulceration, and coadministration of gut protectants did not reduce this effect.[89] Gut ulceration as a side effect of GC use may be more prominent in dogs, because meta-analyses studies in people have not found the same results.[90]

Delay and Obstruction in Making a Definitive Diagnosis

GC will have effects on test results and owner perception of pet well-being as outlined above. GC also affect the ability of contrast agent to cross the blood-brain barrier and reduce edema (see above) meaning that their use can be obstructive to diagnosis on MR imaging. Similarly, they have a specific antitumor effect on lymphoma, meaning that this condition can be more difficult to diagnose after GC administration.

Muscle Wasting

Muscle wasting may occur in ~10% of human brain tumor patients[91] but is thought to be less common when using nonfluorinated GC (such as prednisolone or hydrocortisone),[92] and the effects vary depending on the muscle type; fast twitch fibers are more severely affected (in rats). The effects are probably mediated through reduction in production of muscle proteins, can be reversible when the steroid therapy is terminated, and may be ameliorated by exercise programs.[28]

SUMMARY

GC are powerful drugs that have widespread effects throughout the body and would ideally be used only after a definitive diagnosis that indicates their use (ie, immune-mediated, noninfectious inflammatory conditions, or [for edema relief] CNS tumors).

However, veterinarians frequently must make pragmatic decisions in the face of incomplete knowledge and will often be tempted to reach for the GC bottle. To avoid detrimental consequences of this decision, it would be sensible to first ask the following:

1. Will the owner subsequently change their mind and wish to have further diagnostic workup performed and seek definitive treatment? If so, it is highly preferable to avoid GC therapy at this stage.
2. Could the use of GC cause detrimental effects in this patient? Is it at high risk of overwhelming infection (especially fungal disease)? Will GC be likely to cause gut ulceration? Might this dose of GC cause muscle weakness?

REFERENCES

1. Singh N, Rieder MJ, Tucker MJ. Mechanisms of glucocorticoid-mediated anti-inflammatory and immunosuppressive action. Paediatr Perinat Drug Ther 2004;6:107–15.
2. Ferguson DC, Dirikolu L, Hoenig M. Glucocorticoids, mineralocorticoids, and adrenolytic drugs. In: Riviere JE, Papich MG, editors. Veterinary pharmacology and therapeutics. 9th edition. Hoboken (NJ): Wiley-Blackwell; 2013. p. 771–887 Chapter 30.
3. Krieger S, Sorrells SF, Nickerson M, et al. Mechanistic insights into corticosteroids in multiple sclerosis: war horse or chameleon? Clin Neurol Neurosurg 2014;119:6–16.
4. De Bosscher K, Vanden Berghe W, Haegeman G, et al. Mechanisms of anti-inflammatory action and of immunosuppression by glucocorticoids: negative interference of activated glucocorticoid receptor with transcription factors. J Neuroimmunol 2000;109:16–22.
5. Presman DM, Ogara MF, Stortz M, et al. Live cell imaging unveils multiple domain requirements for in vivo dimerization of the glucocorticoid receptor. PLoS Biol 2014;12:e1001813.
6. Sedwick C. Wanted: a new model for glucocorticoid receptor transactivation and transrepression. PLoS Biol 2014;12:e1001814.
7. Kunicka JE, Talle MA, Denhardt GH, et al. Immunosuppression by glucocorticoids: inhibition of production of multiple lymphokines by in vivo administration of dexamethasone. Cell Immunol 1993;149:39–49.
8. Tobler A, Meier R, Seitz M, et al. Glucocorticoids downregulate gene expression of GM-CSF, NAP-1/IL-8, and IL-6, but not of M-CSF in human fibroblasts. Blood 1992;79:45–51.
9. AyanlarBatuman O, Ferrero AP, Diaz A, et al. Regulation of transforming growth factor-beta 1 gene expression by glucocorticoids in normal human T lymphocytes. J Clin Invest 1991;88:1574–80.
10. Almawi WY, Saouda MS, Stevens AC, et al. Partial mediation of glucocorticoid antiproliferative effects by lipocortins. J Immunol 1996;157:5231–9.

11. Franchimont D, Galon J, Gadina M, et al. Inhibition of Th1 immune response by glucocorticoids: dexamethasone selectively inhibits IL-12-induced Stat4 phosphorylation in T lymphocytes. J Immunol 2000;164:1768–74.
12. Haller J, Mikics E, Makara GB. The effects of non-genomic glucocorticoid mechanisms on bodily functions and the central neural system. A critical evaluation of findings. Front Neuroendocrinol 2008;29:273–91.
13. Zen M, Canova M, Campana C, et al. The kaleidoscope of glucorticoid effects on immune system. Autoimmun Rev 2011;10:305–10.
14. Jonat C, Rahmsdorf HJ, Park KK, et al. Antitumor promotion and antiinflammation: down-modulation of AP-1 (Fos/Jun) activity by glucocorticoid hormone. Cell 1990;62:1189–204.
15. Meleo K. Management of insuloma patients with refractory hypoglycemia. Probl Vet Med 1990;2:602–9.
16. Shaw WA, Issekutz TB, Issekutz B Jr. Gluconeogenesis from glycerol at rest and during exercise in normal, diabetic, and methylprednisolone-treated dogs. Metabolism 1976;25:329–39.
17. Kadowitz PJ, Yard AC. Influence of hydrocortisone on cardiovascular responses to epinephrine. Eur J Pharmacol 1971;13:281–6.
18. Whitworth JA, Schyvens CG, Zhang Y, et al. The nitric oxide system in glucocorticoid-induced hypertension. J Hypertens 2002;20:1035–43.
19. Hammer F, Stewart PM. Cortisol metabolism in hypertension. Best Pract Res Clin Endocrinol Metab 2006;20:337–53.
20. Lindvall-Axelsson M, Hedner P, Owman C. Corticosteroid action on choroid plexus: reduction in Na+-K+-ATPase activity, choline transport capacity, and rate of CSF formation. Exp Brain Res 1989;77:605–10.
21. Sato O, Hara M, Asai T, et al. The effect of dexamethasone phosphate on the production rate of cerebrospinal fluid in the spinal subarachnoid space of dogs. J Neurosurg 1973;39:480–4.
22. Vela AR, Carey ME, Thompson BM. Further data on the acute effect of intravenous steroids on canine CSF secretion and absorption. J Neurosurg 1979;50: 477–82.
23. Johnston I, Gilday DL, Hendrick EB. Experimental effects of steroids and steroid withdrawal on cerebrospinal fluid absorption. J Neurosurg 1975;42:690–5.
24. Schweingruber N, Reichardt SD, Lühder F, et al. Mechanisms of glucocorticoids in the control of neuroinflammation. J Neuroendocrinol 2012;24:174–82.
25. Elovaara I, Lällä M, Spåre E, et al. Methylprednisolone reduces adhesion molecules in blood and cerebrospinal fluid in patients with MS. Neurology 1998;51: 1703–8.
26. Smith KJ, McDonald WI. The pathophysiology of multiple sclerosis: the mechanisms underlying the production of symptoms and the natural history of the disease. Philos Trans R Soc Lond B Biol Sci 1999;354:1649–73.
27. Groeneweg FL, Karst H, de Kloet ER, et al. Rapid non-genomic effects of corticosteroids and their role in the central stress response. J Endocrinol 2011;209: 153–67.
28. Dietrich J, Rao K, Pastorino S, et al. Corticosteroids in brain cancer patients: benefits and pitfalls. Expert Rev Clin Pharmacol 2011;4:233–42.
29. Miller JD, Sakalas R, Ward JD, et al. Methylprednisolone treatment in patients with brain tumors. Neurosurgery 1977;1:114–7.
30. Kim H, Lee JM, Park JS, et al. Dexamethasone coordinately regulates angiopoietin-1 and VEGF: a mechanism of glucocorticoid-induced stabilization of blood-brain barrier. Biochem Biophys Res Commun 2008;372:243–8.

31. Förster C, Silwedel C, Golenhofen N, et al. Occludin as direct target for glucocorticoid-induced improvement of blood-brain barrier properties in a murine in vitro system. J Physiol 2005;565:475–86.
32. Pitzalis C, Pipitone N, Perretti M. Regulation of leukocyte-endothelial interactions by glucocorticoids. Ann N Y Acad Sci 2002;966:108–18.
33. Boumpas DT, Chrousos GP, Wilder RL, et al. Glucocorticoid therapy for immune-mediated diseases: basic and clinical correlates. Ann Intern Med 1993;119: 1198–208.
34. Villeneuve J, Galarneau H, Beaudet MJ, et al. Reduced glioma growth following dexamethasone or anti-angiopoietin 2 treatment. Brain Pathol 2008;18:401–14.
35. Sur P, Sribnick EA, Patel SJ, et al. Dexamethasone decreases temozolomide-induced apoptosis in human gliobastoma T98G cells. Glia 2005;50:160–7.
36. Zhang C, Beckermann B, Kallifatidis G, et al. Corticosteroids induce chemotherapy resistance in the majority of tumour cells from bone, brain, breast, cervix, melanoma and neuroblastoma. Int J Oncol 2006;29:1295–301.
37. Tipold A, Jaggy A. Steroid responsive meningitis-arteritis in dogs: long-term study of 32 cases. J Small Anim Pract 1994;35:311–6.
38. Tipold A, Stein VM. Inflammatory diseases of the spine in small animals. Vet Clin North Am Small Anim Pract 2010;40:871–9.
39. Behr S, Cauzinille L. Aseptic suppurative meningitis in juvenile boxer dogs: retrospective study of 12 cases. J Am Anim Hosp Assoc 2006;42:277–82.
40. Lowrie M, Penderis J, McLaughlin M, et al. Steroid responsive meningitis-arteritis: a prospective study of potential disease markers, prednisolone treatment, and long-term outcome in 20 dogs (2006-2008). J Vet Intern Med 2009; 23:862–70.
41. Rose JH, Harcourt-Brown TR. Screening diagnostics to identify triggers in 21 cases of steroid-responsive meningitis-arteritis. J Small Anim Pract 2013;54:575–8.
42. Adamo PF, Adams WM, Steinberg H. Granulomatous meningoencephalomyelitis in dogs. Compend Contin Educ Vet 2007;29:678–90.
43. Granger N, Smith PM, Jeffery ND. Clinical findings and treatment of non-infectious meningoencephalomyelitis in dogs: a systematic review of 457 published cases from 1962 to 2008. Vet J 2010;184:290–7.
44. Higginbotham MJ, Kent M, Glass EN. Noninfectious inflammatory central nervous system diseases in dogs. Compend Contin Educ Vet 2007;29:488–97.
45. Barber RM, Porter BF, Li Q, et al. Broadly reactive polymerase chain reaction for pathogen detection in canine granulomatous meningoencephalomyelitis and necrotizing meningoencephalitis. J Vet Intern Med 2012;26:962–8.
46. Zarfoss M, Schatzberg S, Venator K, et al. Combined cytosine arabinoside and prednisone therapy for meningoencephalitis of unknown aetiology in 10 dogs. J Small Anim Pract 2006;47:588–95.
47. Coates JR, Barone G, Dewey CW, et al. Procarbazine as adjunctive therapy for treatment of dogs with presumptive antemortem diagnosis of granulomatous meningoencephalomyelitis: 21 cases (1998-2004). J Vet Intern Med 2007;21: 100–6.
48. Flegel T, Boettcher IC, Matiasek K, et al. Comparison of oral administration of lomustine and prednisolone or prednisolone alone as treatment for granulomatous meningoencephalomyelitis or necrotizing encephalitis in dogs. J Am Vet Med Assoc 2011;238:337–45.
49. Muñana KR, Luttgen PJ. Prognostic factors for dogs with granulomatous meningoencephalomyelitis: 42 cases (1982-1996). J Am Vet Med Assoc 1998;212: 1902–6.

50. Dubey JP, Carpenter JL, Speer CA, et al. Newly recognized fatal protozoan disease of dogs. J Am Vet Med Assoc 1988;192:1269–85.
51. Lewis RM. Immune-mediated muscle disease. Vet Clin North Am Small Anim Pract 1994;24:703–10.
52. Allgoewer I, Blair M, Basher T, et al. Extraocular muscle myositis and restrictive strabismus in 10 dogs. Vet Ophthalmol 2000;3:21–6.
53. Aktas M, Auguste D, Lefebvre HP, et al. Creatine kinase in the dog: a review. Vet Res Commun 1993;17:353–69.
54. Shelton GD, Cardinet GH 3rd, Bandman E. Canine masticatory muscle disorders: a study of 29 cases. Muscle Nerve 1987;10:753–66.
55. Khaleeli AA, Edwards RH, Gohil K, et al. Corticosteroid myopathy: a clinical and pathological study. Clin Endocrinol (Oxf) 1983;18:155–66.
56. Rossmeisl JH Jr, Jones JC, Zimmerman KL, et al. Survival time following hospital discharge in dogs with palliatively treated primary brain tumors. J Am Vet Med Assoc 2013;242:193–8.
57. Mariani CL, Schubert TA, House RA, et al. Frameless stereotactic radiosurgery for the treatment of primary intracranial tumours in dogs. Vet Comp Oncol 2013. http://dx.doi.org/10.1111/vco.12056.
58. Greenstein S, Ghias K, Krett NL, et al. Mechanisms of glucocorticoid-mediated apoptosis in hematological malignancies. Clin Cancer Res 2002;8:1681–94.
59. Kfir-Erenfeld S, Sionov RV, Spokoini R, et al. Protein kinase networks regulating glucocorticoid-induced apoptosis of hematopoietic cancer cells: fundamental aspects and practical considerations. Leuk Lymphoma 2010;51:1968–2005.
60. Allenspach K, Bergman PJ, Sauter S, et al. P-glycoprotein expression in lamina propria lymphocytes of duodenal biopsy samples in dogs with chronic idiopathic enteropathies. J Comp Pathol 2006;134:1–7.
61. Mealey KL, Bentjen SA, Gay JM, et al. Dexamethasone treatment of a canine, but not human, tumour cell line increases chemoresistance independent of P-glycoprotein and multidrug resistance-related protein expression. Vet Comp Oncol 2003;1:67–75.
62. Price GS, Page RL, Fischer BM, et al. Efficacy and toxicity of doxorubicin/cyclophosphamide maintenance therapy in dogs with multicentric lymphosarcoma. J Vet Intern Med 1991;5:259–62.
63. Yetgin S, Cetin M. The dose related effect of steroids on blast reduction rate and event free survival in children with acute lymphoblastic leukemia. Leuk Lymphoma 2003;44:489–95.
64. Zandvliet M, Rutteman GR, Teske E. Prednisolone inclusion in a first-line multidrug cytostatic protocol for the treatment of canine lymphoma does not affect therapy results. Vet J 2013;197:656–61.
65. Northington JW, Brown MJ, Farnbach GC, et al. Acute idiopathic polyneuropathy in the dog. J Am Vet Med Assoc 1981;179:375–9.
66. Shelton GD, Lindstrom JM. Spontaneous remission in canine myasthenia gravis: implications for assessing human MG therapies. Neurology 2001;57:2139–41.
67. Cuddon PA. Acquired canine peripheral neuropathies. Vet Clin North Am Small Anim Pract 2002;32:207–49.
68. Jeffery ND, Talbot CE, Smith PM, et al. Acquired idiopathic laryngeal paralysis as a prominent feature of generalised neuromuscular disease in 39 dogs. Vet Rec 2006;158:17.
69. Murawska-Ciałowicz E, Szychowska Z, Trebusiewicz B. Nitric oxide production during bacterial and viral meningitis in children. Int J Clin Lab Res 2000;30:127–31.

70. Brouwer MC, McIntyre P, Prasad K, et al. Corticosteroids for acute bacterial meningitis. Cochrane Database Syst Rev 2013;(6):CD004405.
71. Sykes JE, Sturges BK, Cannon MS, et al. Clinical signs, imaging features, neuropathology, and outcome in cats and dogs with central nervous system cryptococcosis from California. J Vet Intern Med 2010;24:1427–38.
72. Finn MJ, Stiles J, Krohne SG. Visual outcome in a group of dogs with ocular blastomycosis treated with systemic antifungals and systemic corticosteroids. Vet Ophthalmol 2007;10:299–303.
73. Vandevelde M, Zurbriggen A. The neurobiology of canine distemper virus infection. Vet Microbiol 1995;44:271–80.
74. Thomas WB. Inflammatory diseases of the central nervous system in dogs. Clin Tech Small Anim Pract 1998;13:167–78.
75. Monteiro-Steagall BP, Steagall PV, Lascelles BD. Systematic review of nonsteroidal anti-inflammatory drug-induced adverse effects in dogs. J Vet Intern Med 2013;27:1011–9.
76. Roelofs PD, Deyo RA, Koes BW, et al. Non-steroidal antiinflammatory drugs for low back pain. Cochrane Database Syst Rev 2008;(1):CD000396. Available at: http://dx.doi.org/10.1002/14651858.CD000396.pub3.
77. Jeffery ND, Levine JM, Olby NJ, et al. Intervertebral disk degeneration in dogs: consequences, diagnosis, treatment, and future directions. J Vet Intern Med 2013;27:1318–33.
78. Quraishi NA. Transforaminal injection of corticosteroids for lumbar radiculopathy: systematic review and meta-analysis. Eur Spine J 2012;21:214–9.
79. Friedly JL, Comstock BA, Turner JA, et al. A randomized trial of epidural glucocorticoid injections for spinal stenosis. N Engl J Med 2014;371:11–21.
80. Johnson M, Neher JO, St Anna L. How effective – and safe – are systemic steroids for acute low back pain? J Fam Pract 2011;60:297–8.
81. Hall ED, Braughler JM, McCall JM. Antioxidant effects in brain and spinal cord injury. J Neurotrauma 1992;9(Suppl 1):S165–72.
82. Hoerlein BF, Redding RW, Hoff EJ, et al. Evaluation of dexamethasone, DMSO, mannitol and solcoseryl in acute spinal cord trauma. J Am Anim Hosp Assoc 1983;19:216–26.
83. Bracken MB, Shepard MJ, Collins WF, et al. (NASCIS-2) A randomized, controlled trial of methylprednisolone or naloxone in the treatment of acute spinal-cord injury. N Engl J Med 1990;322:1405–11.
84. Hurlbert RJ. The role of steroids in acute spinal cord injury: an evidence-based analysis. Spine (Phila Pa 1976) 2011;26:S39–46.
85. Short DJ, El Masry WS, Jones PW. High dose methylprednisolone in the management of acute spinal cord injury - a systematic review from a clinical perspective. Spinal Cord 2000;38:273–86.
86. Coates JR, Sorjonen DC, Simpson ST, et al. Clinicopathologic effects of a 21-aminosteroid compound (U74389G) and high-dose methylprednisolone on spinal cord function after simulated spinal cord trauma. Vet Surg 1995;24:128–39.
87. Roberts I, Yates D, Sandercock P, et al, CRASH Trial Collaborators. Effect of intravenous corticosteroids on death within 14 days in 10008 adults with clinically significant head injury (MRC CRASH trial): randomised placebo-controlled trial. Lancet 2004;364:1321–8.
88. Galgut BI, Janardhan KS, Grondin TM, et al. Detection of Neospora caninum tachyzoites in cerebrospinal fluid of a dog following prednisone and cyclosporine therapy. Vet Clin Pathol 2010;39:386–90.

89. Hanson SM, Bostwick DR, Twedt DC, et al. Clinical evaluation of cimetidine, sucralfate, and misoprostol for prevention of gastrointestinal tract bleeding in dogs undergoing spinal surgery. Am J Vet Res 1997;58:1320-3.

90. Conn HO, Poynard T. Corticosteroids and peptic ulcer: meta-analysis of adverse events during steroid therapy. J Intern Med 1994;236:619-32.

91. Dropcho EJ, Soong SJ. Steroid-induced weakness in patients with primary brain tumors. Neurology 1991;41:1235-9.

92. Kelly FJ, McGrath JA, Goldspink DF, et al. A morphological/biochemical study on the actions of corticosteroids on rat skeletal muscle. Muscle Nerve 1986;9:1-10.

Canine Hereditary Ataxia

Ganokon Urkasemsin, DVM, PhD[a],
Natasha J. Olby, VetMB, PhD, MRCVS[b],*

KEYWORDS

- Cerebellar abiotrophy • Spinocerebellar • Purkinje neuron
- Granuloprival degeneration

KEY POINTS

- Hereditary ataxias are a heterogeneous group of neurodegenerative diseases characterized clinically by cerebellar ataxia.
- Classification of the disorders in veterinary medicine has been based on neuropathologic changes into cerebellar cortical degeneration, spinocerebellar degeneration, canine multiple system degeneration, cerebellar ataxias without significant neurodegeneration, and episodic ataxia.
- Genetic tests for these diseases are emerging and will help to reduce prevalence of disease, make a definitive diagnosis, and identify potential therapies.

INTRODUCTION

The hereditary ataxias are a large group of diseases that have inherited cerebellar or spinocerebellar dysfunction at their core. Although each individual disease is rare, as a group they are an important cause of movement disorders in purebred dogs.[1] The recent rapid increase in our understanding of their genetic basis has culminated in the availability of genetic tests for certain diseases, with the potential to reduce prevalence or eliminate them in the near future. This article outlines the current classification system in veterinary medicine and compares it with the system used in human medicine. Key clinical and diagnostic features of well-described diseases are highlighted and, where known, the genetic basis is described. There are several other neurodegenerative disease processes that target the cerebellum. Most notably, these include many lysosomal storage diseases as well as neuroaxonal dystrophies and spongy degeneration of the cerebellum but these diseases are classified separately and are not discussed here.

The authors have nothing to disclose.
[a] Department of Pre-Clinic and Applied Animal Science, Faculty of Veterinary Science, Mahidol University, 999 Phuttamonthon Sai 4 Road, Salaya, Phuttamonthon, Nakhon Pathom 73170, Thailand; [b] Department of Clinical Sciences, College of Veterinary Medicine, North Carolina State University, 1060 William Moore Drive, Raleigh, NC 27607, USA
* Corresponding author.
E-mail address: natasha_olby@ncsu.edu

CLASSIFICATION

In human medicine, hereditary ataxia is currently classified according to the mode of inheritance and genetic cause or locus (**Box 1**).[2–4] However, the current human classification system evolved from a neuropathologic classification divided into olivopontocerebellar atrophy, cerebellar cortical atrophy, and spinocerebellar degeneration in the early twentieth century, through a combination of clinical presentation and genetic mapping in the 1980s[5] to the current twenty-first century system. This evolution was vital because a purely neuropathologic classification led to incorrect diagnoses and incomplete understanding of the disease mechanisms. Genetic mapping of these disorders in humans has revolutionized the understanding of this group of diseases and highlighted the ability of diverse underlying defects to produce the same neuropathologic endpoint. For example, autosomal dominant spinocerebellar ataxia (SCA) can be caused by a mutation in a growth factor gene (FGF14), a gene for a cytoskeletal component (β-III spectrin) or an ion channel (*CACNA1A*, a calcium channel).[3] Conversely, one mutation can produce extremely diverse clinical phenotypes in

---

Box 1
Classification of hereditary ataxias in humans

Autosomal dominant ataxias

  Spinocerebellar ataxias:

- Thirty-seven different genetic subtypes recognized to date; this number increases steadily

  Episodic ataxias:

- Six different episodic ataxias are currently recognized

Autosomal recessive ataxias

- Friedreich ataxia
- Ataxia telangiectasia
- Autosomal recessive ataxia with oculomotor apraxia type1
- Autosomal recessive ataxia with oculomotor apraxia type2
- Autosomal recessive spastic ataxia of Charlevoix-Saguenay
- Ataxia with isolated vitamin E deficiency
- Marinesco-Sjögren syndrome
- Autosomal recessive ataxias due to POLG mutations (MIRAS, SANDO)
- Cerebrotendinous xanthomatosis
- Refsum disease
- Abetalipoproteinemia
- Other autosomal recessive ataxias

X-linked ataxias

- Fragile X–associated tremor/ataxia syndrome
- Other X-linked ataxias

Ataxias due to mitochondrial mutations

The primary categorization is based on the mode of inheritance and then subdivided by pathology, clinical syndrome, or mutation.
  Data from Jayadev S, Bird TD. Hereditary ataxias: overview. Genet Med 2013;15:673–83.

different individuals. For example, a calcium channelopathy in SCA6 can cause cerebellar degeneration, episodic ataxia, or familial hemiplegic migraine, sometimes with all phenotypes expressed in a single family.[2]

The underlying genetic cause of these disorders is much less well defined in veterinary medicine, although it is currently expanding rapidly. As a result, the classification still relies on neuropathologic features, but it is important to appreciate that this should and will evolve over the next decade as our knowledge of genetic basis of these diseases grows. It is noticeable when reading the veterinary literature that many different terms are used to describe these diseases, and in some instances (eg, the Russell Terrier group) at least 2 clinically similar, but genetically distinct disorders occur, leading to an extremely confusing clinical picture.[6–9] In this article, the authors attempt to place the most well-described diseases into consistent categories to limit confusion. The categories of diseases included under the term "hereditary ataxia" in this article are as follows:

- *Cerebellar cortical degeneration* (also known as cerebellar abiotrophies, cerebellar ataxias, cerebellar degeneration, and cerebellar cortical degeneration) in which neurodegeneration is largely limited to the cerebellar cortex. Cerebellar abiotrophy is the term that has been used most frequently historically.[1] The term "abiotrophy" means lack of nutritive substance but it is now known that many of these diseases can result from abnormalities that are not metabolic in origin. Thus, the term "cerebellar cortical degeneration" is preferred. These disorders can be further divided into diseases primarily affecting the Purkinje neurons or the granular neurons (known as *granuloprival degeneration*).
- *Spinocerebellar degeneration* in which there is also involvement of the medulla and/or spinal cord with or without involvement of the cerebellum.
- *Canine multiple system degeneration (CMSD)* in which there is also involvement of the olivary nuclei, substantia nigra, putamen, and caudate nuclei.
- *Cerebellar ataxias without significant neurodegeneration* in which there are obvious signs of cerebellar dysfunction without any microscopic histopathologic changes.
- *Episodic ataxias* in which there are episodes of profound ataxia, again without histopathologic changes. Affected individuals are neurologically normal between episodes.

A large number of sporadic cases have been reported that may or may not represent hereditary diseases and these are included in **Table 1**.

CLINICAL APPROACH TO HEREDITARY ATAXIA

A hereditary ataxia should be suspected whenever a veterinarian encounters a patient with symmetric, progressive signs of cerebellar ataxia. A careful history should be taken to include details of littermates and other related dogs and a detailed physical and neurologic examination should be performed. Because more subtle ataxias can be overlooked in a patient that is anxious, it is important to observe them moving freely in an environment where there are small obstacles for them to encounter and move around. Diagnosis of a neurodegenerative disease is typically one of exclusion of other causes and so other disease processes should be considered and systematically investigated. Different disease processes tend to have different presenting histories, progression, and localization (**Table 2**). This process implies routine blood analysis (to identify metabolic abnormalities and evidence of inflammatory or infectious disease) and, ideally, magnetic resonance imaging (MRI) of the brain to identify structural

Table 1
Summary of breeds for which there are reports of hereditary ataxia

	Cerebellar Cortical Degeneration: Primary Loss of Purkinje Neurons				
Familial reports	**Age of onset**	**Progression**	**Gene/Locus**	**Mode of inheritance**	**Genetic test**
Beagles[17,21]	2–3 wk	Rapid	SPTBN2	Autosomal recessive	Yes
Finnish Hound[15]	4–12 wk	Rapid	SEL1L	Autosomal recessive	Yes
Rhodesian Ridgeback[16]	2 wk	Rapid	—	Autosomal recessive	—
Portuguese Podenco[20]	2–3 wk	Rapid	—	—	—
Gordon Setter[12,13,22]	6–10 mo	Slow	RAB24	Autosomal recessive	Yes
Old English Sheepdog[11,12]	6–40 mo	Slow	RAB24	Autosomal recessive	Yes
Scottish Terrier[14,23,28]	2–84 mo	Slow	—	Autosomal recessive	—
Australian Kelpie[18,25]	5–12 wk	Rapid	CFA3	Autosomal recessive	—
Sporadic reports					
Papillon[54]	5 mo	Slow	—	—	—
Miniature Poodle[55]	Neonatal	Rapid	—	—	—
Miniature Schnauzer[56]	3.25 mo	Rapid	—	—	—
English Bulldog[24]	10–12 wk	Rapid	—	—	—
Labrador Retriever[36,37]	7–17 wk	Slow/Rapid	—	—	—
Boxers[57]	40 mo	N/A	—	—	—
Lagotto Romagnolo[31]	5 wk	Slow	—	—	—

Cerebellar Cortical Degeneration: Granuloprival Degeneration

	Age of onset	Progression	Gene/Locus	Mode of inheritance	Genetic test
Familial reports					
Border Collie[30]	4 mo	Rapid	—	—	—
Sporadic reports					
Bavarian mountain dog[35]	3 mo	Slow	—	—	—
Italian Hound[34]	3 mo	Rapid	—	—	—
Australian Kelpie[32]	6 wk	Rapid	—	—	—
Lagotto Romagnolo[31]	13 wk	Rapid	—	—	—
Labrador Retriever[32]	13 mo	Rapid	—	—	—
Coton de Tulear[33]	7–8 wk	Rapid	—	—	—
Ataxia Without Neurodegeneration					
Familial reports					
Coton de Tulear[44,45]	2 wk	Stable	GRM1	Autosomal recessive	Yes
Episodic Ataxia					
Sporadic reports					
Bichon Frise[52]	4 mo	Slow	—	—	—
Spinocerebellar Degeneration					
Familial reports					
Parson Russell Terrier[9]	6–12 mo	Variable	CAPN1	Polygenic model	Yes
Jack Russell Terrier[6–8]	2–12 mo	Variable	KCNJ10	Polygenic model	Yes
Smooth-haired Fox Terrier[40,41]	4–6 mo	Rapid and slow	—	Autosomal recessive	—
Brittany Spaniel[39]	5–10.7 y	Slow	—	—	—
Canine Multiple System Degeneration					
Familial reports					
Kerry Blue Terrier[48,50,51]	9–16 wk	Rapid	SERAC1	Autosomal recessive	Yes
Chinese crested dog[49,51]	3–6 mo	Rapid	SERAC1	Autosomal recessive	Yes

Data from Refs. 6–9,11–18,20–25,28,30–37,39–41,44,45,48–52,54–57

Table 2
Typical presenting histories and clinical courses for different disease processes

Disease Process	Onset	Progression	Localization
Vascular	Peracute, most commonly older animals	Signs improve if self-limiting (ischemic), deteriorate rapidly if ongoing disease (eg, bleeding disorder)	Focal, often asymmetric neurologic signs
Infectious/ Inflammatory	Acute to subacute, any age but most commonly young adults	Progressive deterioration, often rapid	Focal or multifocal, asymmetric neurologic signs
Neoplasia	Subacute or chronic, most commonly older animals	Progressive deterioration	Focal, often asymmetric neurologic signs
Congenital	At birth	Nonprogressive	Symmetric neurologic signs
Neurodegenerative	Insidious onset, any age but most commonly less than 3 y of age	Progressive deterioration	Symmetric neurologic signs

changes and inflammation, followed by cerebrospinal fluid (CSF) analysis to identify inflammatory or infectious disease. Other infectious or metabolic disease testing may be indicated based on these results.

Routine laboratory testing is normal in dogs with hereditary ataxia, as is CSF analysis. However, neurodegenerative processes can result in brain atrophy and dogs that have hereditary ataxia frequently exhibit atrophy of the cerebellum on MRI images.[10] Sagittal T2-weighted images are especially useful because they highlight the increase in CSF volume around the atrophied cerebellar folia (**Fig. 1**). An MRI index of cerebellar atrophy (ratio of the cross-sectional area of the brainstem to the cerebellum on midsagittal images) has been developed and tested across several different breeds of dog with cerebellar cortical degeneration. A ratio of the brainstem to cerebellar cross-sectional area of greater than 89% had 100% sensitivity and specificity for detecting affected individuals.[10] The sensitivity in detecting other forms of hereditary ataxia is unknown.

Unfortunately, in many instances, owners are reluctant to perform an MRI, either because of concern about general anesthesia or because of the cost. In such cases,

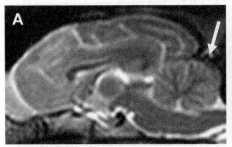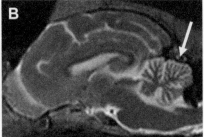

Fig. 1. Midsagittal T2-weighted MRI of the brain of a normal 5-year-old Labrador Retriever (*A*) and a Scottish Terrier with cerebellar cortical degeneration (*B*). The *white arrows* point to the cerebellum. Note that atrophy of the cerebellar cortex in (*B*) results in detailed outlining of cerebellar folia by the hyperintense (*white*) CSF signal.

it is reasonable to compare the constellation of clinical signs, the age of onset, and rate of progression with published reports of breed-specific diseases. In addition, genetic tests are increasingly available and it may be possible to confirm a diagnosis with a genetic test. There are various easily accessible and frequently updated online resources that list available genetic tests (eg, http://www.akcchf.org/canine-health/health-testing/). It is also notable that new syndromes can emerge in breeds and be described in detail on breed-specific health websites long before appearing in the scientific literature (eg, idiopathic head tremors have been recognized, described, and illustrated with videos online in English Bulldogs for many years, but the first veterinary publication describing the disease appeared in 2014). Although it is important to review such material with care, canine health websites can be considered a useful up-to-date source of information on emerging breed-specific problems. Details of well-described canine hereditary ataxias follow, grouped according to the neuropathologic classification.

CEREBELLAR CORTICAL DEGENERATION

This group of diseases is defined by postnatal degeneration of the cerebellar cortex and accounts for most of the reports in the veterinary literature. Most of the familial syndromes reported thus far are inherited by an autosomal recessive mode including the Old English Sheepdog (OES),[11,12] Gordon Setter,[12,13] Scottish Terrier,[14] Finnish Hound,[15] Rhodesian Ridgeback,[16] Beagle,[17] and Australian Kelpie.[18] An X-linked disorder has been reported in the English Pointer.[19] In addition, there are numerous sporadic reports of cerebellar degeneration in different breeds that may be hereditary (**Table 1**).

Clinical signs reflect cerebellar dysfunction including a wide-based stance, dysmetria producing a hypermetric gait, truncal sway, and intention tremor, as well as limb spasticity, absent menace response, spontaneous nystagmus, and opsoclonus. Onset of signs can be neonatal or as early as 2 to 4 weeks of age with rapid progression and early euthanasia.[15,16,20,21] Juvenile onset of signs (between 2 and 12 months) with slow progression over several years has been described in Gordon Setters[13,22] and Old English Sheepdogs.[11] Onset of signs in Scottish Terriers usually occurs in this juvenile period, but in many dogs, progression is slow and signs stabilize resulting in a lifelong mild phenotype.[14,23] A more rapid progression has been reported in the English Bulldog[24] and Australian Kelpie.[18,25] In some breeds (eg, Scottish Terriers[14] and Old English Sheepdogs[11]), signs may first appear during adulthood (more than 3 years of age) with slow progression. Details of both familial and sporadic reports of this disorder are summarized in **Table 1**.

Neuropathologic findings include gross atrophy of the cerebellum resulting from loss of Purkinje neurons, atrophy of the molecular and granular layers, and associated white matter atrophy and gliosis (**Fig. 2**). Neuronal degeneration in the deep cerebellar nuclei may be identified although, most commonly, the Purkinje neuron is the primary target of the disease. Detailed examination in OES and Gordon setters reveals large intracytoplasmic ubiquitin inclusions in the cerebellar cortex and axonal spheroids in the cerebellar white matter that contain autophagy vacuoles.[12,26,27] Although these changes are typical of a neurodegenerative process, not all breeds show the same findings. For example, increased numbers of polyglucosan bodies are found in the molecular layer in the Scottish Terrier.[28] Morphometric study of the cerebellum in Scottish Terriers revealed that the ventral part of the cerebellum is less severely affected[28] and this feature has also been reported in several breeds, such as Finnish Hounds, Beagles,[21] Old English Sheepdogs, and Gordon

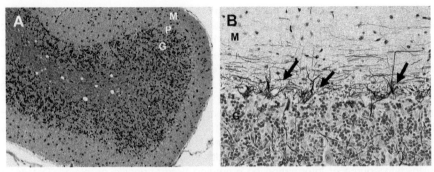

Fig. 2. (*A*) A transverse section of the cerebellar hemisphere of an Old English Sheepdog with cerebellar cortical degeneration showing atrophy of the molecular layer (M), depletion of neurons in the granular layer (G), and absence of Purkinje neurons, which should be visible as large neurons at the interface of the molecular and granular layers (P). Vacuolation is also visible in the white matter (hematoxylin and eosin; 10×). (*B*) A transverse section of cerebellar hemisphere from a Scottish Terrier with cerebellar cortical degeneration. Processes from basket cells that terminate on Purkinje neurons are stained dark brown by the Bielskowsky silver stain showing sites where Purkinje neurons have died (*black arrows*) (Bielskowsky; 20×).

Setters,[12] although the significance of this differential susceptibility to the neurodegenerative process is unclear.

In some breeds, neuronal degeneration primarily targets the granular layer of the cerebellar cortex with relative sparing of Purkinje neurons; this is known as *granuloprival degeneration* and has been reported in Jack and Parson Russell Terriers[29] and a family of Border Collies with rapidly progressive disease.[30] Sporadic cases of granuloprival degeneration have been reported in Lagotto Romagnolo dogs,[31] Labrador Retrievers,[32] Australian Kelpies,[32] Coton de Tulears,[33] the Italian Hound,[34] and Bavarian mountain dogs.[35] Age of onset ranges from 2 to 13 months. The loss of granular neurons described in the Coton de Tulears is presumed to be immune-mediated based on extensive infiltration of the cerebellar cortex by T cells. The investigators hypothesize that this disease could represent a genetically determined immune disorder.[33]

It is important to note that both forms of degeneration—Purkinje neuron versus granular neuron—can be found within the same breed, including Lagotto Romagnolo dogs,[31] Labrador Retrievers,[32,36,37] and Australian Kelpies.[18,25,32] It is unclear whether these histopathologic differences represent different diseases or simply different expression of the same disease but on a different genetic background.

The molecular cause of these diseases has been described in 3 dog breeds to date (**Table 3**).

SEL1

A *SEL1* mutation has been described in Finnish Hounds with hereditary ataxia.[15] SEL1L is a transmembrane glycoprotein located in the endoplasmic reticulum (ER) that plays an important role in ER-associated degradation (ERAD). ERAD is responsible for targeting misfolded or unassembled polypeptides, transferring them to the cytoplasm and marking them for proteasome-dependent degradation. The investigators reported an upregulation in ER stress responsive genes, supporting the proposal that this mutation does cause dysfunction of the ERAD machinery resulting in neuronal degeneration.[15]

Table 3
Summary of genetic tests offered for canine hereditary ataxias

Breed	Gene	Laboratory Link
Finnish Hound	SEL1	www.mydogdna.com
Beagle	SPBNT2	http://www.aht.org.uk/cms-display/genetics_canine.html
Coton de Tulear	GRM1	http://www.offa.org/dna_alltest.html
Gordon Setter, Old English Sheepdog	RAB24	http://www.ncstatevets.org/genetics/
Russell Group Terrier	KCNJ10	http://www.offa.org/dna_alltest.html http://www.aht.org.uk/cms-display/genetics_canine.html
Parson Russell Terrier	CAPN1	http://www.aht.org.uk/cms-display/genetics_canine.html http://www.offa.org/dna_alltest.html
Kerry Blue Terrier	SERAC1	http://www.offa.org/dna_alltest.html
Chinese crested dog	SERAC1	http://www.offa.org/dna_alltest.html
Italian Spinone	Unknown	http://www.aht.org.uk/cms-display/genetics_canine.html

RAB24

Along similar pathologic lines, a mutation in *RAB24* has been reported in OES and Gordon Setters with hereditary ataxia.[12] *RAB24* encodes a protein believed to play a role in late stages of autophagy, particularly in the fusion of the autophagosome with lysosome in which long-lived proteins and cellular organelles are degraded. Defects in neuronal autophagy may result in an inability to remove abnormal or dysfunctional proteins or organelles and cause cell death or dysfunction.[12] The fact that 2 different canine hereditary ataxias have been associated with potential defects in protein disposal is potentially an important observation in the field of neurodegenerative disease.

SPTBN2

An 8 bp deletion in *SPTBN2* has been described in Beagles with neonatal onset cerebellar cortical degeneration.[17] SPTBN2 encodes β-III spectrin, a CNS cytoskeletal protein that is expressed at high levels in Purkinje neurons and is important in maintaining a variety of critical structures including sodium channel density, the localization of the glutamate transporter (EAAT4), and trafficking of vesicles. Mutations in the same gene have been described in human SCA type 5.[3,38]

Mapped diseases

Finally, a locus on chromosome 3 has been associated with the cerebellar cortical degeneration in the Australian Kelpie,[18] and a linkage test is available for the disease in Italian Spinones (see **Table 3**), although details of the chromosomal mapping of the disease in this breed have not been published.

SPINOCEREBELLAR DEGENERATION

Spinocerebellar degeneration has been reported in Brittany Spaniels,[39] Jack Russell Terriers, Parson Russell Terriers,[6–9] and Smooth-haired Fox Terriers (also known as Russell Terrier Group) (see **Table 1**).[40,41] Brittany Spaniels suffer from late-onset (5–10.7 years) spinocerebellar degeneration.[39] Affected dogs develop dramatic neurologic deficits that begin with subtle thoracic limb spasticity and hypermetria and progress over a period of months to classic cerebellar signs affecting all 4 limbs plus truncal ataxia and intention tremors. With further progression, progressive neck extension and a "saluting" gait in the thoracic limbs develop, and dogs ultimately move with their neck extended to hold their head held close to the ground; the thoracic limbs are lifted over the head with each step. Lesions are confined to cerebellum, medulla oblongata, and spinal cord. There is massive loss of Purkinje neurons; neuronal loss in the deep cerebellar nuclei; axonal spheroids, and polyglucosan bodies in the cerebellum; neuronal degeneration in the gracile and cuneate nuclei; and axonal degeneration in the dorsal columns and lateral and ventromedial areas of the spinal cord.[39] The genetic cause and mode of inheritance has not been identified.

The Terrier group presents with a very diverse range of signs and only recently, with the identification of 2 different mutations, has it become clear that there are at least 2 different diseases causing hereditary ataxia in these breeds. The Russell Terrier group includes Jack Russell, Parson Russell, and Russell Terriers, all believed to be descended from dogs owned by one breeder. The first important phenotype is one of cerebellar ataxia combined with myokymia (rippling involuntary muscle contractions), neuromyotonia (sustained muscle contractions), and seizures.[6,42,43] Onset of ataxia is between 2 and 10 months of age and typically there is obvious progression over a few weeks, then stabilization with intermittent periods of deterioration. Dogs exhibit a hypermetric, spastic gait, with postural reaction and proprioceptive placing deficits localizing to the cervical spinal cord. In one group of dogs, the predominant sign was ataxia, with approximately one-third of dogs also developing seizures[6] and a few dogs developing respiratory distress (that can be fatal). In another report, dogs developed signs of ataxia followed by myokymia and neuromyotonia.[42,43] Brainstem auditory evoked responses (BAERs) are frequently abnormal in affected dogs. Most dogs are euthanized because of the disease at a mean of 1 year after onset[6]; although milder, more slowly progressive, phenotypes are also recognized.

Pathologic findings of an axonopathy are most severe in the spinal cord, but are present throughout the brain. There is gliosis, swollen axons, and loss of myelinated fibers in the spinocerebellar tracts, plus the lateral lemniscus, cochlea nuclei, and trapezoid bodies, thus accounting for the abnormal BAERs. This group of dogs is now identified using the term *SAMS* (spinocerebellar ataxia with myokymia, seizures, or both),[8] and the fact that they have different phenotypic expressions of the same disease has been confirmed by the identification of a mutation in the gene *KCNJ10*. The *KCNJ10* gene encodes the inwardly rectifying potassium (K+) channel Kir4.1 that is expressed by glial cells. Kir4.1 is responsible for the negative resting membrane potential of astrocytes and the large K+ conductance across astrocyte membranes. These properties allow astrocytes to buffer fluctuations in extracellular potassium caused by axonal depolarization, and dysfunction of these channels causes an increase in extracellular K+, resulting in hyperexcitability. Glutamate transporters also rely on this high K+ conductance to remove glutamate from synapses, therefore dysfunction of Kir4.1 may also induce hyperexcitability through failure to remove glutamate. Furthermore, Kir4.1 is also important in the maintenance of myelin in the CNS, although the underlying mechanisms remain unclear.[8] This autosomal recessive disease can now be confirmed by genetic testing (see **Table 3**).

The second hereditary ataxia that segregates in Parson Russell Terriers causes a pure SCA with an age of onset ranging from 6 to 12 months (referred to as late-onset ataxia in older publications). This disease has been associated with a missense mutation in *CAPN1*.[9] The *CAPN1* gene encodes an intracellular calcium-dependent cysteine protease called calpain 1. Although the exact function of calpain 1 is unknown, it is proposed to play a role in neuronal maintenance and remodeling; this represents a third disorder in which potential defects in disposal of proteins results in neuronal degeneration. This autosomal recessive disorder can also be diagnosed by means of a genetic test (see **Table 3**).

To confound the picture in the Terrier group further, a very early-onset (<2 weeks) granuloprival ataxia has been described in Parson Russell Terriers[29] and the SCA has been described in Fox Terriers[40,41]; these may or may not fall under the categories of the 2 SCAs described earlier and further delineation of these diseases by investigation of their genetic cause will be invaluable.

ATAXIAS WITHOUT NEURODEGENERATION

Bandera's neonatal ataxia or neonatal ataxia without neuronal degeneration has been identified as an autosomal recessive trait in Coton de Tulears.[44] Affected dogs are identified when their littermates start to move in a coordinated fashion. They exhibit intention tremors, titubation, and inability to stand or walk. They can move around by propelling themselves in sternal recumbency, but intermittently they become laterally recumbent with paddling and adoption of a decerebellate posture. Their righting reflexes are delayed and they have abnormal postural reactions. They have a menace deficit (once old enough to develop a menace response), and ocular motor abnormalities include fine vertical tremors at rest, saccadic dysmetria, and vertical nystagmus (when placed on their back). Their signs remain static. There is no observed abnormality on both gross and microscopic pathology, but on ultrastructural examination, synaptic abnormalities are evident affecting the Purkinje cell dendritic spines in the molecular layer.[44]

A mutation in *GRM1* was identified in affected dogs.[45] This gene encodes the metabotropic glutamate receptor (mGluR1) that regulates intracellular Ca^{2+} levels and neuronal excitability. It is highly expressed in the cerebellum and crucial for the neonatal development of the cerebellar cortex. It is also essential for cerebellar and hippocampal synaptic plasticity, learning, and memory.[46] There is a genetic test available for this mutation (see **Table 3**).

CANINE MULTIPLE SYSTEM DEGENERATION (CMSD)

Multiple system degeneration is analogous to multiple system atrophy (MSA) in humans; these diseases are subdivided into MSA-P (Parkinsonian) and MSA-C (cerebellar) in humans depending on their pattern of lesions and may not be hereditary.[47] MSA-C but not MSA-P is commonly placed under the Hereditary Ataxia umbrella. The authors have provided a description of these diseases in 2 breeds of dogs because their initial presentation is typically one of cerebellar ataxia and there are obvious cerebellar lesions.

CMSD is described in Kerry Blue Terriers and Chinese crested dogs and the 2 breeds appear to have an identical disorder.[48,49] Age of onset of signs ranges from 9 weeks to 6 months[48–50] and clinical signs progress rapidly. Affected dogs exhibit a goose-stepping gait, dysmetria, truncal ataxia, spasticity, intention tremor, wide-base stance, delayed postural reactions, and falling. In the cerebellum, there is degeneration of Purkinje neurons, axons and myelin in the folia and medullary white matter, and swollen axons in the cerebellar nuclei. There is also degeneration of neurons in the olivary nuclei, the substantia nigra, and the basal nuclei (caudate nucleus and putamen) as well as degeneration of extrapyramidal nuclei.[48–50] Genetically, a locus on chromosome 1 has been linked to CMSD in both Kerry Blue Terriers and Chinese crested dogs,[49] and recently different mutations in *SERAC1* have been identified in affected dogs from each breed.[51] *SERAC1* encodes a protein that is located at the interface of mitochondria and ER where it mediates phospholipid exchange. It is vital for mitochondrial function and cholesterol trafficking. In humans, mutations in this gene cause the well-described childhood syndrome of 3-methylglutaconic aciduria with deafness, encephalopathy, and Leigh-like syndrome. Genetics tests for both breeds have been developed (see **Table 3**).

EPISODIC ATAXIA

A single case of episodic ataxia has been reported in a Bichon Frise with onset of episodes at 4 months of age (see **Table 1**).[52] Clinical signs included episodes of hypermetria and spasticity in all 4 limbs with frequent falling, a wide-based stance, truncal sway, head bobbing, and absent menace response. The ataxia episodes lasted several minutes to hours and the severity slowly increased until the dog was presented for evaluation at 4 years of age. The dog responded to 4-aminopyridine (4-AP), a potassium channel blocker, with nearly complete resolution of all signs unless triggered by strenuous exercise or long car rides. The episodic signs and successful response to treatment with 4-AP are comparable to that of episodic ataxia type 2 in humans[53] but the genetic cause has not yet been investigated. Although this is clearly an extremely rare disorder, it is possible that it has simply not been recognized to date. Episodes of falling and ataxia are frequently placed in the category of idiopathic vestibular disease and are not investigated fully.

SUMMARY

This summary highlights the fact that there are numerous descriptions of different autosomal recessive neurodegenerative diseases in purebred dogs that produce cerebellar ataxia and categorizes them by lesion patterns. However, the discovery of 8 different mutations associated with these diseases is starting to provide a more specific means of identifying different disorders. Three of the mutations relate to protein disposal (*SEL1* in Finnish Hounds; *RAB24* in Gordon Setters and Old English Sheepdogs, and *CAPN1* in Parson Russell Terriers). Two mutations influence cation fluxes (*Kir4* in Russell Terrier Group and *GRM1* in Coton de Tulear), whereas the remaining mutations affect mitochondrial function (2 different mutations in *SERAC1* in Kerry Blue and Chinese crested Terriers) and cytoskeleton integrity (*SPTBN2* in Beagles). As more mutations are identified classification may change to revolve around the underlying pathologic mechanism. When faced with a purebred dog exhibiting slowly progressive, symmetric signs of ataxia, veterinarians should consult online resources on the availability of genetic tests for specific breeds exhibiting compatible signs. Appropriate genetic testing will allow veterinarians to definitively diagnose affected dogs and breeders to screen for carriers so as to reduce the prevalence of hereditary disease. In addition, once disease-causing pathways are known, therapeutic agents can be developed targeting downstream cascades and signals, such as drugs stimulating the fusion of the autophagosome with lysosome in neuronal autophagy or augmenting proteasome-based degradation in neuronal degeneration. We are entering an exciting era in the field of neurodegenerative disease, thanks largely to advances in genetics. It is possible that the next decade will bring new screening tests and treatments for canine neurodegenerative disease.

REFERENCES

1. de Lahunta A. Abiotrophy in domestic animals: a review. Can J Vet Res 1990; 54(1):65–76.

2. Klockgether T, Paulson H. Milestones in ataxia. Mov Disord 2011;26(6):1134–41.
3. Jayadev S, Bird TD. Hereditary ataxias: overview. Genet Med 2013;15:673–83.
4. De Michele G, Coppola G, Cocozza S, et al. A pathogenetic classification of hereditary ataxias: is the time ripe? J Neurol 2004;251(8):913–22.
5. Harding AE. Classification of the hereditary ataxias and paraplegias. Lancet 1983;321(8334):1151–5.
6. Wessmann A, Goedde T, Fischer A, et al. Hereditary ataxia in the Jack Russell Terrier–clinical and genetic investigations. J Vet Intern Med 2004;18(4):515–21.
7. Simpson K, Eminaga S, Cherubini GB. Hereditary ataxia in Jack Russell terriers in the UK. Vet Rec 2012;170(21):548.
8. Gilliam D, O'Brien DP, Coates JR, et al. A homozygous KCNJ10 mutation in Jack Russell terriers and related breeds with spinocerebellar ataxia with myokymia, seizures, or both. J Vet Intern Med 2014;28(3):871–7.
9. Forman OP, De Risio L, Mellersh CS. Missense mutation in CAPN1 is associated with spinocerebellar ataxia in the Parson Russell terrier dog breed. PLoS One 2013;8(5):1–8.
10. Thames RA, Robertson ID, Flegel T, et al. Development of a morphometric magnetic resonance image parameter suitable for distinguishing between normal dogs and dogs with cerebellar atrophy. Vet Radiol Ultrasound 2010;51(3):246–53.
11. Steinberg HS, Van Winkle T, Bell JS, et al. Cerebellar degeneration in old english sheepdogs. J Am Vet Med Assoc 2000;217(8):1162–5.
12. Agler C, Nielsen DM, Urkasemsin G, et al. Canine hereditary ataxia in old english sheepdogs and gordon setters is associated with a defect in the autophagy gene encoding RAB24. PLoS Genet 2014;10(2):e1003991.
13. de Lahunta A, Fenner WR, Indrieri RJ, et al. Hereditary cerebellar cortical abiotrophy in the Gordon Setter. J Am Vet Med Assoc 1980;177(6):538–41.
14. Urkasemsin G, Linder KE, Bell JS, et al. Hereditary cerebellar degeneration in Scottish terriers. J Vet Intern Med 2010;24(3):565–70.
15. Kyöstilä K, Cizinauskas S, Seppälä E, et al. A SEL1L mutation links a canine progressive early-onset cerebellar ataxia to the endoplasmic reticulum-associated protein degradation (ERAD) machinery. PLoS Genet 2012;8(6):e1002759.
16. Chieffo C, Stalis IH, Van Winkle TJ, et al. Cerebellar Purkinje's cell degeneration and coat color dilution in a family of Rhodesian Ridgeback dogs. J Vet Intern Med 1994;8(2):112–6.
17. Forman OP, De Risio L, Stewart J, et al. Genome-wide mRNA sequencing of a single canine cerebellar cortical degeneration case leads to the identification of a disease associated SPTBN2 mutation. BMC Genet 2012;13:55.
18. Shearman JR, Cook RW, McCowan C, et al. Mapping cerebellar abiotrophy in Australian Kelpies. Anim Genet 2011;42(6):675–8.
19. O'Brien D. Hereditary cerebellar ataxia. From the Proceedings 11th ACVIM Forum. Washington, DC: 1993. p. 546–9.
20. van Tongern SE, van Vonderen IK, van Nes JJ, et al. Cerebellar cortical abiotrophy in two Portuguese Podenco littermates. Vet Q 2000;22(3):172–4.
21. Kent M, Glass E, deLahunta A. Cerebellar cortical abiotrophy in a beagle. J Small Anim Pract 2000;41(7):321–3.
22. Steinberg HS, Troncoso JC, Cork LC, et al. Clinical features of inherited cerebellar degeneration in Gordon setters. J Am Vet Med Assoc 1981;179(9):886–90.
23. van der Merwe LL, Lane E. Diagnosis of cerebellar cortical degeneration in a Scottish terrier using magnetic resonance imaging. J Small Anim Pract 2001;42(8):409–12.

24. Gandini G, Botteron C, Brini E, et al. Cerebellar cortical degeneration in three English bulldogs: clinical and neuropathological findings. J Small Anim Pract 2005;46(6):291–4.

25. Thomas JB, Robertson D. Hereditary cerebellar abiotrophy in Australian kelpie dogs. Aust Vet J 1989;66(9):301–2.

26. Tiemeyer MJ, Singer HS, Troncoso JC, et al. Synaptic neurochemical alterations associated with neuronal degeneration in an inherited cerebellar ataxia of gordon setters. J Neuropathol Exp Neurol 1984;43:580–91.

27. Troncoso JC, Cork LC, Price DL. Canine inherited ataxia: ultrastructural observations. J Neuropathol Exp Neurol 1985;44:165–75.

28. Urkasemsin G, Linder KE, Bell JS, et al. Mapping of Purkinje neuron loss and polyglucosan body accumulation in hereditary cerebellar degeneration in Scottish terriers. Vet Pathol 2012;49(5):852–9.

29. Coates JR, Carmichael KP, Shelton GD, et al. Preliminary characterization of a cerebellar ataxia in Jack Russell Terriers. J Vet Intern Med 1996;10:176.

30. Sandy JR, Slocombe RE, Mitten RW, et al. Cerebellar abiotrophy in a family of Border Collie dogs. Vet Pathol 2002;39(6):736–8.

31. Jokinen TS, Rusbridge C, Steffen F, et al. Cerebellar cortical abiotrophy in Lagotto Romagnolo dogs. J Small Anim Pract 2007;48(8):470–3.

32. Huska J, Gaitero L, Snyman HN, et al. Cerebellar granuloprival degeneration in an Australian kelpie and a Labrador retriever dog. Can Vet J 2013;54(1):55–60.

33. Tipold A, Fatzer R, Jaggy A, et al. Presumed immune-mediated cerebellar granuloprival degeneration in the Coton de Tulear breed. J Neuroimmunol 2000; 110(1–2):130–3.

34. Cantile C, Salvadori C, Modenato M, et al. Cerebellar granuloprival degeneration in an Italian hound. J Vet Med A Physiol Pathol Clin Med 2002;49(10):523–5.

35. Flegel T, Matiasek K, Henke D, et al. Cerebellar cortical degeneration with selective granule cell loss in Bavarian mountain dogs. J Small Anim Pract 2007;48(8):462–5.

36. Perille AL, Baer K, Joseph RJ, et al. Postnatal cerebellar cortical degeneration in Labrador Retriever puppies. Can Vet J 1991;32(10):619–21.

37. Bildfell RJ, Mitchell SK, de Lahunta A. Cerebellar cortical degeneration in a Labrador retriever. Can Vet J 1995;36(9):570–2.

38. Hersheson J, Haworth A, Houlden H. The inherited ataxias: genetic heterogeneity, mutation databases, and future directions in research and clinical diagnostics. Hum Mutat 2012;33(9):1324–32.

39. Higgins RJ, LeCouteur RA, Kornegay JN, et al. Late-onset progressive spinocerebellar degeneration in Brittany Spaniel dogs. Acta Neuropathol 1998;96(1):97–101.

40. Rohdin C, Ludtke L, Wohlsein P, et al. New aspects of hereditary ataxia in smooth-haired fox terriers. Vet Rec 2010;166(18):557–60.

41. Bjorck G, Dyrendhal S, Olsson SE. Hereditary ataxia in smooth-haired fox terriers. Vet Record 1957;69:871–6.

42. Bhatti SF, Vanhaesebrouck AE, Van Soens I, et al. Myokymia and neuromyotonia in 37 Jack Russell terriers. Vet J 2011;189(3):284–8.

43. Vanhaesebrouck AE, Bhatti SF, Franklin RJ, et al. Myokymia and neuromyotonia in veterinary medicine: a comparison with peripheral nerve hyperexcitability syndrome in humans. Vet J 2013;197(2):153–62.

44. Coates JR, O'Brien DP, Kline KL, et al. Neonatal cerebellar ataxia in Coton de Tulear dogs. J Vet Intern Med 2002;16(6):680–9.

45. Zeng R, Farias FH, Johnson GS, et al. A truncated retrotransposon disrupts the GRM1 coding sequence in Coton de Tulear Dogs with Bandera's neonatal ataxia. J Vet Intern Med 2011;25(2):267–72.

46. Guergueltcheva V, Azmanov DN, Angelicheva D, et al. Autosomal-recessive congenital cerebellar ataxia is caused by mutations in metabotropic glutamate receptor 1. Am J Hum Genet 2012;91(3):553–64.
47. Lin DJ, Hermann KL, Schmahmann JD. Multiple system atrophy of the cerebellar type: clinical state of the art. Mov Disord 2014;29(Suppl 3):294–304.
48. deLahunta A, Averill DR Jr. Hereditary cerebellar cortical and extrapyramidal nuclear abiotrophy in Kerry Blue Terriers. J Am Vet Med Assoc 1976;168(12):1119–24.
49. O'Brien DP, Johnson GS, Schnabel RD, et al. Genetic mapping of canine multiple system degeneration and ectodermal dysplasia loci. J Hered 2005;96(7): 727–34.
50. Deforest ME, Eger CE, Basrur PK. Hereditary cerebellar neuronal abiotrophy in a Kerry Blue Terrier dog. Can Vet J 1978;19(7):198–202.
51. O'Brien DP, Zeng R, Schnabel RD, et al. Identification of two breed-specific mutations associated with canine multiple system degeneration using whole genome resequencing. Proc ACVIM Forum. 2013.
52. Hopkins AL, Clarke J. Episodic cerebellar dysfunction in a bichon frise: a canine case of episodic ataxia? J Small Anim Pract 2010;51(8):444–6.
53. Strupp M, Kalla R, Claassen J, et al. A randomized trial of 4-aminopyridine in EA2 and related familial episodic ataxias. Neurology 2011;77(3):269–75.
54. Nibe K, Kita C, Morozumi M, et al. Clinicopathological features of canine neuroaxonal dystrophy and cerebellar cortical abiotrophy in Papillon and Papillon-related dogs. J Vet Med Sci 2007;69(10):1047–52.
55. Cummings JF, de Lahunta A. A study of cerebellar and cerebral cortical degeneration in miniature poodle pups with emphasis on the ultrastructure of Purkinje cell changes. Acta Neuropathol 1988;75(3):261–71.
56. Berry ML, Blas-Machado U. Cerebellar abiotrophy in a miniature schnauzer. Can Vet J 2003;44(8):657–9.
57. Gumber S, Cho DY, Morgan TW. Late onset of cerebellar abiotrophy in a boxer dog. Vet Med Int 2010;2010:406275.

Canine Paroxysmal Movement Disorders

Ganokon Urkasemsin, DVM, PhD[a], Natasha J. Olby, VetMB, PhD, MRCVS[b],*

KEYWORDS

- Episodic movement disorders • Hypertonicity • Episodic falling
- Hyperkinetic episode • Paroxysmal dyskinesia • Scottie cramp

KEY POINTS

- Paroxysmal dyskinesias form a heterogeneous group of disorders recognized with increasing frequency in dogs and characterized by episodic, involuntary, abnormal movements.
- Classification of these disorders in veterinary medicine has not been attempted, but most seem to be comparable to paroxysmal nonkinesigenic dyskinesia in humans.
- Hypertonicity of limbs characterized by sustained flexion (dystonia) and brief flexion (chorea) of muscles are common clinical signs.
- During an episode, affected animals do not exhibit autonomic signs, electroencephalographic abnormalities, or change in consciousness.
- Clinical signs do not usually respond to antiepileptic drugs.

INTRODUCTION

Movement disorders are a heterogeneous group of diseases in humans and animals characterized by involuntary movements without changes in consciousness. Episodic or paroxysmal movement disorders can be broadly classified into paroxysmal dyskinesias and episodic ataxias; episodic ataxias are usually grouped with hereditary ataxias and will not be considered further in this review. The paroxysmal dyskinesias are a fascinating group of central nervous system diseases that produce dramatic and often puzzling clinical signs, canine examples of which have been described in veterinary medicine from as early as the 1940s.[1] However, it is only recently that these diseases have been grouped together under the label of paroxysmal dyskinesia and their genetic causes investigated in detail. They are characterized by episodic hyperkinesis

The authors have nothing to disclose.
[a] Department of Pre-Clinic and Applied Animal Science, Faculty of Veterinary Science, Mahidol University, 999 Phuttamonthon Sai 4 Road, Salaya, Phuttamonthon, Nakhon Pathom 73170, Thailand; [b] Department of Clinical Sciences, College of Veterinary Medicine, North Carolina State University, 1060 William Moore Drive, Raleigh, NC 27607, USA
* Corresponding author.
E-mail address: natasha_olby@ncsu.edu

impairing posture and locomotion without loss of consciousness.[2] Chorea, dystonia, ballism, and athetosis are all signs of hyperkinesis that are common to the phenomenology of this group of diseases (**Box 1**). They are differentiated from seizures because, during episodes, consciousness and electroencephalography (EEG) are normal and there is a lack of autonomic signs. However, differentiation from seizures can be difficult, and now that the underlying genetic mutations are described in humans, it is becoming clear that specific mutations in dyskinesia patients may also be associated with seizures (eg, familial infantile convulsions with paroxysmal choreoathetosis) or a high frequency of seizure disorders in their families.[3]

Paroxysmal dyskinesias (PDs) can be primary, secondary, or part of more complex neurologic syndromes.[3] This review focuses on the primary PDs, in which patients are normal between episodes; however, it is important to note that an example of a secondary dyskinesia has been described in veterinary patients.[4] In humans, classification of PDs has evolved over time. Initially, they were described by their clinical signs, leading to terms such as paroxysmal choreoathetosis. More recently, a clinically useful classification system has been developed in which patients are categorized by the precipitants, age of onset and duration of attacks.[5] There are 3 main forms: (1) Paroxysmal kinesigenic dyskinesia (PKD), in which episodes are precipitated by sudden movements; (2) paroxysmal nonkinesigenic dyskinesia (PNKD), in which episodes are not triggered by movements, but may be associated with stress, alcohol, or caffeine; and (3) paroxysmal exertion-induced dyskinesia, in which heavy exercise produces signs.[5] A fourth form known as paroxysmal hypnogenic dyskinesia in which episodes occur during sleep has been reclassified as a frontal lobe epilepsy and removed from the classification system. Key features of each type of dyskinesia are listed in **Table 1**. Note also that the genetic causes described to date are listed and show that, although the clinical categorization is useful, genetic definition of the disorders shows crossover between types, and new classification systems in which the disease is first assigned to a category as described, and then assigned to a genetic category, are emerging.[3]

In veterinary medicine, paroxysmal dyskinesia has been used as a broad term to describe an abnormal, sudden, involuntary contraction of a group of skeletal muscles that recurs episodically.[6] This group of diseases is not well categorized and names

---

Box 1
Terms used to describe involuntary movements in human medicine

- Hyperkinesis: General term for increased muscle activity.
- Dyskinesia: Impairment of voluntary movements
- Chorea: Brief muscle contractions producing rapid movements similar to those seen during dancing. Frequently accompanied by athetosis giving rise to the term choreoathetosis.
- Dystonia: Sustained muscle contractions producing abnormal movements and postures
- Ballism: Flailing limb movements
- Athetosis: Writhing movements produced by sustained contraction of the trunk muscles. This is frequently accompanied by chorea.
- Movements affecting 1 side of the body are identified by the prefix "hemi"

Although the term dystonia is commonly used in canine reports, and ballism is occasionally reported, the terms chorea and athetosis are rarely used. This may reflect species differences or a failure to recognize these signs in dogs.

Data from Bhatia KP. Paroxysmal dyskinesias. Mov Disord 2011;26(6):1157–65.

Table 1
Comparison of key features in the 3 main categories of human paroxysmal dyskinesia

	PKD	PNKD	PED
Trigger	Sudden movements	Caffeine, alcohol, strong emotion	Prolonged exercise
Duration of signs	<2 min	10 min to 12 h, usually <4 h	Mean 2–5 min, ≤2 h
Age of onset	1–20 y	Early childhood, mean 8 y	2–30 y; mean, 5 y
Frequency of signs	Multiple attacks a day, improves and may resolve with age	Clusters several times a year	Dependent on exercise
Known genetic causes	PRRT2	PRRT2, MR-1, KCNMA1	GLUT1, MR-1
Treatment	Respond to antiepileptic drugs and carbamazepine	Avoid triggers; clonazepam effective in majority of patients; haloperidol, gabapentin, and L-dopa may be of benefit	Ketogenic diet, gabapentin.

Abbreviations: GLUT1, glucose transporter type 1 gene (also known as SLC2A1); KCNMA1, calcium-activated potassium channel, subfamily M, alpha member 1; MR-1, myofibrillogenesis regulator 1 (the function of this gene is poorly understood); PED, paroxysmal exertion-induced dyskinesia; PKD, paroxysmal kinesigenic dyskinesia; PNKD, paroxysmal nonkinesigenic dyskinesia; PRRT2, proline-rich transmembrane protein 2 gene (defects in this transmembrane protein are thought to destabilize synapses and alter neuronal excitability but the pathophysiologic basis requires more investigation).

given to different disorders include hypertonicity syndrome, episodic falling, hyperkinetic episodes, and dyskinesia. Similar to their human counterparts, they are distinguished from seizures by an absence of autonomic signs, EEG abnormalities, or changes in consciousness during episodes. Affected animals are normal between episodes. Nevertheless, when faced with a patient exhibiting episodic neurologic signs, a careful workup is needed to rule out other disorders. Transient, self-limiting, involuntary movements can be a result of disorders of the central nervous system (PDs, epileptic seizures, episodic ataxia), vestibular dysfunction, disease of muscle (eg, muscle cramps from a variety of causes), or peripheral nerve hyperexcitability (eg, hypocalcemia, myokymia, neuromyotonia). A logical approach to these cases is provided in **Fig. 1**.

Hereditary paroxysmal dyskinesias have been described in Scottish Terriers,[7] Cavalier King Charles Spaniels,[8] Chinooks[9] and Border terriers.[10] Episodic head tremors are recognized as hereditary or breed-associated disorders in the Doberman pinscher[11] and the English bulldog[12] and may represent a form of paroxysmal dyskinesia. Sporadic cases have been reported in a variety of breeds, the details of which are summarized in **Table 2**.[6,13]

INHERITED DISEASES
Episodic Falling in Cavalier King Charles Spaniels

Cavalier King Charles spaniels suffer from familial paroxysmal exercise-induced dyskinesia, also known as episodic falling, which has been recognized within the breed since the 1960s, but was first reported in the 1980s,[8] at which time it was suspected to be a myopathy.[14,15] It is also known as sudden collapse, muscle hypertonicity, and hyperekplexia, although the latter term is misleading because "hyperekplexia"

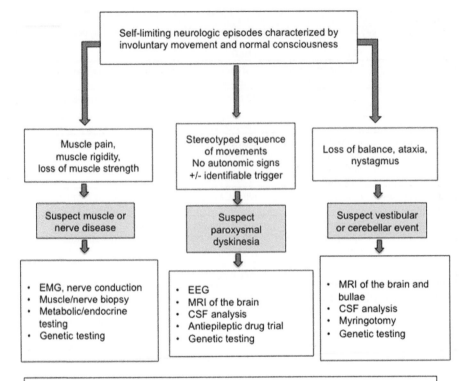

Fig. 1. Logical approach to a dog with an involuntary movement disorder.

describes startle disorders that are triggered by unexpected stimuli such as noise and touch and classically caused by mutations in the genes involved in glycinergic synaptic transmission.[16] The age of onset of episodic falling episodes ranges from 3 to 48 months.[8] Episodes are triggered by exercise, excitement, and stress, and as such it may be more accurately classified as a PNKD. Affected dogs exhibit progressive muscular hypertonicity during an episode during which there is marked dystonia of the pelvis or all 4 limbs. Typically, an episode is characterized by lowering of the head, arching of the lumbar spine, stiffness of the limbs that creates a 'deer-stalking' posture, and falling over.[8,15] The duration of episodes varies among cases ranging from a few seconds to several minutes[8,15] and they are self-limiting or can be limited by interaction with the owner.[8] There is no loss of consciousness during the period of collapse. There are no significant clinical or neurologic abnormalities and no spontaneous discharges on electromyography in between episodes.[15] The benzodiazepine, clonazepam (0.5 mg/kg every 8 hours), has been used to treat episodic falling effectively[17] and acetazolamide is also reported to be beneficial. An autosomal-recessive mode of inheritance has been demonstrated.[18] On postmortem examination, a variety of changes have been described in skeletal muscle, such as enlargement and proliferation of the sarcoplasmic reticulum, but these are likely to be secondary to excessive muscle contractions.[14,15,19] Recently, this dramatic condition has been linked to a deletion in the gene *BCAN*[18,19] that encodes a protein called brevican. This protein is a component of the extracellular matrix proteoglycan complex and is found at high levels in the central nervous system as part of the perineuronal network. In particular, it is found at the nodes of Ranvier in large-diameter axons and is thought to play a role in homoeostasis of the microenvironment in the face of fluctuating ion concentrations. It is proposed that disruption of these extracellular complexes results in alterations in nerve conduction and in synaptic stability.[19] As is typical for all genetic disease, there is phenotypic variability and both research groups that described the mutation identified dogs homozygous for the mutation, but with no reported clinical signs. They theorized that these dogs may simply not have exerted themselves to the point of producing signs, but it is important to note that mouse *BCAN* knockouts are clinically normal. Moreover, compensatory pathways involving upregulation of other proteoglycans may occur and account for the observation that some dogs can become clinically normal after a period of years.[18] This genetic test is offered at http://www.aht.org.uk/cms-display/genetics_canine.html.

PNKD in Chinooks

Familial PNKD has been reported in the Chinook with the age of onset ranging from 2 to 60 months, but the majority of dogs first developing signs by 3 years of age.[9] Initially, these episodes were known as Chinook seizures, but closer examination revealed that the episodes were not epileptic. Episodes are not triggered by sudden movements or exercise, and can last between 1 and 60 minutes. The frequency of occurrence also varies widely from several episodes per day to a handful of episodes in the dog's entire lifetime. The phenomenology as described by owners in questionnaires was remarkably consistent between cases and includes flailing or kicking (ballism), sustained limb flexion combined with repetitive small limb movements and, occasionally, head tremor. The dogs remain fully conscious and responsive throughout the episode, although owners report they may be lethargic afterward. A video of an episode is available at: http://www.canine-epilepsy.net/Chinook/chinook.html. Dogs are neurologically normal between episodes and interictal analysis including pre and post exercise lactate and pyruvate levels, EEG, magnetic resonance imaging, and cerebrospinal fluid examination from 2 affected dogs, was unremarkable.[9] An autosomal-recessive mode of inheritance has been identified by segregation analysis and it is interesting to note that epilepsy also occurs in the same family lines, and even coincidentally with PNKD in 2 dogs. The causative genetic disorder has not yet been determined.

Scottie Cramp in Scottish Terriers

PNKD in Scottish Terriers, also known as Scottie cramp, hyperkinetic episodes, and hypertonicity syndrome has been recognized since the 1940s[1] and was investigated extensively in the 1970s.[7,20–23] Age of onset of ranges from 1 to 84 months, but in most cases clinical signs start early in life (approximately 6 months). Episodes are

Table 2
Summary of clinical manifestations of paroxysmal dyskinesias in dogs

Canine Breed	Disease	Triggers	Age of Onset (mo)	Duration (min)	Frequency	Progression	Clinical Signs	Treatment
Inherited disorders (autosomal recessive)								
Cavalier King Charles spaniel[8,18,19]	Episodic falling	Exercise, stress, excitement	3–48 (most cases at 3–4 mo)	Seconds to minutes	Depends on triggers	Frequency and duration of episodes decreased with age and treatment	Dystonia of hind limbs or all 4 limbs, lowering of the head close to the ground, arching of the lumbar spine, stiffening of limbs, increasing of muscle tone, developing the deer-stalking posture, falling over	Clonazepam
Scottish terrier[7,20–26]	Scottie cramp	Stress, excitement, exercise	1–84 (most cases <12 mo)	5–20	Depends on triggers	Severity and frequency decreased with time	Dystonia of hind limbs or all 4 limbs, lowering of the head close to the ground, arching of the lumbar spine, stiffening of limbs, increasing of muscle tone, developing the deer-stalking posture, falling over	Fluoxetine, diazepam
Chinook[9]	Paroxysmal nonkinesigenic dyskinesia	Unidentified	2–60 (most cases <36 mo)	1–60	Several per day to few per year	NR	Flexion of limb(s), repetitive, small range movements of limb(s) and ballism, head tremors	NR
Border terrier[10]	Canine epileptoid cramping syndrome	Vary: waking up, excitement, stress, hot/cold temperature	2.5–84 (most cases <36 mo)	0.5–150	Several per day to per months or years	NR	Inability to stand or walk, involuntary flexion or extension of 1 or multiple limbs, mild tremor, dystonia, borborygmi	Diet change

Sporadic reports

Wheaton terrier[13]	Paroxysmal dyskinesia	N/A	12–24	NR	Several per day to few per year; tend to cluster	NR	Prolonged pelvic limb flexion, rigidity, and back spasms with variable involvement of thoracic limbs	Diazepam
Bichon Frise[27]	Paroxysmal dyskinesia	Random	46.5	NR	10 times per day to 1 time per week	Unchanged within 1 year	Hyperflexion of 1 limb with progression to other limbs, dystonia, rapid flexion and extension of limb, hyperflexion of thoracic spine	NR
Boxer[28]	Paroxysmal dyskinesia	Unidentified, possibly excitement	2	1–5	10 episodes per day to 2 episodes per 6 mo	Frequency and duration of episodes decreased with age	Briefly sustained hyperflexion of a single thoracic or pelvic limb, unilateral dystonia of the neck, face, and trunk	NR
German shorthaired pointer[29]	Paroxysmal dyskinesia	Excitement, prolonged activity or exercise	12	10–30, 180	Trigger dependent	NR	Arching the lumbar spine, flexion of both hind limbs	Phenobarbital
Springer spaniel[13]	Paroxysmal dyskinesia	Excitement, exercise	3	NR	NR	NR	Hind limbs rigidity, arching the lumbar spine, fore limbs hypertonicity, falling	NR

The episodic head tremor syndromes are not included in this table.
Abbreviation: NR, not reported.
Data from Refs.[7–10,13,18–29]

triggered by excitement, stress, and exercise. The phenomenology is remarkably similar to that exhibited by Cavalier King Charles spaniels with episodic falling although the authors have worked with several dogs in which mild signs of hind limb spasticity and bunny hopping occur. Episodes last between 5 and 20 minutes. In the majority of dogs, signs decrease in severity with time, with behavior modification or a change in the level of activity and, in those that require medication, fluoxetine and diazepam have been reported to be beneficial.[21,24] Electromyography revealed an increase in interference patterns during episodes but no abnormal spontaneous discharges at rest.[7] No macroscopic or microscopic lesions have been found in the nervous system and muscle of affected dogs, consistent with a primarily functional disorder.[21] A potential role for serotonin in producing episodes is intriguing. Depletion of serotonin with drugs such as methysergide or methionine induces clinical signs, whereas increasing serotonin with fluoxetine, tryptophan, and nialamide reduces or prevents episodes.[23,25,26] However, quantification of brain serotonin content shows no difference between affected and normal dogs,[23,26] and it is unclear whether serotonin has a primary or secondary role in the pathophysiology. Scottie cramp is reported to be inherited as an autosomal-recessive trait.[21] An identical syndrome has also been reported anecdotally in Cairn terriers, Norwich terriers, and West Highland White Terriers, and may be caused by the same genetic disorder given the common lineage of these breeds. Currently, the causative genetic mutation has not been identified, although sequencing of *BCAN* is normal in this breed (Ganokon Urkasemsin and Natasha J. Olby, unpublished observations).

Canine Epileptoid Cramping in Border Terriers

This paroxysmal movement disorder initially went by the name of Spike's disease after the first dog in which it was recognized and is now classified as a paroxysmal dyskinesia.[10] Similar to the condition in Chinooks, episodes do not seem to be triggered by sudden movements or exertion, although some owners report an association with stress or excitement and others report signs during waking from sleep. Age of onset varies widely ranging from 2.5 months to 7 years; typically, events happen in clusters, sometimes separated by months. Episode phenomenology includes difficulty walking that progresses to difficulty standing; dystonia of the limbs, head, and neck; and tremors. Air licking and stretching are also reported. Videos of these episodes can be found at http://www.borderterrier-cecs.com/cecs_videos.htm. A possible link to gastrointestinal disease is intriguing in these dogs. Many owners report borborygmi during an episode and some dogs have episodes of vomiting and diarrhea immediately before or after an episode. This possible association with an autonomic sign may indicate that these episodes are more like seizures in their etiology. Because of discussion about the possible role of food intolerance in this syndrome, most owners alter their dog's diet to a hypoallergenic diet, although there is no evidence that this has any beneficial effect. Treatment with antiepileptic or antispasmodic drugs is ineffective.

Episodic Head Tremor Syndrome

This syndrome is recognized as a suspected hereditary disorder in English bulldogs,[11] and Doberman pinschers[12] and occurs sporadically in a wider population of dogs. Signs typically first appear in young dogs (<2 years of age), but onset can be as late as 9 years of age. There are no specific triggers noted for English bulldogs, although owners usually report their dogs as being quiet when signs appear. Triggers reported in the Doberman pinscher include stress, fatigue, illness, and excitement. Duration of episodes varies from a few seconds to up to 3 hours and frequency ranges from multiple per day to clusters every few months. The phenomenology of episodes is essentially the same for both breeds of dog; dogs nod their head repetitively horizontally or vertically or both at a frequency of 5 to 8 Hz. They may show mild dystonia of the neck during an episode and, although fully conscious, may show signs of anxiety, irritation, or discomfort, and may yawn, bark, or press their heads against solid surfaces. Numerous videos of these events can be found on the internet simply by searching the term "head bobbing." At least 66% of dogs can be distracted out of the episodes using treats or other interactions and signs are typically not responsive to antiepileptic drugs.[11,12] Approximately 50% of dogs seem to grow out of the condition with time. This disease has been tentatively classified as a paroxysmal dyskinesia, but such isolated head tremors have not been described in people with PD.

SPORADIC REPORTS

Paroxysmal Dyskinesia in a Bichon Frise

Episodic dyskinesia has been described in a 4-year-old Bichon Frise with a 6-week history of episodes.[27] Episodes were unpredictable and occurred at rest, when excited, and with exercise with a frequency ranging from 10 times per day to once a week. The clinical signs were hyperflexion of 1 limb that could progress to additional limbs while disappearing in the first affected limb. Dystonia and rapid flexion and extension of limb were also observed. During the episode, the dog had no change in consciousness. The dog was clinically normal between episodes and brain magnetic resonance imaging and cerebrospinal fluid analysis were normal. Treatment was attempted with phenobarbital but was not effective.

Paroxysmal Dyskinesia in the Boxer

Two litters of boxers were examined for a paroxysmal dyskinesia.[28] Episodes consisted of briefly sustained hyperflexion of a single thoracic or pelvic limb, with unilateral dystonia of the neck, face, and trunk. Dogs would fall if the episode occurred during movement. The age of onset was 2 months and the frequency of episodes ranged from 10 episodes per day to 2 episodes per 6 months. Episodes were more severe and more frequent in males than females. Excitement seemed to trigger some episodes, but they could also occur randomly. The episodes lasted for 1 to 5 minutes and frequency and duration decreased with age. During the episodes, the dogs remained conscious and responded when the owner called their name. Stroking and calmly talking to the dog shortened the duration of episodes. There was a rapid recovery and no neurologic deficits between episodes.

Paroxysmal Dyskinesia Reported in Other Breeds

There are brief clinical descriptions of paroxysmal dyskinesias affecting Springer spaniels and Wheaton terriers.[13] In Springer spaniels, the age of onset was 3 months and the triggers were exercise or excitement. The clinical signs of progressive hypertonicity were characterized by pelvic limb rigidity, arching of lumbar spine, thoracic limb hypertonicity, and falling. Resting helped to resolve the signs. In Wheaton terriers, signs started around 1 to 2 years of age. The main clinical signs included sustained flexion or rigidity of hind limbs and back spasms. Diazepam may have reduced severity of clinical signs.

Phenobarbital-Responsive Paroxysmal Dyskinesia

Most dogs affected by paroxysmal dyskinesia do not respond to antiepileptic drugs. However, a rapid reduction of frequency and severity of clinical signs were reported in a German shorthaired pointer with suspected paroxysmal dyskinesia after phenobarbital administration.[29] This dog exhibited typical muscle hypertonicity, including arching of the lumbar spine and flexion of both hind limbs that was triggered by excitement and prolonged exercise. Episodes lasted from 10 minutes to 3 hours. The dog had symmetric signs in both pelvic limbs and was conscious during episodes, although partial seizure activity was not ruled out with EEG.

Phenobarbital-Induced Dyskinesia

There are few reports of acquired dyskinesias in veterinary medicine, but there is a description of a dyskinesia associated with phenobarbital therapy in an epileptic Chow Chow.[4] The dog showed progressive twitching of the facial, neck, and shoulder muscles, impairing its ability to walk and worsening as the dose of phenobarbital increased. EEG evaluation during an episode was normal and withdrawal of phenobarbital resulted in complete resolution of the signs.

OTHER INVOLUNTARY MOVEMENT DISORDERS

Jack and Parson Russell terriers suffer from a complex cluster of hereditary neurologic conditions including hereditary ataxia, myokymia and seizures (see elsewhere in this issue by Urkasemsin and Olby). Because of the variation in clinical manifestations, classification of this syndrome has been compared with hyperkinetic movement disorders and peripheral nerve hyperexcitability syndromes in humans.[30] Myokymia is characterized by rhythmic undulating muscle contractions producing vermicular movement of the overlying skin or rippling muscles, and accompanied by spontaneous discharges on EMG originating from the motor neuron. The clinical signs may progress to cause collapse and generalized rigidity (neuromyotonia). Affected Jack Russell terriers develop hyperthermia from sustained muscle contractions that can be life threatening.[31] Based on the recent discovery mutation in *KCNJ10* gene in a group of Jack Russell terriers (age of onset between 2 to 12 months) affected by cerebellar ataxia with or without myokymia, seizure, or both,[32] this clinical complex is now classified as a hereditary ataxia.

Startle disease or hyperekplexia has been reported in 2 Irish wolfhound littermates.[33] This dramatic disorder is characterized by muscle rigidity that can be severe enough to cause apnea. In humans, these diseases are caused by abnormal glycinergic neurotransmission. Clinical signs in the puppies started from 5 to 7 days after birth and were triggered by noise, touch, and handling. Nursing caused cyanosis. Affected dogs were normal at rest. A mutation in *SLC6A5* gene encoding presynaptic glycine transporter GlyT2 was identified.[33] Thus, besides the different types of triggers, age of onset, and duration of signs, genetic investigation is also useful to distinguish hyperekplexia from paroxysmal dyskinesias.

SUMMARY

Paroxysmal dyskinesias are being described with increasing frequency in dogs and may start to fall into groups based on clinical signs, triggers, progression, duration, and frequency of episodes. Precipitating factors and duration of episodes are central to categorizing paroxysmal dyskinesias in the human and are helpful in therapeutic decisions.[3,5] None of the canine disorders described seem to fit well into the human category of paroxysmal kinesigenic dyskinesia, and sometimes triggers are hard to identify in dogs. As more syndromes are described, clinically useful categories of disease may start to be developed based on clinical presentation. However, with the rapid increase in our understanding of the genetic basis of canine neurologic disorders, it is reasonable to hope that these diseases will be classified according to their mutation and the pathophysiologic mechanism underlying them in the near future. To date, only a single mutation in the gene *BCAN* has been identified as a cause of canine PNKD. Genetic investigations in other breeds are ongoing and will likely revolutionize our ability to understand and treat these disorders.

REFERENCES

1. Klarenbeek A. An intermittently appearing disturbance in the regulation of the leg tonus observed in Scottish Terriers. Tijdschr Diergeneeskd 1942;69:14–21.
2. Bhatia KP. Paroxysmal dyskinesias. Mov Disord 2011;26(6):1157–65.
3. Erro R, Sheerin UM, Bhatia KP. Paroxysmal dyskinesias revisited: a review of 500 genetically proven cases and a new classification. Mov Disord 2014. http://dx. doi.org/10.1002/mds.25933.
4. Kube SA, Vernau KM, LeCouteur RA. Dyskinesia associated with oral phenobarbital administration in a dog. J Vet Intern Med 2006;20(5):1238–40.
5. Jankovic J, Demirkiran M. Classification of paroxysmal dyskinesias and ataxias. Adv Neurol 2002;89:387–400.
6. de Lahunta A, Glass E. Veterinary neuroanatomy and clinical neurology. St Louis (MO): Saunders Elsevier; 2009. p. 363–9.
7. Meyers KM, Dickson WM, Lund JE, et al. Muscular hypertonicity. Episodes in Scottish terrier dogs. Arch Neurol 1971;25(1):61–8.
8. Herrtage ME, Palmer AC. Episodic falling in the cavalier King Charles spaniel. Vet Rec 1983;112(19):458–9.
9. Packer RA, Patterson EE, Taylor JF, et al. Characterization and mode of inheritance of a paroxysmal dyskinesia in Chinook dogs. J Vet Intern Med 2010;24(6):1305–13.
10. Black V, Garosi L, Lowrie M, et al. Phenotypic characterisation of canine epileptoid cramping syndrome in the Border terrier. J Small Anim Pract 2013. http://dx. doi.org/10.1111/jsap.12170.
11. Guevar J, De Decker S, Van Ham LM, et al. Idiopathic head tremor in English bulldogs. Mov Disord 2014;29(2):191–4.
12. Wolf M, Bruehschwein A, Sauter-Louis C, et al. An inherited episodic head tremor syndrome in Doberman pinscher dogs. Mov Disord 2011;26(13):2381–6.
13. Shelton GD. Muscle pain, cramps and hypertonicity. Vet Clin North Am Small Anim Pract 2004;34(6):1483–96.
14. Wright JA, Smyth JB, Brownlie SE, et al. A myopathy associated with muscle hypertonicity in the Cavalier King Charles Spaniel. J Comp Pathol 1987;97(5):559–65.
15. Wright JA, Brownlie SE, Smyth JB, et al. Muscle hypertonicity in the cavalier King Charles spaniel–myopathic features. Vet Rec 1986;118(18):511–2.
16. Bhidayasiri R, Truong DD. Startle syndromes. Handb Clin Neurol 2011;100: 421–30.
17. Garosi LS, Platt SR, Shelton GD. Hypertonicity in Cavalier King Charles spaniels. J Vet Intern Med 2002;16:330.
18. Forman OP, Penderis J, Hartley C, et al. Parallel mapping and simultaneous sequencing reveals deletions in BCAN and FAM83H associated with discrete inherited disorders in a domestic dog breed. PLoS Genet 2012;8(1):e1002462.
19. Gill JL, Tsai KL, Krey C, et al. A canine BCAN microdeletion associated with episodic falling syndrome. Neurobiol Dis 2012;45(1):130–6.
20. Meyers KM, Lund JE, Padgett G, et al. Hyperkinetic episodes in Scottish Terrier dogs. J Am Vet Med Assoc 1969;155:129–33.
21. Meyers KM, Padgett GA, Dickson WM. The genetic basis of a kinetic disorder of Scottish terrier dogs. J Hered 1970;61:189–92.

22. Clemmon RM, Peters RI, Meyers KM. Scotty cramp: a review of cause, characteristics, diagnosis, and treatment. Compend Contin Educ Vet 1980;2:385–8.
23. Peters RI Jr, Meyers KM. Precursor regulation of serotonergic neuronal function in Scottish Terrier dogs. J Neurochem 1977;29:753–5.
24. Geiger KM, Klopp LS. Use of a selective serotonin reuptake inhibitor for treatment of episodes of hypertonia and kyphosis in a young adult Scottish Terrier. J Am Vet Med Assoc 2009;235:168–71.
25. Roberts DD, Hitt ME. Methionine as a possible inducer of Scotty Cramp. Canine practice 1986;13:29–31.
26. Meyers KM, Schab B. The relationship of serotonin to a motor disorder of Scottish Terrier dogs. Life Sci 1974;14:1895–906.
27. Penderis J, Franklin RJ. Dyskinesia in an adult bichon frise. J Small Anim Pract 2001;42(1):24–5.
28. Ramsey IK, Chandler KE, Franklin RJ. A movement disorder in boxer pups. Vet Rec 1999;144(7):179–80.
29. Harcourt-Brown T. Anticonvulsant responsive, episodic movement disorder in a German shorthaired pointer. J Small Anim Pract 2008;49(8):405–7.
30. Vanhaesebrouck AE, Bhatti SF, Franklin RJ, et al. Myokymia and neuromyotonia in veterinary medicine: a comparison with peripheral nerve hyperexcitability syndrome in humans. Vet J 2013;197(2):153–62.
31. Bhatti SF, Vanhaesebrouck AE, Van Soens I, et al. Myokymia and neuromyotonia in 37 Jack Russell terriers. Vet J 2011;189(3):284–8.
32. Gilliam D, O'Brien DP, Coates JR, et al. A homozygous KCNJ10 mutation in Jack Russell terriers and related breeds with spinocerebellar ataxia with myokymia, seizures, or both. J Vet Intern Med 2014;28(3):871–7.
33. Gill JL, Capper D, Vanbellinghen JF, et al. Startle disease in Irish wolfhounds associated with a microdeletion in the glycine transporter GlyT2 gene. Neurobiol Dis 2011;43(1):184–9.

Status Epilepticus and Cluster Seizures

Edward (Ned) E. Patterson, DVM, PhD

KEYWORDS

- Dog • Epilepsy • Seizures • Diazepam • Phenobarbital • Levetiracetam

KEY POINTS

- First-line (emergent initial) therapy for dogs or cats with prolonged (>5 min) seizures or seizures without recovery between should be initiated as soon as possible with a benzodiazepine drug at home (dogs) or in the veterinary hospital.
- Following first-line therapy, urgent therapy with parenteral loading doses or miniloading doses of a long-acting antiepileptic drug such as phenobarbital, levetiracetam (LEV), or bromide (dogs only) should be given to rapidly attain therapeutic levels of a chronic therapy drug.
- The etiology of status epilepticus (SE) should be diagnosed and treated as soon as possible.
- For companion animal patients failing to respond to first line therapy, second-line therapy should be attempted with nonanesthetizing doses of intravenous phenobarbital and/or intravenous LEV and/or a constant rate infusion (CRI) of diazepam or midazolam.
- Companion animals in refractory SE because they have failed to respond to first- and second-line treatments should be anesthetized with a CRI of propofol or pentobarbital or other anesthetic as third-line therapy.

DEFINITIONS

Status Epilepticus

Status epilepticus (SE) in the current veterinary and human literature is most often defined as a single seizure lasting 5 minutes or longer, or 2 or more seizures without recovery between.[1] Previous definitions had often been seizure activity lasting for at least 30 minutes due to the clear-cut potential for permanent damage at that point. The rational for a shorter duration for the definition has been the need for urgent and aggressive treatment early in the process well before the 30-minute mark.[2]

Generalized Seizure

This type of seizure is one in which the first clinical changes indicate the initial involvement of both cerebral hemispheres.[3]

Department of Veterinary Clinical Sciences, College of Veterinary Medicine, University of Minnesota, 1352 Boyd Avenue, St Paul, MN 55108, USA
E-mail address: patte037@umn.edu

Vet Clin Small Anim 44 (2014) 1103–1112
http://dx.doi.org/10.1016/j.cvsm.2014.07.007
0195-5616/14/$ – see front matter © 2014 Elsevier Inc. All rights reserved.

Focal Seizure

A focal seizure is one that originates within neuronal networks limited to 1 hemisphere. Such networks may include cortical and subcortical structures.[4]

Convulsive Status Epilepticus

Convulsive SE (CSE) is SE with convulsions that are associated with rhythmic jerking of the extremities such as generalized tonic–clonic movements and/or mental status, impairment and/or neurologic deficits.[5]

Nonconvulsive SE

Nonconvulsive SE (NCSE) is defined as prolonged seizure activity seen on electroencephalography (EEG) without the clinical findings associated with CSE, with either a wandering and confused patient or a patient with severely impaired mental status.[5] Although NCSE could be common, it has rarely been recognized in veterinary patients to date; therefore this article will not address NCSE beyond this section. Continuous intensive care unit (ICU) EEG monitoring is routinely done for human SE patients. Similar monitoring for NCSE has been done in some canine and feline patients and proposed to be further investigated,[6] but it is not standard practice in veterinary ICUs at this time.

Acute Repetitive Seizures and Cluster Seizures

Acute repetitive seizures (ARS) in people have been variably defined, but an accepted definition is 3 or more seizures in the 5 to 12 hours prior to presentation.[7–10] In dogs, frequent seizures (ie, ARS) have usually been defined as cluster seizures (CS). Definitions of CS in dogs have been inconsistent between publications, but they generally have been defined as a bout of multiple seizures occurring over a short period of time that is different from the patient's typical seizure pattern. A useful clinical definition of CS is 2 or more seizures occurring within a 24-hour period, in which the patient regains consciousness between the seizures.[11]

Refractory SE

Refractory SE (RSE) in people is defined as continuation of either clinical or EEG-defined seizures after receiving adequate doses of initial benzodiazepines followed by a second acceptable antiepileptic drug (AED).[5] Patients with RSE usually require anesthetic agents at anesthetic doses as third-line treatment.

Super RSE (SRSE)

Super RSE (SRSE) is SE that goes on 24 hours or more after the onset of anesthesia[12]; because of financial constraints and other considerations, companion animals are often euthanized before SRSE occurs.

Recently, several definitions regarding seizures in companion animals have been proposed (**Box 1**).[1] These proposed definitions are based on, but not identical to current definitions for people.

INTRODUCTION

Most seizures in dogs and cats are self-limiting and last a couple of minutes or less. Seizures that last more than a few minutes or occur back-to-back without recovery between are emergencies and should be treated promptly, aggressively, and with a systematic plan. If 30 to 60 minutes of continuous seizure activity occur, irreversible neuronal damage begins, mainly because of excitotoxic cell injury related to excessive glutamate release.[13] Resulting autonomic and endocrine dysfunction can lead

---

Box 1
Proposed definitions for companion animal seizures[1] that relate to seizure emergencies

Status Epilepticus:

- A seizure that persists for greater than 5 minutes or
- Recurrent seizures without interictal resumption of baseline central nervous system function

Cluster Seizure

- Two or more seizures within a 24-hour period.

Duration

- Time between the beginning of initial seizure manifestations and the cessation of observed seizure activity. Does not include prodrome or postictal states but might include aura.

Data from Mariani CL. Terminology and classification of seizures and epilepsy in veterinary patients. Top Companion Anim Med 2013;28:34–41.

---

to loss of normal brain homeostasis, kindling, functional and structural hippocampal changes, neurodegeneration, and altered distribution of ion channels and neurotransmitter receptors on a cellular level.[6] Systemically, prolonged or frequent seizures can result in hyperglycemia, hypertension[11] neuronal necrosis, hyperthermia, cardiac arrhythmias, kidney damage, metabolic acidosis, disseminated intravascular coagulation, cardiorespiratory failure, and a predisposition to further seizure episodes.[4] Consequently, aggressive and safe early intervention is important.

About 40% to 60% of dogs with genetic (idiopathic, primary) epilepsy suffer CS or SE,[11,14–17] and CS can evolve into SE.

In people, SE and ARS are common reasons for presentation to emergency rooms, with approximately 152,000 cases per year and 42,000 annual deaths in the United States.[18,19] Reported mortality rates in people range from 8% to 38%, depending on the underlying cause and patient age, with an overall mortality rate of 22%.[18,20]

To date, several detailed retrospective studies evaluating SE and CS in dogs have been published.[14–17] Although the designs differed, particularly for the underlying cause of SE, many similar conclusions were reached:

- The incidence of CS in dogs with genetic (idiopathic) epilepsy has been reported to be as high as 41%.[16]
- The prevalence of SE in dogs admitted for seizures has been documented to be 16%.[14]
- The incidence of SE in dogs with primary epilepsy was found to be 2.5%[16] in 1 study, whereas in another study it was found to be up to 59%.[15]
- Overall mortality rates (mostly from euthanasia) for dogs with episodes of SE were 23%,[14] 32%[15] and 38%,[17] with death occurring in a relatively small number of cases (2%–5%) (these estimates of morbidity and mortality are roughly comparable to those reported in studies in people).
- The underlying causes identified were genetic (idiopathic) epilepsy (26.8%–37.5%), structural (symptomatic, secondary) epilepsy (35.1%–39.8%), and reactive epileptic seizures (6.7%–22.7%).[14,17]

THERAPY OF SE
General Considerations for SE Care for Companion Animals

The initial management of SE should utilize basic principles of life support and drug administration to stop the seizures. Sedating antiseizure drugs can lead to loss of pharyngeal tone and risk of aspiration. Oral or nasal administration of oxygen is therefore needed in some patients, and when anesthetic drugs are used, intubation and ventilator support are required. Intravenous access should be obtained as soon as possible and blood collected for glucose measurement and therapeutic monitoring in patients already on AED therapy. Temperature, pulse oximetry, electrocardiogram (ECG), and blood pressure should be monitored, and any abnormalities, such as hyperthermia, hypoglycemia, or hypocalcemia should be quickly treated.[11] As the SE is being treated with drugs, efforts should also be made to diagnose the etiology as quickly as possible and start treatment for any causes with specific therapies.

CURRENT AND HISTORICAL DRUG THERAPY FOR SE
Human SE

In the 19th century, starting in the 1860s, bromides were given hypodermally, rectally, or orally. Intravenous barbiturates, including phenobarbital, were introduced in the 1920s. Phenytoin was first used by intravenous injection in 1958. Benzodiazepines were introduced for SE in 1965, and the therapy of SE remained mainly unchanged for more than 40 years until the recent introduction of intravenous levetiracetam (LEV), intravenous valproate, and intravenous lacosamide.[21]

Despite the high levels of morbidity and mortality associated with human SE (HSE), there is a relative paucity of prospective, controlled research to determine the optimum treatment regimens for people. To date, 4 prospective, randomized, double-masked studies have been performed for first-line therapy for HSE. The most notable findings are:

- Intravenous lorazepam is superior to intravenous diazepam for first-line treatment.[22]
- Intravenous lorazepam is superior to intravenous phenytoin alone and is comparable to intravenous phenobarbital treatment and combination intravenous diazepam with intravenous phenytoin treatment.[23]
- Intramuscular midazolam is equivalent to intravenous lorazepam in prehospital treatment by paramedics.[24]

The most current published guidelines for HSE by a panel of experts[5] indicate

- **First-line (initial emergent) therapy for HSE**. When available, intravenous therapy is preferred with intravenous lorazepam. When intravenous access is not available, midazolam is the preferred intramuscular agent (and can also be given nasally or buccally), and diazepam is the preferred drug for rectal administration.
- **Urgent control**. Additional antiepileptic drug (AED) treatment should be given following benzodiazepines unless the immediate cause of HSE is known and corrected. The goal is rapid attainment of therapeutic levels of an AED and continued dosing for maintenance therapy.
- **Second-line therapy for HSE for patients who continue to have motor or EEG seizures**. The preferred agents include intravenous fosphenytoin/phenytoin, intravenous valproate sodium, intravenous phenobarbital, intravenous LEV, or CRI of midazolam. Of these agents, fosphenytoin may be preferred for most patients, with the exception of patients, particularly children, with a history of primary generalized epilepsy, in whom valproate would be the best choice.
- **Third-line therapy for (human) RSE (induction of general anesthesia)**. AEDs most often recommended for use as a continuous infusion are midazolam,

propofol, and pentobarbital; in some countries, thiopental is also used. At present, there are insufficient data to suggest whether midazolam, propofol, or pentobarbital is the preferred agent. Alternatives for RSE include inhalant anesthesia, corticosteroids, ketamine, hypothermia, and neuromodulation.[5]

Canine SE

Although there are some recommended guidelines for the emergency treatment of seizures for companion animals, only 1 prospective controlled study in dogs evaluating the efficacy of AEDs for SE has been published to date.[25] Current treatment recommendations for seizure emergencies in dogs and cats are based on clinical experience and the results of human or rodent studies. One published algorithm[26] recommends diazepam as first-line therapy followed by phenobarbital as second-line therapy. Additional recommended medications are diazepam or midazolam CRI, and/or general anesthesia with pentobarbital, propofol, thiopental (if available), or inhalant anesthesia.[2] Other treatment options include mannitol for elevated intracranial pressure, and ketamine has been used in some refractory cases.[27] In addition to in-hospital therapy, at-home therapy with rectal (1.0–2.0 mg/kg, 2.0 mg/kg if on phenobarbital)[28] and intranasal administration of diazepam (0.5 mg/kg) have also been recommended. The pharmacokinetics of intranasal midazolam (0.2–0.5 mg/kg) and intranasal lorazepam (0.2 mg/kg) have also been studied in dogs. It should be noted that lorazepam per rectum may not be useful AED therapy because of rapid conversion to inactive metabolites and first pass hepatic metabolism,[29] and that there is erratic systemic availability of midazolam when given per rectum.[30]

General Standard of Practice for Companion Animal SE (Box 2)

There has not yet been an expert panel consensus statement for the treatment of companion animal SE. There does seem, however, to be fairly similar recommendations from a number of sources[11,26,31] that can be generally summarized as

First-line therapy should be with a benzodiazepine, which is most often is intravenous diazepam, but can be by other routes and/or with midazolam, or lorazepam. There have not been any published studies comparing the benzodiazepines to each other in dogs or cats as there has been for people. Shortly after the benzodiazepine, there should be intravenous loading or mini loading doses of intravenous phenobarbital or intravenous LEV to start chronic therapy, for when the short acting benzodiazepines wear off.

In second-line therapy for continuing seizure activity, intravenous phenobarbital or intravenous LEV or a CRI of diazepam or midazolam should be given. The author has found that 2 or more of these second-line therapies can potentially be given to the same patient.

Third-line therapy of RSE to induce general anesthesia can be with intravenous propofol or pentobarbital. In some instances, IV ketamine or inhalant anesthesia has been administered.

Feline SE

Most of the data and studies for SE in companion animals have been performed in dogs. The same general recommendations, with some exceptions (**Box 2**), are generally valid for cats at this time, but more retrospective analysis and prospective studies are needed in cats to be able to confidently make specific recommendations for treating feline SE.

Box 2
Generally recommended doses and staged plan for parenteral AED therapy for canine SE

First-line (initial emergent) therapy[a]

Diazepam 0.5–2.0 mg/kg intravenously up to 3 times,[11] intranasally,[32] per rectum[28]

or

Midazolam 0.06–0.3 mg/kg intravenously, intramuscularly,[33] 0.2 mg/kg intranasally[34] not per rectum

or

Lorazepam 0.2 mg/kg intravenously,[29] intranasally[35] not per rectum

Second-line therapy

Phenobarbital 2–6 mg/kg intravenously,[33] every 20 to 30 minutes to effect; maximum dose 24 mg/kg[33]

or

Diazepam CRI 0.1–0.5 mg/kg/h, 0.5–2.0 mg/kg/h.[33] Use with caution, as diazepam can crystallize in solution and adsorb to polyvinyl chloride tubing, or midazolam 0.1–0.2 mg/kg/h

or

LEV 30–60 mg/kg intravenously in dogs,[25] 20 mg/kg intravenously in cats[36]

Third-line therapy for RSE by induction of general anesthesia.

Propofol 1–4 mg/kg intravenous bolus slowly to effect[33]

   0.1–0.6 mg/kg/h CRI[37,38]

or

Pentobarbital 3–15 mg/kg intravenously to effect[33]

   0.5–4 mg/kg/h CRI[37]

Other anesthetic therapies

Isoflurane 1%–2% minimum alveolar concentration[31]

or

Ketamine 2–8 mg/kg intravenous bolus[27]

Other drugs with very little published data to date

Bromide 3% sodium bromide 800 mg/kg/24 h intravenous loading[39] (not cats)

Fosphenytoin 15 mg/kg phenytoin equivalent (PE) intravenously, dog[40]

LEV 60 mg/kg subcutaneously at home, dog[2,41]

Lacosamide 3 mg/kg/15 min[39] intravenous loading dose, dog only

   [a] Be sure to load or miniload with a long-term chronic AED soon after initial therapy.
   Data from Refs.[2,11,27–29,31–37,39–41]

Recent Prospective Studies of SE in Dogs

Levetiracetam

LEV was approved in the United States in 1998 for the oral treatment of partial-onset seizures in adult people. An intravenous formulation was approved in 2006 for use as bridge therapy in people.[25] Since that time, there have been increasing reports of the off-label use of LEV in people for the treatment of seizure emergencies with variable response rates. In adults, success rates for the treatment of HSE have ranged from 44% to 71% with LEV with few reported adverse effects.[42–45] A wide safety margin and minimal drug-drug interactions have led to LEV use in children, the elderly, and critically ill patients with SE. The author's group completed a randomized controlled trial of LEV for SE and CS for dogs in 2012 indicating that 30 to 60 mg/kg LEV intravenously for second-line therapy may be safe and effective.[25]

Fosphenytoin

Fosphenytoin is the most often-used second-line agent in people. The author's group has published that intravenous fosphenytoin at 15/mg/kg intravenous PE at a rate of 50 mg/min PE infusion is generally well tolerated in normal dogs, with minor vomiting in some dogs.[40] The author and colleagues have just completed a randomized clinical trial of diazepam and placebo versus diazepam and 15 mg/kg PE of fosphenytoin for canine SE in 31 cases.[46] The results of this study are in preparation for article submission, and the author expects they should be published in the coming year. Based on the full results of this study and possibly other future studies, fosphenytoin might be a possible additional nonanesthetizing choice for second-line therapy of SE for dogs.

CS Recommendations

Because of the lack of consistent definitions of CS for companion animals, and lack of published information, there are not clear-cut recommendations that can be unequivocally made for monitoring and treatment of CS. In the author's experience, dogs or cats with 2 or more generalized seizures with recovery between within a 12- to 24-hour period should at a minimum be monitored carefully, and can be given per rectum or intranasal diazepam at home by the owner to try to prevent the need for hospitalization. If benzodiazepines are ineffective at home, and/or the seizures continue, then in-hospital monitoring and possible treatment as for SE are recommended. It has been advocated by a number of specialists to give an extra dose or doses of chronic therapy drugs such as phenobarbital, zonisamide, or levetiracetam at home when the patient is awake enough to swallow safely, in order to break cluster seizures. There are not any published studies of this strategy in dogs, although reasonable additional doses of chronic AEDs are unlikely to cause significant harm, and future studies of pulse therapy in dogs are indicated to determine if this practice is truly helpful for cluster seizures prior to possible hospitalization.

Open Question—Single-Agent Versus Combined Therapy for Initial Treatment of SE?

It has been suggested by some that first-line therapy be with 2 nonanesthetizing drugs immediately rather than benzodiazepines first and then second-line therapy. Synergy between LEV and diazepam has been shown in both rodent models of SE, and in a clinical population of human patients with acute repetitive or prolonged seizures. In rats with electrical stimulation-induced SE, the combination of LEV and diazepam as first-line therapy was superior to either drug alone, even when plasma concentrations were well below the therapeutic range of either drug alone.[47] Two reasons for possibly utilizing intravenous LEV combined with benzodiazepines as first-line therapy are the high safety profile of LEV and favorable pharmacokinetics. Compared with all other AEDs, LEV has the widest safety margin of an AED.[48] Doses as high as 1200 mg/kg/d by mouth have been shown to cause only mild adverse effects in long-term oral dosing studies in dogs.[49] Future controlled prospective trials are needed to determine whether early combination therapy might be more effective and still safe compared with benzodiazepine therapy only.

FUTURE POSSIBILITIES

In the last 10 years there have been evolving potential therapies for SE beyond the benzodiazepines, which open the hope for new treatments, and if successful would be paradigm shifts; these include but are not limited to neurosteroids,[50] gene therapy, optogenetics (light control of neurons through light-sensitive proteins), use of antagomirs (inhibitors of micro RNAs that affect gene expression),[21] and new biochemical targets such as adenosine.[51]

FINAL SUMMARY

SE in companion animals is an emergency and should be quickly treated by recommended first-line (emergent) therapy with benzodiazepines followed by loading doses of chronic therapy drugs, and then second-line, and third-line (refractory) therapy when needed. CS can evolve into SE, and therefore at-home treatment with per rectum or intranasal benzodiazepines and longer-acting oral AEDs for dogs is often recommended, and if not effective, then hospitalization for observation and treatment as for SE are recommended.

REFERENCES

1. Mariani CL. Terminology and classification of seizures and epilepsy in veterinary patients. Top Companion Anim Med 2013;28:34–41.
2. Hardy BT. Injectable levetiracetam use in the dog [MS thesis]. University of Minnesota Graduate School. 2012. Available at: http://conservancy.umn.edu/bitstream/122959/1/Hardy_Brian_March2012.pdf. Accessed December 1, 2013.
3. Proposal for revised clinical and electroencephalographic classification of epileptic seizures. From the Commission on Classification and Terminology of the International League against epilepsy. Epilepsia 1998;22:489–501.
4. Berg AT, Berkovic SF, Brodie MJ, et al. Revised terminology and concepts for organization of seizures and epilepsies: report of the ILAE commission on classification and terminology, 2005-2009. Epilepsia 2010;51:676–85.
5. Brophy GM, Bell R, Classen J, et al. Guidelines for the evaluation and management of status epilepticus. Neurocrit Care 2012;17:3–23.
6. Raith K, Steinberg T, Fischer A. Continuous electroencephalographic monitoring of status epilepticus in dogs and cats: 10 patients (2004-2005). J Vet Emerg Crit Care (San Antonio) 2010;20(4):446–55.
7. Bleck TP. Management approaches to prolonged seizures and status epilepticus. Epilepsia 1999;40:s59–63.
8. Lowenstein DH, Bleck T, MacDonald RL. It's time to revise the definition of status epilepticus. Epilepsia 1999;40(1):120–2.
9. Beran RG. An alternative perspective on the management of status epilepticus. Epilepsy Behav 2008;12(3):349–53.
10. Gilad RN, Izkovitz N, Dabby R, et al. Treatment of status epilepticus and acute repetitive seizures with i.v. valproic acid vs phenytoin. Acta Neurol Scand 2008;118(5):296–300.
11. Thomas W. Idiopathic epilepsy in dogs and cats. Vet Clin North Am Small Anim Pract 2010;40(1):161–79.
12. Shorvon S, Ferlisi M. The outcome of therapies in refractory and super-refractory convulsive status epilepticus and recommendations for therapy. Brain 2012; 135:2314–28.

13. Huff JS, Fountain NB. Pathophysiology and definitions of seizures and status epilepticus. Emerg Med Clin North Am 2011;29(1):1–13.
14. Bateman SW, Parent JM. Clinical findings, treatment, and outcome of dogs with status epilepticus or cluster seizures: 156 cases (1990-1995). J Am Vet Med Assoc 1998;215(10):1463–8.
15. Saito M, Muñana KR, Sharp NJ, et al. Risk factors for development of status epilepticus in dogs with idiopathic epilepsy and effects of status epilepticus on outcome and survival time: 32 cases (1990-1996). J Am Vet Med Assoc 2001;219(5):618–23.
16. Monteiro R, Adams V, Keys D, et al. Canine idiopathic epilepsy: prevalence, risk factors and outcome associated with cluster seizures and status epilepticus. J Small Anim Pract 2012;53(9):526–30.
17. Zimmermann R, Hulsmeyer VI, Sauter-Louis C, et al. Status epilepticus and epileptic seizures in dogs. J Vet Intern Med 2009;23(5):970–6.
18. DeLorenzo RJ, Hauser WA, Towne AR, et al. A prospective, population-based epidemiologic study of status epilepticus in Richmond, Virginia. Neurology 1996;46(4):1029–35.
19. Fountain NB. Status epilepticus: risk factors and complications. Epilepsia 2000; 41(Suppl 2):S23–30.
20. Chin RF, Neville BG, Scott RC. A systematic review of the epidemiology of status epilepticus. Eur J Neurol 2004;11(12):800–10.
21. Shorvon S. The historical evolution of, and the paradigms shifts in, the therapy of convulsive status epilepticus over the past 150 years. Epilepsia 2013; 54(Suppl 6):64–7.
22. Leppik IE, Derivan AT, Homan RW, et al. Double-blind study of lorazepam and diazepam in status epilepticus. JAMA 1983;249(11):1452–4.
23. Treimam DM, Meyer PD, Walton NY, et al. A comparison of four treatments for generalized convulsive status epilepticus. Veterans Affairs Status Epilepticus Cooperative Study Group. N Engl J Med 1998;339(12):792–8.
24. Silbergleit R, Durkalski V, Lowenstein D, et al. Intramuscular versus intravenous therapy for pre-hospital status epilepticus. N Engl J Med 2012;366(7):591–600.
25. Hardy BT, Patterson EE, Cloyd JM, et al. Double-masked, placebo-controlled study of intravenous levetiracetam for the treatment of status epilepticus and acute repetitive seizures in dogs. J Vet Intern Med 2012;26:334–40.
26. Podell M. Antiepileptic drug therapy. Clin Tech Small Anim Pract 1998;13(3): 185–92.
27. Serrano SD, Hughes D, Chandler K. Use of ketamine for the management of refractory status epilepticus in a dog. J Vet Intern Med 2006;20(1):194–7.
28. Podell M. The use of diazepam per rectum at home for the acute management of cluster seizures in dogs. J Vet Intern Med 1995;9(2):68–74.
29. Podell M, Wagner SO, Sams RA. Lorazepam concentrations in plasma following its intra- venous and rectal administration in dogs. J Vet Pharmacol Ther 1998; 21:158–60.
30. Schwartz M, Muñana KR, Nettifee-Osborne JA, et al. The pharmacokinetics of midazolam after intravenous, intramuscular, and rectal administration in healthy dogs. J Vet Pharmacol Ther 2013;36(5):471–7.
31. Platt S, Garosis L. Small animal neurological emergencies. London: Manson Publishing; 2012. p. 425–6 Google eBook.
32. Platt SR, Randell SC, Scott KC, et al. Comparison of plasma benzodiazepine concentrations following intranasal and intravenous administration of diazepam to dogs. Am J Vet Res 2000;61(6):651–4.

33. Platt SR. Status epilepticus: life after diazepam. Proceedings 26th Annual ACVIM Forum. San Antonio (TX), June 4–7, 2008.
34. Eagleson JS, Platt SR, Elder Strong DL, et al. Bioavailability of a novel midazolam gel after intranasal administration in dogs. Am J Vet Res 2012;73:539–45.
35. Mariani CL, Clemmons RM, Lee-Ambrose L, et al. A comparison of intranasal and intravenous lorazepam in normal dogs [abstract]. J Vet Intern Med 2003; 17:402.
36. Carnes MB, Axlund TW, Boothe DM. Pharmacokinetics of levetiracetam after oral and intravenous administration of a single dose to clinically normal cat. Am J Vet Res 2011;72(9):1247–52.
37. Dewey CW. Anticonvulsant therapy in dogs and cats. Vet Clin Small Anim 2006; 36:1107–27.
38. Steffen F, Grasmueck S. Propofol for treatment of refractory seizures in dogs and a cat with intracranial disorders. J Small Anim Pract 2000;41(11):496–9.
39. Podell M. Antiepileptic drug therapy and monitoring. Top Companion Anim Med 2013;28:59–66.
40. Leppik IE, Patterson EE, Coles LD, et al. Canine status epilepticus: a translational platform for human therapeutic trials. Epilepsia 2011;52(Suppl 8):31–4.
41. Hardy BT, Patterson EE, Cloyd JM. Subcutaneous administration of levetiracetam in healthy dogs [abstract]. J Vet Intern Med 2011;25:635.
42. Eue S, Grumbt M, Müller M, et al. Two years of experience in the treatment of status epilepticus with intravenous levetiracetam. Epilepsy Behav 2009;15(4): 467–9.
43. Gamez-Leyva G, Aristin JL, Fernadez E, et al. Experience with intravenous levetiracetam in status epilepticus: a retrospective case series. CNS Drugs 2009;23(11):983–7.
44. Moddel G, Bunten S, Dobis C, et al. Intravenous levetiracetam: a new treatment alternative for refractory status epilepticus. J Neurol Neurosurg Psychiatry 2009; 80(6):689–92.
45. Alvarez V, Januel JM, Burnand B, et al. Second-line status epilepticus treatment: comparison of phenytoin, valproate, and levetiracetam. Epilepsia 2011;52(7): 1292–6.
46. Patterson E, Coles L, Cloyd J, et al. The canine translational platform; proof of concept study of fosphenytoin for status epilepticus in canine clinical patients. Presented at the American Epilepsy Society Annual Meeting. Washington, DC, December 6–10, 2013.
47. Mazarati AM, Baldwin R, Klitgaard H, et al. Anticonvulsant effects of levetiracetam and levetiracetam-diazepam combinations in experimental status epilepticus. Epilepsy Res 2004;58(2–3):167–74.
48. Patterson EE, Goel V, Cloyd JC, et al. Intramuscular, intravenous and oral levetiracetam in dogs: safety and pharmacokinetics. J Vet Pharmacol Ther 2008; 31(3):253–8.
49. Available at: http://www.accessdata.fda.gov/drugsatfda_docs/nda/99/21035_ Keppra_pharmr_P2.pdf. Accessed December 1, 2013.
50. Rogowksi M, Loya CM, Reddy K, et al. Neuroactive steroids for the treatment of status epilepticus. Epilepsia 2013;54(Suppl 6):93–8.
51. Bolson D. Role of adenosine in status epilepticus: a potential new target? Epilepsia 2013;54(Suppl 6):20–2.

Aging in the Canine and Feline Brain

Charles H. Vite, DVM, PhDª, Elizabeth Head, MA, PhDᵇ,*

KEYWORDS

- β-Amyloid • Cat • Dog • Cognitive dysfunction • Neuron loss • Tau

KEY POINTS

- Brain atrophy, neuron loss, decreased neurogenesis, and oxidative stress but few tau-associated disorders are observed in aging dog brains.
- Cerebrovascular pathology can be extensive in canine brain aging.
- β-Amyloid protein, associated with Alzheimer disease in humans, is increased with age in the dog brain and is linked to signs of learning and memory impairments.
- Lysosomal storage diseases in dogs are associated with similar types of neuropathology as are observed with aging and Alzheimer disease.
- Few studies describe the neurobiology of aging in cats but interesting similarities and differences from dogs have been reported.
- Feline Niemann-Pick type C disease has several neuropathologic and clinical similarities to Alzheimer disease.

INTRODUCTION

This article reviews canine and feline brain aging. Several key features are discussed and compared, including general aging characteristics and neuropathology. Aging dogs and cats show many similarities in terms of brain changes but also some important differences. Several research groups have been working with aging dogs and cats to test various theories of aging and to develop therapeutics that will be beneficial to both species.

Research reported in this publication was supported by the National Institute on Aging of the National Institutes of Health under award number R01AG031764 (E. Head) and R01NS073661 and P40-02512 (C.H. Vite, Mark Haskins), and the Ara Parseghian Medical Research Foundation (C.H. Vite). The content is solely the responsibility of the authors and does not necessarily represent the official views of the National Institutes of Health.

ª Department of Clinical Studies, School of Veterinary Medicine, University of Pennsylvania, Section of Neurology & Neurosurgery, Department of Clinical Studies - Philadelphia, 3900 Delancey Street, Philadelphia, PA 19104, USA; ᵇ Department of Pharmacology & Nutritional Sciences, Sanders-Brown Center on Aging, University of Kentucky, 800 South Limestone Street, 203 Sanders Brown Building, Lexington, KY 40515, USA
* Corresponding author.
E-mail address: elizabeth.head@uky.edu

Vet Clin Small Anim 44 (2014) 1113–1129
http://dx.doi.org/10.1016/j.cvsm.2014.07.008   **vetsmall.theclinics.com**
0195-5616/14/$ – see front matter © 2014 Elsevier Inc. All rights reserved.

The median life span of dogs varies as a function of breed, with larger breeds typically having shorter life spans than smaller breeds.[1–3] For the purposes of this article, several studies that are described have been collected in purpose-bred beagles and additional companion animals and clinical data are shared when available. Beagles have a median life span of 13.9 years, with no significant differences between males and females.[4] A young beagle less than 5 years old is similar to humans who are less than 40 years old.[3] Middle-aged beagles between 5 and 9 years are similar to humans between 40 and 60 years and beagles more than 9 years old are similar to humans more than 60 years old. However, the larger the breed of dog, the shorter the life span and thus biological age may vary across breeds given a specific age.[1]

In a laboratory setting and in the veterinary clinic, studies of aging dogs report that some but not all aged dogs are impaired on different measures of learning and memory (see Refs.[5–7]). Not all old dogs are impaired and not all types of learning and memory are equally affected. Neurobiological changes, as described later, can account for some, but not all, of the clinical signs of cognitive decline in aging dogs.

NEUROBIOLOGY OF AGING IN THE DOG

This article describes several neurobiological changes associated with aging in dogs (**Table 1**).

Brain Atrophy

Old dogs often show marked ventriculomegaly at postmortem examination associated with thinning of the cerebral cortex and the subcortical white matter.[8] Magnetic resonance imaging (MRI) studies performed on aged beagle and German shepherd

Table 1
Comparison of dog and cat neurologic neurodegenerative features

Neurobiological Outcome Measures	Canine	Feline	NCL or MPSI	NPC Disease
Brain atrophy	Yes	NA	Yes	Yes
β-Amyloid	Yes	Yes	Yes	Yes
Tau	Yes	Yes	NA	Yes
Cerebral amyloid angiopathy	Yes	Yes	NA	NA
Infarcts	Yes	NA	NA	NA
Vascular disease	Yes	NA	Yes	NA
Lipofuscin accumulation	Yes	Yes	Yes	NA
Caspase activation	Yes	NA	Yes	Yes
DNA fragmentation	Yes	NA	NA	NA
Neuron loss: hippocampus	Yes	NA	Yes	Yes
Neuron loss: caudate	NA	Yes	Yes	Yes
Neuron loss: locus coeruleus	Yes	Yes	NA	NA
Neuron loss: Purkinje cerebellar cells	Yes	NA	Yes	Yes
White matter degeneration	Yes	NA	Yes	Yes
Inflammation	Yes	NA	Yes	Yes
Oxidative damage	Yes	NA	Yes	Yes
Gliosis	Yes	NA	Yes	Yes

Abbreviations: MPSI, mucopolysaccharidosis type I; NA, not available; NCL, neuronal ceroid lipofuscinoses; NPC, Niemann-Pick type C.

dogs show that cortical atrophy, identified as widened sulci, thinned parenchyma,[9] and ventricular dilatation,[9–11] progresses with age and is a consistent feature of canine brain aging. Furthermore, MRI studies suggest differential vulnerabilities of specific brain areas to aging. For example, in aging beagle dogs, the prefrontal cortex loses tissue volume at an earlier age (approximately 8–11 years) than does the hippocampus (after 11 years).[12] An MRI study by Hasegawa and colleagues[13] (2005) suggested that although interthalamic adhesion thickness was smaller in older dogs, those showing age-related cognitive decline and a single dog with GM1 gangliosidosis also had a significant decrease in the thickness.

Periventricular white matter signal abnormalities are frequently seen in MRI of various dog breeds greater than 12 years of age that are evaluated for seizures, vestibular disease, or behavioral abnormalities. These bilaterally symmetric T2-weighted hyperintensities of the internal capsule are suspected to be caused by wallerian degeneration, demyelination, and accompanying gliosis.[14]

Selective Neuron Loss

Atrophy may result from neuron loss or changes in neuronal density, as reported in normal human brain aging,[15,16] although more extensive neuronal loss occurs in Alzheimer disease (AD).[17,18] When neurons were counted using unbiased stereological methods within individual subfields of the hippocampus of young (3.4–4.5 years) and old (13.0–15.0 years) dogs, the aged dogs had significantly ($\sim$30%) fewer neurons in the hilus of the dentate gyrus.[19] A study by Pugliese and colleagues[20] (2007) showed that cognitive deficits correlated with loss of Purkinje cells in the cerebellum. More recently, a study by Insua and colleagues[21] (2010) examined noradrenergic neurons in the locus coeruleus of aged canines, a group of neurons that are implicated in AD in humans.[22,23] Dogs that are cognitively impaired show a significant reduction in noradrenergic neurons. Reduced neurogenesis in the mature brain may also contribute to reduced neuron numbers and age-associated cognitive decline, resulting in slower replacement of dying neurons. In the hippocampus of beagles, a 90% to 95% decline in neurogenesis was measured in aged dogs.[24] Similar reductions in neurogenesis in aged dogs have been reported by other investigators.[25]

Senile Plaques (β-Amyloid) in Dogs

A key feature of canine brain aging was the observation in 1956, by Braumühl, who reported Alzheimer-like senile plaques in aged dogs (reviewed in Ref.[26]). Senile plaque accumulation in the aged canine brain has been well described.[26] Senile plaques are composed of β-amyloid (Aβ) protein, and are one of 2 key types of neurologic pathologies observed in the AD brain.[27] The Aβ peptide is produced by the sequential cleavage of the amyloid precursor protein (APP) by beta-secretase and gamma-secretase.[28,29] Cleavage by gamma-secretase results in differing lengths of Aβ, with the 42 amino acid form, $A\beta_{1-42}$ making up most of the insoluble deposits found in the AD brain.[30] One of the reasons why the canine brain has been examined extensively for Aβ neurologic disorder is that dogs and humans share an identical amino acid sequence of the protein.[31,32] Aβ is thought to be a causative factor for AD in people.[33] The observation of brain Aβ first stimulated interest in the use of the dog to model human aging and disease.[34] Diffuse plaques are the predominant subtype of Aβ in the aging dog brain (**Fig. 1**).[35–40] Specific brain regions are differentially vulnerable to Aβ.[36,41–46] When cortical regions are sampled for Aβ deposition, each region shows a different age of Aβ onset.[43] In the dog, Aβ deposition occurs earliest in the prefrontal cortex (see **Fig. 1**C, D) and later in the temporal cortex, hippocampus (see **Fig. 1**A, B), and occipital cortex.[45]

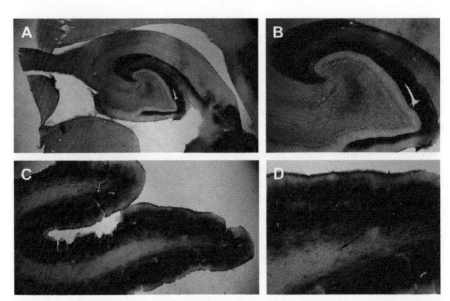

Fig. 1. Aβ immunostaining (brown) in the brain of a 14-year-old border collie (Martha) with signs of cognitive dysfunction syndrome. Aβ was detected using the 6E10 antibody that binds Aβ 1 to 16. (A) Low-power magnification (1.5×) of extensive Aβ deposition in the hippocampus. (B) Aβ is primarily found in the outer molecular layer of the dentate gyrus, which contains neuron terminals originating from the entorhinal cortex (4×). (C) The prefrontal cortex also shows extensive Aβ deposition that appears most dense in layers II and V of the cortex and is less apparent in the white matter (1.5×). (D) At high magnification (4×), the differential deposition of Aβ in the 6 cortical layers can be seen as well as extensive white matter cerebral amyloid angiopathy (arrow). Sections have been counterstained with cresyl violet (blue).

Beagles that show learning and memory impairments in a laboratory setting with systematic cognitive tests also show higher levels of Aβ plaques than those old dogs without cognitive impairments.[47–50] For example, dogs with prefrontal cortex–dependent reversal learning deficits show significantly higher amounts of Aβ in this brain region.[48,49] As in laboratory beagles, the extent of Aβ plaques varies as a function of age in companion dogs (including a wide variety of breeds and mixed breeds).[50–52] Further, the extent of Aβ plaques correlates with behavior changes and this association remains significant even if age is removed as a covariate.[47,50] Case report 1 and **Figs. 1** and **2** show a case study of cognitive decline and age-associated Aβ neurologic disorder in a border collie.

The focus in AD pathogenesis has recently shifted from Aβ plaques to considering smaller, soluble forms of Aβ assemblies called Aβ oligomers. Oligomers are highly toxic and impair synaptic function.[53] Furthermore, increased oligomer levels are strongly associated with cognitive dysfunction.[53–55] A recent study by Pop and colleagues,[56] examined the accumulation of oligomeric Aβ in the temporal lobe of canines. This study provided evidence that canines, like humans, experience an increase in toxic oligomers with age.

Vascular Disorders, Cerebrovascular Amyloid Angiopathy

Cerebrovascular amyloid angiopathy (CAA) is the deposition of Aβ in association with the cerebrovasculature (see **Fig. 1**D). In dogs with CAA, the blood vessels of the brain

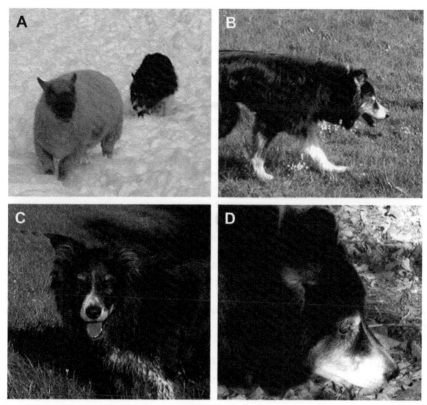

Fig. 2. Aging and canine cognitive dysfunction in a border collie (Martha). (*A*) Martha competing in sheep dog trials when she was young, and (*B*) still active around the age of 10 years. As she reached 11 years of age she struggled to complete commands issued by her owner (*C*). At 14 years of age, Martha was generally in good health except for arthritis but would not make eye contact with her owner (*D*).

typically contain the shorter, 40 amino acid–long species of Aβ.[57–59] The occipital cortex seems to be particularly vulnerable to CAA in the aged dog brain. Vascular Aβ may compromise the blood-brain barrier, disrupt vessel wall viability,[60] and cause microhemorrhages.[61]

Aged dogs may also show lacunar infarcts of the caudate nucleus and thalamus with most dogs showing no causative metabolic, endocrine, or hypertensive disease.[62,63] In a longitudinal study, these lesions were shown to increase in number with advancing age.[64] Lacunar infarcts of the caudate nucleus have been induced experimentally in beagle dogs by proximal middle cerebral artery occlusion.[65] The cause of naturally occurring lacunar infarcts in dogs remains unidentified.

Tau Neuropathology

Unlike humans but like many other animal species, canines do not develop full-blown neurofibrillary tangles,[32,37,39,40] which is the second neuropathologic characteristic of AD. However, aged dogs show the accumulation of several phosphorylated tau epitopes that are consistent with AD in humans and observations in aged cats (described later).[66] In a study of cognitively impaired pet dogs that included a variety of breeds, intracellular phosphorylated tau was observed that was similar to the AD brain.[67]

Oxidative Damage and Mitochondrial Dysfunction

Aging and the production of free radicals can lead to oxidative damage to proteins, lipids, and nucleotides that, in turn, may cause neuronal dysfunction and ultimately neuronal death. In the aging dog, the brain accumulates carbonyl groups, which are a measure of oxidative damage to proteins.[68,69] Carbonyl groups are associated with reduced endogenous antioxidant enzyme activity or protein levels, including those of glutamine synthetase and superoxide dismutase (SOD).[68,70–72] In addition, increased oxidative damage to proteins can be measured by the end products of lipid peroxidation (oxidative damage to lipids), including 4-hydroxynonenal,[50,52,72,73] lipofuscin,[50] lipofuscinlike pigments,[52,73] or malondialdehyde.[68] In addition, oxidative damage to DNA or RNA may be increased in the aged dog brain.[5,50]

Oxidative damage may also be associated with behavioral decline in dogs. Increased oxidative end products in the aged companion dog brain are correlated with more severe behavioral changes.[50,52,69] In laboratory studies of aging beagles, higher protein oxidative damage (3-nitrotyrosine) and lower endogenous antioxidant capacity (SOD and glutathione-S-transferase activities) are associated with poorer prefrontal-dependent and spatial learning.[71] Mitochondria are sources of free radicals that damage proteins, lipids, and DNA/RNA.[74] In a study of aged beagles, isolated mitochondria showed increased reactive oxygen species production in aged animals relative to young animals.[75] Thus, aged dogs show mitochondrial dysfunction and oxidative damage, consistent with humans with age-related neurologic dysfunction.

Correlates of Brain Aging Found in Lysosomal Storage Diseases

Cross-sectional studies of brain aging are negatively influenced by interindividual variations in brain size and structure, as well as by differing rates of atrophy. Longitudinal studies may be limited by repeated access to aged animals and to subject attrition.[64] Insight into mechanisms of brain aging can also be obtained through the study of breeding colonies of dogs with naturally occurring hereditary metabolic disorders, including mitochondrial disorders, lysosomal storage diseases, and leukodystrophies, which have clinical, neuropathologic, and biochemical changes similar to those found in old dogs. These disorders allow both cross-sectional and longitudinal studies of disease progression in related animals with short life spans.[76,77] For example, more than 40 inherited lysosomal storage diseases (LSDs) have been identified, with many characterized by progressive cognitive decline, memory loss, brain atrophy, loss of myelin, and region-specific loss of neurons as are seen in aging.[78,79] Two well-studied diseases are examples of what has been learned by studying affected dogs. The neuronal ceroid lipofuscinoses (NCLs) are characterized by seizures, motor dysfunction, impaired vision, progressive cognitive decline, impaired memory, behavioral problems, brain degeneration, selective neuronal loss that is most severe in the cerebral cortex, white matter atrophy, neuronal accumulation of protein and lipid, and premature death.[80,81] Both human patients and affected dogs show various ages of onset, disease course, and neuropathology.[80–82] The juvenile-onset form of the disease, known as Batten disease, has naturally occurring analogous disease in English setters, Tibetan terriers, and border collies.[83] Biochemical analysis of the brain shows that storage of subunit c of the mitochondrial ATP synthase complex occurs; subunit c is an essential membrane component of the proton channel of the ATP synthase complex, which generates ATP by oxidative phosphorylation.[81] Although not fully characterized, the neuronal loss seen in Batten disease is postulated to be caused by mitochondrial dysfunction and energy-linked excitotoxicity.[83] Synaptic loss and glial activation also occur in this disease, although the mechanism and contribution of these abnormalities to disease progression are not yet understood.[80]

The T-maze reversal learning task has been used to evaluate progressive cognitive decline in the dachshund model of late-infantile NCL, which is caused by a mutation in the gene encoding the enzyme tripeptidyl-peptidase 1 (TTP1).[84] This model system is particularly interesting because intrathecal administration of TTP1 results in decreased lysosomal storage.[85] It is likely that a better understanding of how mitochondrial dysfunction and neuronal loss develop in the NCLs, as well as how they may be reversed with therapy, will shed light on similar mechanisms postulated to occur in brain aging.

Mucopolysaccharidosis type I (MPSI; Hurler syndrome) is another LSD characterized by progressive cognitive decline, including impaired memory and intelligence, in human patients.[86] Affected humans and dogs show progressive cortical atrophy, ventricular enlargement, and white matter loss.[87] Cardiovascular disease and accumulation of intracellular $A\beta$ are also described in affected patients.[88,89] In human patients with MPSI, MRI showed that corpus callosum volume and fractional anisotropy correlated with neuropsychological testing.[86] In dogs with MPSI, imaging studies showed corpus callosum volumes to be smaller in affected dogs compared with unaffected dogs; no cognitive studies have yet been performed. Similar to the late-infantile NCL, this disease is amenable to either whole-brain therapy by intrathecal enzyme replacement therapy or to regional gene therapy allowing for the assessment of therapeutic effect.[90,91] When treated with intrathecal alpha-iduronidase, the enzyme that is deficient in MPSI, corpus callosum volumes in affected dogs were no longer distinguishable from those in unaffected dogs. These studies indicate the usefulness of quantitative imaging to study brain atrophy over time as well as the effectiveness of therapy in ameliorating the atrophy.

NEUROBIOLOGY OF AGING IN THE CAT

Cats are considered to be old, or senior, starting around the age of 7 to 10 years but consistently after 12 years, depending on the individual animal. Aging cats show several behavioral changes that can be of concern to a pet owner and that are not related to systemic illness or disease.[92] Whether there is cognitive decline in aging cats as observed in dogs is still being studied but there are behavioral changes that have been reported clinically.[93] There are fewer studies of the aging cat brain compared with aging dogs in the literature, highlighting the significant gaps in knowledge regarding feline brain aging. Several reviews have been written describing feline age-associated neurologic disorder and some of those observations are summarized here.[92,93]

Neuron Loss and Atrophy

There are several studies suggesting that the caudate nucleus of aging cats is affected by aging, including reduced neuronal numbers and reduction in the density of synapses.[94–97] These losses may lead to impairments in motor function.[94] The locus coeruleus, a key nucleus responsible for producing the neurotransmitter acetylcholine, which is associated with learning and memory, also shows neuronal losses with age in cats.[98]

$A\beta$

$A\beta$ is typically observed in cats more than the age of 10 years,[99–103] although there is a report of 7.5-year-old animal showing $A\beta$ disorder.[102] Feline $A\beta$ deposition seems to be different from that of dogs and humans in several respects. Unlike human and dog brain, plaques in the cat brain are primarily made up of $A\beta1$-42 without $A\beta1$-40 and the peptide is not posttranslationally modified (suggesting a more rapid turnover) in cats compared with dogs and humans.[66,99] Further, truncated Aβ (AβpN3) was absent in aged cat brain.[104] Blood vessels in aging cat brains are positive for Aβ1-40, the shorter more soluble form of Aβ.[66] To our knowledge, there are few reports of the link between behavioral dysfunction and the extent of Aβ disorder as reported in dogs. Although cats that show signs of behavioral dysfunction tend to also have Aβ plaques,[100] the severity of behavioral changes does not seem to correlate well with the extent of Aβ disorder.[66]

Tau Phosphorylation

An interesting feature of the aging cat brain is the detection of phosphorylated tau protein, which is consistent with reports in human AD.[105,106] Cats show multiple isoforms of tau protein, as do humans.[107] Not all studies consistently observe tau neuropathology in cats[101,108,109] and this may be because of methodological challenges. In addition, when using sensitive immunohistochemical methods, phosphorylated tau is not as frequently observed as Aβ plaques, but the epitopes on tau that are phosphorylated overlap with those observed in dogs and humans.[66] The morphology of neurons that show an accumulation of intracellular phosphorylated tau suggests a sprouting response, which is also similar to human brain.[66] Tau phosphorylation is also more frequently associated with the presence of seizures in aging cats.[100]

Neuronal Loss in Feline Niemann-Pick Type C Disease and Similarities to AD

Niemann-Pick type C (NPC) disease is another example of how LSDs may contribute to the understanding of neuronal loss, oxidative stress, Aβ deposition, and tau neuropathology in the aging brain. NPC disease is caused by dysfunction of either of 2 proteins, NPC1 or NPC2, which result in lysosomal storage of cholesterol and glycosphingolipids.[110] How dysfunction of these proteins results in the dementia and neuronal loss associated with disease has been difficult to determine. A feline model of NPC1 disease exists and has been critical for understanding disease pathogenesis and evaluating therapy.[110–115] As disease-modifying therapies are evaluated, clinicians hope to gain insight into the relative contributions of each of the following factors in causing cognitive decline and brain atrophy.

Autophagy, the degradation or recycling of damaged intracellular organelles and aggregated-proteins, is necessary for cellular homeostasis. NPC1 has been implicated in mediating membrane-tethering events between autophagosomes and late endosomes that subsequently fuse with lysosomes to degrade their contents.[116] When NPC1 is defective, autophagy is impaired. Because impaired basal autophagy has been found to cause neurodegeneration,[117,118] it is postulated that impaired autophagy in NPC1 disease may contribute to the observed neuronal loss as a consequence of the buildup of dysfunctional mitochondria and the accumulation of misfolded proteins, resulting in cell death. Altered autophagosomal-lysosomal function has similarly been implicated in brain aging.[119,120]

Oxidative stress and the generation of reactive oxygen species have also been proposed as contributing factors for neuronal loss in NPC disease.[121] In vitro studies showed increased oxidative stress in cultured neurons and fibroblasts.[122] Evaluation of serum from patients with NPC showed decreased fractions of reduced coenzyme Q10 and decreased Trolox-equivalent antioxidant capacity.[121] Evaluation of plasma and cerebrospinal fluid from patients and affected cats showed accumulation of cholesterol oxidation products, and, in cats, these oxysterols decreased in response to a disease-modifying therapy.[122]

In addition, both NPC1 disease and AD are marked by dementia and abnormal cholesterol metabolism; however, they also share abnormalities in Aβ processing and the presence of neurofibrillary tangles.[110,123] First, in both affected humans and cats, relative Aβ peptide distributions differ from those found in unaffected individuals, with lower relative levels of Aβ1-37, Aβ1-38 and Aβ1-39 in cats with NPC1 compared with controls.[124] Second, neurofibrillary tangles composed of paired helical filaments of phosphorylated microtubular protein accumulate in NPC disease as they do in AD.[110] Third, apolipoprotein E4, the isoform associated with increased risk for developing AD, has also been found to be associated with early onset of disease and with increased NPC1 disease severity.[123] Other deficits seen in NPC1 disease, including peroxisomal dysfunction,[125] abnormal sphingosine metabolism,[126] neuroinflammation,[127] and induction of apoptosis,[128] may also contribute to changes seen in the aging brain.[129]

CLINICAL IMPLICATIONS OF BRAIN AGING IN DOGS AND CATS

Laboratory-based studies of cognition in beagles suggest that there are age-dependent functional changes related to brain disorders. In the clinic, owners of

---

Case report 1

Martha was a female border collie that was a very competent farm dog with what her owner called "lots of sheep savvy." She was also a fully integrated family member and companion to the family when hiking, skiing, and mountain biking. In addition, she successfully competed in sheep dog trials till the age of 10 years (see **Fig. 2A**). She and her handler worked their way through the succession of novice-level trials, winning several, and ultimately competing and placing in the highest level, the Open class, which attests to her skill (see **Fig. 2B**).

By the time Martha was 11 years old she was nearly deaf and slow enough that she could no longer trial. She started to show some confusion with commands at which she was expert. For example, one day her owner took her out in the field and gave her a command to go counter clockwise around the sheep and she went clockwise. Further, when her owner next said "OK, go clockwise" she reversed her direction, when she should have continued the clockwise direction (see **Fig. 2C**). The next time her owner was working with her, a normally benign ewe turned around to face Martha and stomped her foot. Martha, who would normally have politely stood her ground until the sheep backed down, promptly turned away and left the field. The owner at this time thought, "Well that is proof that Martha is fully retired now." Not long after the incident with the ewe, the sheep began to act as if Martha did not even exist.

Over the next 2 years, changes in Martha were subtle and included increasing hearing loss and stubbornness. She also stopped having interest in the sheep, and appeared most fixated with another dog (Ida) in the family. Several behaviors with the other dog appeared abnormal. For example, Martha would stare at Ida, the middle dog, whether they were inside or out walking, and then would stalk Ida, despite a lack of interest from Ida in interacting. The owners had to intervene frequently to prevent a snarling episode, although the two dogs never injured each other.

To her last day, Martha's social skills with human friends persisted. However, she began pacing, panting, and getting stuck under the bedside table at night. During the day when only 1 of the owners was home, Martha was frequently anxious and sometimes clingy, which never used to be the case. She showed signs of disorientation and during walks occasionally lost the younger dogs and her owner although the same daily route was followed. Martha was once found in a road looking up and down as if lost, although she had been walking that direction for years.

Throughout her life Martha had a great appetite and generally excellent health, although she had arthritis in almost every joint in her body and was on high doses of incontinence medication and Rimadyl (a nonsteroidal antiinflammatory drug) for arthritis. For the last year of her life, the owner was unable to get a photograph of Martha looking at her because she was no longer making eye contact (see **Fig. 2D**).

When Martha was 14 years old, the decision was made to euthanize her and the owner donated her brain to the University of Kentucky to determine whether neurologic disorder was present. Aβ neurologic disorder was extensive in Martha (see **Fig. 1**).

geriatric dogs frequently report behavioral changes.[130–132] Some of these behavioral changes may be linked to systemic illness or other health issues (including sensory decline). When ruled out, a subset of older dogs shows evidence of behavioral changes that are now considered to be signs of canine cognitive dysfunction (CCD). The original reports of CCD were by Ruehl and colleagues[133] in the mid 1990s and several reports followed, along with the development of new tools to detect CCD in pet dogs.[6,7,93,134,135] CCD has been linked to brain pathology in pet dogs.[20,136,137] There are reports that CCD can be reduced in aging dogs through treatment with various pharmaceuticals (eg, Anipryl),[134] by dietary intervention using a prescription diet (B/D diet Hills Pet Nutrition[134]; the same diet used in laboratory studies showing a benefit to cognition and neuropathology[138]), and to immunotherapy using anti-Aβ approaches.[139] In cats, there is less evidence of a form of feline cognitive dysfunction syndrome but evidence is accumulating that a similar phenomenon can occur.[66,92,93,100,140]

SUMMARY

Aging dogs and cats show features of brain disorders that can be similar to human aging and AD. Neuropathologic changes with age may be linked to signs of cognitive dysfunction both in the laboratory and in a clinic setting. Less is known about cat brain aging and cognition and this represents an area for further study. Neurodegenerative diseases such as LSDs in dogs and cats also show similar features of aging, suggesting some common underlying pathogenic mechanisms and also suggesting pathways that can be modified to promote healthy brain aging.

ACKNOWLEDGMENTS

The authors are grateful to Virginia Price, DVM, and her stories of Martha and donation of her tissue for research. We thank Judianne Davis-Van Nostrand and Dr William Van Nostrand at Stony Brook University in New York for help with collecting tissue for the study. Ms Katie McCarty collected the Aβ immunostaining data for Martha.

REFERENCES

1. Greer KA, Canterberry SC, Murphy KE. Statistical analysis regarding the effects of height and weight on life span of the domestic dog. Res Vet Sci 2007;82(2): 208–14.
2. Galis F, Van der Sluijs I, Van Dooren TJ, et al. Do large dogs die young? J Exp Zool B Mol Dev Evol 2007;308(2):119–26.
3. Patronek GJ, Waters DJ, Glickman LT. Comparative longevity of pet dogs and humans: implications for gerontology research. J Gerontol A Biol Sci Med Sci 1997;52(3):B171–8.
4. Lowseth LA, Gillett NA, Gerlach RF, et al. The effects of aging on hematology and serum chemistry values in the beagle dog. Vet Clin Pathol 1990;19(1):13–9.
5. Cotman CW, Head E. The canine (dog) model of human aging and disease: dietary, environmental and immunotherapy approaches. J Alzheimers Dis 2008; 15(4):685–707.
6. Landsberg G, Araujo JA. Behavior problems in geriatric pets. Vet Clin North Am Small Anim Pract 2005;35(3):675–98.
7. Landsberg G, Ruehl W. Geriatric behavioral problems. Vet Clin North Am Small Anim Pract 1997;27(6):1537–59.

8. Vandevelde M, Higgins RJ, Oevermann A. Veterinary neuropathology: essentials of theory and practice. West Sussex (United Kingdom): Wiley-Blackwell; 2012.

9. Su MY, Head E, Brooks WM, et al. MR imaging of anatomic and vascular characteristics in a canine model of human aging. Neurobiol Aging 1998;19(5): 479–85.

10. Kimotsuki T, Nagaoka T, Yasuda M, et al. Changes of magnetic resonance imaging on the brain in beagle dogs with aging. J Vet Med Sci 2005;67(10):961–7.

11. Gonzalez-Soriano J, Marin Garcia P, Contreras-Rodriguez J, et al. Age-related changes in the ventricular system of the dog brain. Ann Anat 2001;183(3): 283–91.

12. Tapp PD, Siwak CT, Gao FQ, et al. Frontal lobe volume, function, and beta-amyloid pathology in a canine model of aging. J Neurosci 2004;24(38):8205–13.

13. Hasegawa D, Yayoshi N, Fujita Y, et al. Measurement of interthalamic adhesion thickness as a criteria for brain atrophy in dogs with and without cognitive dysfunction (dementia). Vet Radiol Ultrasound 2005;46(6):452–7.

14. Grossman RI, Yousem DM. Neuroradiology: the requisites. Philadelphia: Mosby; 2003.

15. Simic G, Kostovic I, Winblad B, et al. Volume and number of neurons of the human hippocampal formation in normal aging and Alzheimer's disease. J Comp Neurol 1997;379(4):482–94.

16. West MJ. Regionally specific loss of neurons in the aging human hippocampus. Neurobiol Aging 1993;14:287–93.

17. West MJ, Kawas CH, Martin LJ, et al. The CA1 region of the human hippocampus is a hot spot in Alzheimer's disease. Ann N Y Acad Sci 2000;908: 255–9.

18. Bobinski M, Wegiel J, Tarnawski M, et al. Relationships between regional neuronal loss and neurofibrillary changes in the hippocampal formation and duration and severity of Alzheimer disease. J Neuropathol Exp Neurol 1997; 56(4):414–20.

19. Siwak-Tapp CT, Head E, Muggenburg BA, et al. Region specific neuron loss in the aged canine hippocampus is reduced by enrichment. Neurobiol Aging 2008;29(1):39–50.

20. Pugliese M, Gangitano C, Ceccariglia S, et al. Canine cognitive dysfunction and the cerebellum: acetylcholinesterase reduction, neuronal and glial changes. Brain Res 2007;1139:85–94.

21. Insua D, Suarez ML, Santamarina G, et al. Dogs with canine counterpart of Alzheimer's disease lose noradrenergic neurons. Neurobiol Aging 2008;31(4): 625–35.

22. Dringenberg HC. Alzheimer's disease: more than a 'cholinergic disorder' - evidence that cholinergic-monoaminergic interactions contribute to EEG slowing and dementia. Behav Brain Res 2000;115(2):235–49.

23. Grudzien A, Shaw P, Weintraub S, et al. Locus coeruleus neurofibrillary degeneration in aging, mild cognitive impairment and early Alzheimer's disease. Neurobiol Aging 2007;28(3):327–35.

24. Siwak-Tapp CT, Head E, Muggenburg BA, et al. Neurogenesis decreases with age in the canine hippocampus and correlates with cognitive function. Neurobiol Learn Mem 2007;88(2):249–59.

25. Pekcec A, Baumgartner W, Bankstahl JP, et al. Effect of aging on neurogenesis in the canine brain. Aging Cell 2008;7(3):368–74.

26. Cummings BJ, Head E, Ruehl W, et al. The canine as an animal model of human aging and dementia. Neurobiol Aging 1996;17(2):259–68.

27. Mirra SS, Heyman A, McKeel D, et al. The Consortium to Establish a Registry for Alzheimer's Disease (CERAD). Part II. Standardization of the neuropathologic assessment of Alzheimer's disease. Neurology 1991;41(4):479–86.
28. Murphy MP, LeVine H 3rd. Alzheimer's disease and the amyloid-beta peptide. J Alzheimers Dis 2010;19(1):311–23.
29. Selkoe DJ. Amyloid beta-protein and the genetics of Alzheimer's disease. J Biol Chem 1996;271:18295–8.
30. Selkoe DJ. Alzheimer's disease: genes, proteins, and therapy. Physiol Rev 2001; 81(2):741–66.
31. Johnstone EM, Chaney MO, Norris FH, et al. Conservation of the sequence of the Alzheimer's disease amyloid peptide in dog, polar bear and five other mammals by cross-species polymerase chain reaction analysis. Brain Res Mol Brain Res 1991;10(4):299–305.
32. Selkoe DJ, Bell DS, Podlisny MB, et al. Conservation of brain amyloid proteins in aged mammals and humans with Alzheimer's disease. Science 1987;235(4791): 873–7.
33. Hardy J. Alzheimer's disease: the amyloid cascade hypothesis: an update and reappraisal. J Alzheimers Dis 2006;9(3 Suppl):151–3.
34. Wisniewski HM, Wegiel J, Morys J, et al. Aged dogs: an animal model to study beta-protein amyloidogenesis. In: Maurer K, Riederer P, Beckman H, editors. Alzheimer's disease. Epidemiology, neuropathology, neurochemistry and clinics. New York: Springer-Verlag; 1990. p. 151–67.
35. Cummings BJ, Su JH, Cotman CW, et al. Beta-amyloid accumulation in aged canine brain: a model of early plaque formation in Alzheimer's disease. Neurobiol Aging 1993;14(6):547–60.
36. Giaccone G, Verga L, Finazzi M, et al. Cerebral preamyloid deposits and congophilic angiopathy in aged dogs. Neurosci Lett 1990;114:178–83.
37. Morys J, Narkiewicz O, Maciejewska B, et al. Amyloid deposits and loss of neurones in the claustrum of the aged dog. Neuroreport 1994;5(14):1825–8.
38. Okuda R, Uchida K, Tateyama S, et al. The distribution of amyloid beta precursor protein in canine brain. Acta Neuropathol 1994;87:161–7.
39. Russell MJ, White R, Patel E, et al. Familial influence on plaque formation in the beagle brain. Neuroreport 1992;3(12):1093–6.
40. Uchida K, Tani Y, Uetsuka K, et al. Immunohistochemical studies on canine cerebral amyloid angiopathy and senile plaques. J Vet Med Sci 1992;54(4):659–67.
41. Braak H, Braak E. Neuropathological stageing of Alzheimer-related changes. Acta Neuropathol 1991;82(4):239–59.
42. Braak H, Braak E, Bohl J. Staging of Alzheimer-related cortical destruction. Eur Neurol 1993;33:403–8.
43. Head E, McCleary R, Hahn FF, et al. Region-specific age at onset of beta-amyloid in dogs. Neurobiol Aging 2000;21(1):89–96.
44. Ishihara T, Gondo T, Takahashi M, et al. Immunohistochemical and immunoe-lectron microscopical characterization of cerebrovascular and senile plaque amyloid in aged dogs' brains. Brain Res 1991;548:196–205.
45. Thal DR, Rub U, Orantes M, et al. Phases of A beta-deposition in the human brain and its relevance for the development of AD. Neurology 2002;58(12):1791–800.
46. Wisniewski HM, Johnson AB, Raine CS, et al. Senile plaques and cerebral amyloidosis in aged dogs. Lab Invest 1970;23:287–96.
47. Colle MA, Hauw JJ, Crespeau F, et al. Vascular and parenchymal Ab deposition in the aging dog: correlation with behavior. Neurobiol Aging 2000;21: 695–704.

48. Cummings BJ, Head E, Afagh AJ, et al. Beta-amyloid accumulation correlates with cognitive dysfunction in the aged canine. Neurobiol Learn Mem 1996; 66(1):11–23.
49. Head E, Callahan H, Muggenburg BA, et al. Visual-discrimination learning ability and beta-amyloid accumulation in the dog. Neurobiol Aging 1998;19(5):415–25.
50. Rofina JE, van Ederen AM, Toussaint MJ, et al. Cognitive disturbances in old dogs suffering from the canine counterpart of Alzheimer's disease. Brain Res 2006;1069(1):216–26.
51. Rofina J, van Andel I, van Ederen AM, et al. Canine counterpart of senile dementia of the Alzheimer type: amyloid plaques near capillaries but lack of spatial relationship with activated microglia and macrophages. Amyloid 2003;10(2):86–96.
52. Rofina JE, Singh K, Skoumalova-Vesela A, et al. Histochemical accumulation of oxidative damage products is associated with Alzheimer-like pathology in the canine. Amyloid 2004;11(2):90–100.
53. Selkoe DJ. Soluble oligomers of the amyloid beta-protein impair synaptic plasticity and behavior. Behav Brain Res 2008;192(1):106–13.
54. Tomic JL, Pensalfini A, Head E, et al. Soluble fibrillar oligomer levels are elevated in Alzheimer's disease brain and correlate with cognitive dysfunction. Neurobiol Dis 2009;35(3):352–8.
55. Lacor PN, Buniel MC, Chang L, et al. Synaptic targeting by Alzheimer's-related amyloid beta oligomers. J Neurosci 2004;24(45):10191–200.
56. Pop V, Head E, Berchtold NC, et al. Aβ aggregation profiles and shifts in APP processing favor amyloidogenesis in canines. Neurobiol Aging 2012;33(1): 108–20.
57. Attems J. Sporadic cerebral amyloid angiopathy: pathology, clinical implications, and possible pathomechanisms. Acta Neuropathol 2005;110(4):345–59.
58. Attems J, Jellinger KA, Lintner F. Alzheimer's disease pathology influences severity and topographical distribution of cerebral amyloid angiopathy. Acta Neuropathol 2005;110(3):222–31.
59. Herzig MC, Van Nostrand WE, Jucker M. Mechanism of cerebral beta-amyloid angiopathy: murine and cellular models. Brain Pathol 2006;16(1):40–54.
60. Prior R, D'Urso D, Frank R, et al. Loss of vessel wall viability in cerebral amyloid angiopathy. Neuroreport 1996;7:562–4.
61. Uchida K, Nakayama H, Goto N. Pathological studies on cerebral amyloid angiopathy, senile plaques and amyloid deposition in visceral organs in aged dogs. J Vet Med Sci 1991;53(6):1037–42.
62. Garosi L, McConnell JF, Platt SR, et al. Clinical and topographic magnetic resonance characteristics of suspected brain infarction in 40 dogs. J Vet Intern Med 2006;20(2):311–21.
63. Goncalves R, Carrera I, Garosi L, et al. Clinical and topographic magnetic resonance imaging characteristics of suspected thalamic infarcts in 16 dogs. Vet J 2011;188(1):39–43.
64. Su MY, Tapp PD, Vu L, et al. A longitudinal study of brain morphometrics using serial magnetic resonance imaging analysis in a canine model of aging. Prog Neuropsychopharmacol Biol Psychiatry 2005;29(3):389–97.
65. Liu S, Hu WX, Zu QQ, et al. A novel embolic stroke model resembling lacunar infarction following proximal middle cerebral artery occlusion in beagle dogs. J Neurosci Methods 2012;209(1):90–6.
66. Head E, Moffat K, Das P, et al. Beta-amyloid deposition and tau phosphorylation in clinically characterized aged cats. Neurobiol Aging 2005;26(5): 749–63.

67. Yu CH, Song GS, Yhee JY, et al. Histopathological and immunohistochemical comparison of the brain of human patients with Alzheimer's disease and the brain of aged dogs with cognitive dysfunction. J Comp Pathol 2011;145(1):45–58.

68. Head E, Liu J, Hagen TM, et al. Oxidative damage increases with age in a canine model of human brain aging. J Neurochem 2002;82:375–81.

69. Skoumalova A, Rofina J, Schwippelova Z, et al. The role of free radicals in canine counterpart of senile dementia of the Alzheimer type. Exp Gerontol 2003;38:711–9.

70. Kiatipattanasakul W, Nakamura S, Kuroki K, et al. Immunohistochemical detection of anti-oxidative stress enzymes in the dog brain. Neuropathology 1997;17:307–12.

71. Opii WO, Joshi G, Head E, et al. Proteomic identification of brain proteins in the canine model of human aging following a long-term treatment with antioxidants and a program of behavioral enrichment: relevance to Alzheimer's disease. Neurobiol Aging 2008;29(1):51–70.

72. Hwang IK, Yoon YS, Yoo KY, et al. Differences in lipid peroxidation and Cu,Zn-superoxide dismutase in the hippocampal CA1 region between adult and aged dogs. J Vet Med Sci 2008;70(3):273–7.

73. Papaioannou N, Tooten PC, van Ederen AM, et al. Immunohistochemical investigation of the brain of aged dogs. I. Detection of neurofibrillary tangles and of 4-hydroxynonenal protein, an oxidative damage product, in senile plaques. Amyloid 2001;8:11–21.

74. Shigenaga MK, Hagen TM, Ames BN. Oxidative damage and mitochondrial decay in aging. Proc Natl Acad Sci U S A 1994;91:10771–8.

75. Head E, Nukala VN, Fenoglio KA, et al. Effects of age, dietary, and behavioral enrichment on brain mitochondria in a canine model of human aging. Exp Neurol 2009;220(1):171–6.

76. Kuruppu DK, Matthews BR. Young-onset dementia. Semin Neurol 2013;33(4):365–85.

77. Swain GP, Prociuk M, Bagel JH, et al. Adeno-associated virus serotypes 9 and rh10 mediate strong neuronal transduction of the dog brain. Gene Ther 2014;21(1):28–36.

78. Ellinwood NM, Vite CH, Haskins ME. Gene therapy for lysosomal storage diseases: the lessons and promise of animal models. J Gene Med 2004;6(5):481–506.

79. Raz N, Rodrigue KM, Haacke EM. Brain aging and its modifiers: insights from in vivo neuromorphometry and susceptibility weighted imaging. Ann N Y Acad Sci 2007;1097:84–93.

80. Dolisca SB, Mehta M, Pearce DA, et al. Batten disease: clinical aspects, molecular mechanisms, translational science, and future directions. J Child Neurol 2013;28(9):1074–100.

81. Hofmann SL, Peltonen L. The Neuronal Ceroid Lipofuscinoses. In: Valle D, Beaudet AL, Vogelstein B, et al, editors. OMMBID - The Online Metabolic and Molecular Bases of Inherited Diseases. New York, NY: McGraw-Hill; 2014. http://ommbid.mhmedical.com/content.aspx?bookid=474&Sectionid=45374157. Accessed August 20, 2014.

82. Jolly RD. Comparative biology of the neuronal ceroid-lipofuscinoses (NCL): an overview. Am J Med Genet 1995;57(2):307–11.

83. Jolly RD, Brown S, Das AM, et al. Mitochondrial dysfunction in the neuronal ceroid-lipofuscinoses (Batten disease). Neurochem Int 2002;40(6):565–71.

84. Sanders DN, Kanazono S, Wininger FA, et al. A reversal learning task detects cognitive deficits in a Dachshund model of late-infantile neuronal ceroid lipofuscinosis. Genes Brain Behav 2011;10(7):798–804.

85. Vuillemenot BR, Katz ML, Coates JR, et al. Intrathecal tripeptidyl-peptidase 1 reduces lysosomal storage in a canine model of late infantile neuronal ceroid lipofuscinosis. Mol Genet Metab 2011;104(3):325–37.

86. Shapiro E, Guler OE, Rudser K, et al. An exploratory study of brain function and structure in mucopolysaccharidosis type I: long term observations following hematopoietic cell transplantation (HCT). Mol Genet Metab 2012;107(1–2): 116–21.

87. Vite CH, Nestrasil I, Mlikotic A, et al. Features of brain MRI in dogs with treated and untreated mucopolysaccharidosis type I. Comp Med 2013;63(2):163–73.

88. Pelissier C, Roudier M, Boller F. Factorial validation of the severe impairment battery for patients with Alzheimer's disease. A pilot study. Dement Geriatr Cogn Disord 2002;13(2):95–100.

89. Ferris S, Karantzoulis S, Somogyi M, et al. Rivastigmine in moderately severe-to-severe Alzheimer's disease: severe impairment battery factor analysis. Alzheimers Res Ther 2013;5(6):63.

90. Dierenfeld AD, McEntee MF, Vogler CA, et al. Replacing the enzyme alpha-L-iduronidase at birth ameliorates symptoms in the brain and periphery of dogs with mucopolysaccharidosis type I. Sci Transl Med 2010;2(60):60ra89.

91. Chen A, Vogler C, McEntee M, et al. Glycosaminoglycan storage in neuroanatomical regions of mucopolysaccharidosis I dogs following intrathecal recombinant human iduronidase. APMIS 2011;119(8):513–21.

92. Gunn-Moore D, Moffat K, Christie LA, et al. Cognitive dysfunction and the neurobiology of ageing in cats. J Small Anim Pract 2007;48(10):546–53.

93. Landsberg GM, Denenberg S, Araujo JA. Cognitive dysfunction in cats: a syndrome we used to dismiss as 'old age'. J Feline Med Surg 2010;12(11):837–48.

94. Levine MS, Lloyd RL, Fisher RS, et al. Sensory, motor and cognitive alterations in aged cats. Neurobiol Aging 1987;8:253–63.

95. Levine MS, Adinolfi AM, Fisher RS, et al. Quantitative morphology of medium-sized caudate spiny neurons in aged cats. Neurobiol Aging 1986;7(4):277–86.

96. Levine MS, Adinolfi AM, Fisher RS, et al. Ultrastructural alterations in caudate nucleus in aged cats. Brain Res 1988;440(2):267–79.

97. Levine MS. Neurophysiological and morphological alterations in caudate neurons in aged cats. Ann N Y Acad Sci 1988;515:314–28.

98. Zhang JH, Sampogna S, Morales FR, et al. Age-related changes in cholinergic neurons in the laterodorsal and the pedunculo-pontine tegmental nuclei of cats: a combined light and electron microscopic study. Brain Res 2005;1052(1): 47–55.

99. Cummings BJ, Satou T, Head E, et al. Diffuse plaques contain C-terminal A beta 42 and not A beta 40: evidence from cats and dogs. Neurobiol Aging 1996; 17(4):653–9.

100. Gunn-Moore DA, McVee J, Bradshaw JM, et al. Ageing changes in cat brains demonstrated by beta-amyloid and AT8-immunoreactive phosphorylated tau deposits. J Feline Med Surg 2006;8(4):234–42.

101. Nakamura S, Nakayama H, Kiatipattanasakul W, et al. Senile plaques in very aged cats. Acta Neuropathol 1996;91:437–9.

102. Brellou G, Vlemmas I, Lekkas S, et al. Immunohistochemical investigation of amyloid beta-protein (Abeta) in the brain of aged cats. Histol Histopathol 2005;20(3):725–31.

103. Takeuchi Y, Uetsuka K, Murayama M, et al. Complementary distributions of amyloid-beta and neprilysin in the brains of dogs and cats. Vet Pathol 2008; 45(4):455–66.

104. Chambers JK, Mutsuga M, Uchida K, et al. Characterization of AbetapN3 deposition in the brains of dogs of various ages and other animal species. Amyloid 2011;18(2):63–71.
105. Goedert M, Jakes R, Crowther RA, et al. The abnormal phosphorylation of tau protein at Ser-202 in Alzheimer disease recapitulates phosphorylation during development. Proc Natl Acad Sci U S A 1993;90:5066–70.
106. Braak H, Braak E. Staging of Alzheimer's disease-related neurofibrillary changes. Neurobiol Aging 1995;16(3):271–84.
107. Janke C, Beck M, Stahl T, et al. Phylogenetic diversity of the expression of the microtubule-associated protein tau: implications for neurodegenerative disorders. Brain Res Mol Brain Res 1999;68:119–28.
108. Braak H, Braak E, Strothjohann M. Abnormally phosphorylated tau protein related to the formation of neurofibrillary tangles and neuropil threads in the cerebral cortex of sheep and goat. Neurosci Lett 1994;171:1–4.
109. Kuroki K, Uchida K, Kiatipattanasakul W, et al. Immunohistochemical detection of tau proteins in various non-human animal brains. Neuropathology 1997;17:174–80.
110. Walkley SU, Suzuki K. Consequences of NPC1 and NPC2 loss of function in mammalian neurons. Biochim Biophys Acta 2004;1685(1–3):48–62.
111. March PA, Thrall MA, Brown DE, et al. GABAergic neuroaxonal dystrophy and other cytopathological alterations in feline Niemann-Pick disease type C. Acta Neuropathol 1997;94(2):164–72.
112. Zervas M, Somers KL, Thrall MA, et al. Critical role for glycosphingolipids in Niemann-Pick disease type C. Curr Biol 2001;11(16):1283–7.
113. Somers KL, Brown DE, Fulton R, et al. Effects of dietary cholesterol restriction in a feline model of Niemann-Pick type C disease. J Inherit Metab Dis 2001;24(4):427–36.
114. Ward S, O'Donnell P, Fernandez S, et al. 2-Hydroxypropyl-beta-cyclodextrin raises hearing threshold in normal cats and in cats with Niemann-Pick type C disease. Pediatr Res 2010;68(1):52–6.
115. Ferris S, Cummings J, Christensen D, et al. Effects of donepezil 23 mg on severe impairment battery domains in patients with moderate to severe Alzheimer's disease: evaluating the impact of baseline severity. Alzheimers Res Ther 2013;5(1):12.
116. Sarkar S, Carroll B, Buganim Y, et al. Impaired autophagy in the lipid-storage disorder Niemann-pick type C1 disease. Cell Rep 2013;5(5):1302–15.
117. Hara T, Nakamura K, Matsui M, et al. Suppression of basal autophagy in neural cells causes neurodegenerative disease in mice. Nature 2006;441(7095):885–9.
118. Keller JN, Dimayuga E, Chen Q, et al. Autophagy, proteasomes, lipofuscin, and oxidative stress in the aging brain. Int J Biochem Cell Biol 2004;36(12):2376–91.
119. Komatsu M, Waguri S, Chiba T, et al. Loss of autophagy in the central nervous system causes neurodegeneration in mice. Nature 2006;441(7095):880–4.
120. Kiselyov K, Jennigs JJ Jr, Rbaibi Y, et al. Autophagy, mitochondria and cell death in lysosomal storage diseases. Autophagy 2007;3(3):259–62.
121. Fu R, Yanjanin NM, Bianconi S, et al. Oxidative stress in Niemann-Pick disease, type C. Mol Genet Metab 2010;101(2–3):214–8.
122. Porter FD, Scherrer DE, Lanier MH, et al. Cholesterol oxidation products are sensitive and specific blood-based biomarkers for Niemann-Pick C1 disease. Sci Transl Med 2010;2(56):56ra81.
123. Fu R, Yanjanin NM, Elrick MJ, et al. Apolipoprotein E genotype and neurological disease onset in Niemann-Pick disease, type C1. Am J Med Genet A 2012;158A(11):2775–80.

124. Mattsson N, Olsson M, Gustavsson MK, et al. Amyloid-beta metabolism in Niemann-Pick C disease models and patients. Metab Brain Dis 2012;27(4):573–85.
125. Schedin S, Sindelar PJ, Pentchev P, et al. Peroxisomal impairment in Niemann-Pick type C disease. J Biol Chem 1997;272(10):6245–51.
126. Lloyd-Evans E, Morgan AJ, He X, et al. Niemann-Pick disease type C1 is a sphingosine storage disease that causes deregulation of lysosomal calcium. Nat Med 2008;14(11):1247–55.
127. Baudry M, Yao Y, Simmons D, et al. Postnatal development of inflammation in a murine model of Niemann-Pick type C disease: immunohistochemical observations of microglia and astroglia. Exp Neurol 2003;184(2):887–903.
128. Wu YP, Mizukami H, Matsuda J, et al. Apoptosis accompanied by up-regulation of TNF-alpha death pathway genes in the brain of Niemann-Pick type C disease. Mol Genet Metab 2005;84(1):9–17.
129. van Echten-Deckert G, Walter J. Sphingolipids: critical players in Alzheimer's disease. Prog Lipid Res 2012;51(4):378–93.
130. Houpt KA, Beaver B. Behavioral problems of geriatric dogs and cats. Vet Clin North Am Small Anim Pract 1981;11(4):643–52.
131. Mosier JE. Effect of aging on body systems of the dog. Vet Clin North Am Small Anim Pract 1989;19(1):1–12.
132. Chapman BL, Voith VL. Behavioral problems in old dogs: 26 cases (1984-1987). J Am Vet Med Assoc 1990;196(6):944–6.
133. Ruehl WW, Bruyette DS, DePaoli A, et al. Canine cognitive dysfunction as a model for human age-related cognitive decline, dementia and Alzheimer's disease: clinical presentation, cognitive testing, pathology and response to 1-deprenyl therapy. Prog Brain Res 1995;106:217–25.
134. Landsberg GM, Nichol J, Araujo JA. Cognitive dysfunction syndrome: a disease of canine and feline brain aging. Vet Clin North Am Small Anim Pract 2012;42(4): 749–68, vii.
135. Bosch MN, Pugliese M, Gimeno-Bayon J, et al. Dogs with cognitive dysfunction syndrome: a natural model of Alzheimer's disease. Curr Alzheimer Res 2012; 9(3):298–314.
136. Pugliese M, Geloso MC, Carrasco JL, et al. Canine cognitive deficit correlates with diffuse plaque maturation and S100beta (-) astrocytosis but not with insulin cerebrospinal fluid level. Acta Neuropathol 2006;111(6):519–28.
137. Pugliese M, Mascort J, Mahy N, et al. Diffuse beta-amyloid plaques and hyperphosphorylated tau are unrelated processes in aged dogs with behavioral deficits. Acta Neuropathol 2006;112(2):175–83.
138. Head E, Cotman CW, Zicker SC, et al. The use of dietary antioxidants and mitochondrial co-factors to promote successful aging. Curr Top Nutraceutical Res 2005;3(2):85–94.
139. Bosch MN, Gimeno-Bayon J, Rodriguez MJ, et al. Rapid improvement of canine cognitive dysfunction with immunotherapy designed for Alzheimer's disease. Curr Alzheimer Res 2013;10(5):482–93.
140. Gunn-Moore DA. Cognitive dysfunction in cats: clinical assessment and management. Top Companion Anim Med 2011;26(1):17–24.

Acute Spinal Cord Injury

Tetraplegia and Paraplegia in Small Animals

Nicolas Granger, DVM, PhD, MRCVS*, Darren Carwardine, BVSc

KEYWORDS

- Spinal cord injury • Tetraplegia • Paraplegia • Cellular therapy

KEY POINTS

- Basic neurologic principles, such as the concept of upper motor neuron versus lower motor neuron, are essential in correctly assessing animals following spinal cord injury (SCI).
- Autonomic dysfunction occurs concomitantly with tetraplegia and paraplegia and leads to urinary incontinence and respiratory dysfunction, which are critical in treatment planning for animals with SCI.
- Current evaluation of SCI relies heavily on imaging (by magnetic resonance imaging [MRI]), but new functional tests such as clinical scoring and kinematic analysis are becoming more widely applied.
- Standard of care for animals with acute SCI consists of medical stabilization in the emergency phase of the disease and, where appropriate, surgical decompression, as neuroprotective drugs have not yet reached the clinic.
- Prognosis following severe SCI is best predicted clinically by the presence or absence of pain sensation at the time of injury, but other markers (such as MRI characteristics of the lesion and biomarkers in the cerebrospinal fluid) might help to refine this prognosis.

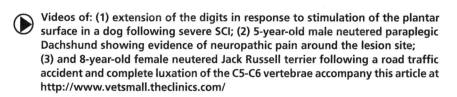

Videos of: (1) extension of the digits in response to stimulation of the plantar surface in a dog following severe SCI; (2) 5-year-old male neutered paraplegic Dachshund showing evidence of neuropathic pain around the lesion site; (3) and 8-year-old female neutered Jack Russell terrier following a road traffic accident and complete luxation of the C5-C6 vertebrae accompany this article at http://www.vetsmall.theclinics.com/

Spinal cord injury (SCI) in animals has been recognized and treated for decades,[1] providing basic knowledge and understanding of the disease, from its pathophysiology to its current management.[2–6] SCI is a common problem in animals (mainly

The School of Veterinary Sciences, University of Bristol, Langford House, Langford, North Somerset BS40 5HU, UK
* Corresponding author.
E-mail address: nicolas.granger@bristol.ac.uk

Vet Clin Small Anim 44 (2014) 1131–1156
http://dx.doi.org/10.1016/j.cvsm.2014.07.013   **vetsmall.theclinics.com**

because of the prevalence of acute disc herniation in dogs[7]) for which treatment aimed at repairing parenchymal lesions is lacking, and information gained from its study has benefit for both companion animals and humans in developing new therapeutic approaches.[8–11] There is a plethora of publications and recent reviews on specific individual aspects of SCI in dogs and cats (including lesion localization,[12] advanced imaging,[13] pathogenesis,[6] traumatic causes of SCI,[3] intervertebral disc herniation [IVDH],[2] and fibrocartilaginous embolic myelopathy[14] causing SCI). The topic seems so vast that it would be almost impossible to summarize it appropriately in a single article. With this in mind, this review provides an overview of the main concepts that are useful for clinicians in assessing companion animals with severe acute SCI. Currently available advanced ancillary tests and those in development are reviewed. In addition, the current standard of care for companion animals following SCI and recent advances in the development of new therapies are presented, and new predictors of recovery discussed.

ETIOLOGY OF SPINAL CORD INJURY

SCI refers to any trauma applied to the spinal cord, although there are numerous possible causes. In dogs, IVDH remains the main cause of SCI (up to 34% in some hospitals[15]), followed by road traffic accidents ($\sim$7% of cases[3,15]). The different types of IVDH (extrusion of the degenerate nucleus or 'type I', protrusion of the degenerating annulus or 'type II', traumatic disc prolapse, or hydrated nucleus pulposus extrusion) have recently been reviewed.[4] However, the proportion of animals presented with the most severe deficits (ie, paraplegia and loss of pain sensation), which constitutes those presenting the greatest clinical problem, is not well defined. In large case series reporting IVDH outcome in dogs (**Table 1**),[16–22] 337 out of 2051 reported cases ($\sim$16%) were presented with the most severe deficits according to a classification by Schulz and colleagues[23]). These data could be an overestimation of the prevalence in the general population because cases with severe signs are more likely to be referred rather than managed in first-opinion practice, or underestimated, because cases with a poor prognosis may be euthanized before referral. Of note, the prevalence in Japan was approximately 25%, which might be a more accurate

Table 1
Prevalence of dogs presented with spinal cord injury classified by clinical grade, as proposed by Schulz and colleagues[23]

Grade 2	Grade 3	Grade 4	Grade 5	Total	Prevalence of grade 5 cases (%)	Reference
108	56	70	25	259	10	Brisson et al,[18] 2004
79	53	54	16	202	8	Brisson et al,[17] 2011
28	12	16	7	63	11	Macias et al,[20] 2002
10	68	167	36	281	13	Necas,[21] 1999
N/A	N/A	N/A	25	250	10	Ruddle et al,[22] 2006
47	32	63	17	165	10	Itoh et al,[19] 2008
274	180	161	211	831	25	Aikawa et al,[16] 2012
		Totals	337	2051	16	

Grade 2: mild ataxia with motor function adequate for weight support; grade 3: severe ataxia with motor function inadequate for weight support; grade 4: no apparent motor function but intact pain response; grade 5: no pain perception.
Abbreviation: N/A, no data available.
Data from Refs.[16–22]

representation of the true prevalence of severe SCI because dogs are rarely euthanized there,[16] although toy breeds form a higher proportion of this population.

In cats, a review of 205 cases with spinal cord disease found that the main cause of acute SCI is external trauma (15 cats, ie, ~7%) followed by IVDH (8 cats, ie, ~4%) and penetrating wounds (5 cats, ie, ~2%).[24] In this case series, clinical signs associated with SCI were not specifically presented but the lesions more commonly affected the thoracic and lumbar spine. Marioni-Henry[5] also summarized findings in 44 cats and found an increased prevalence of IVDH at T12-L1 and L4-L6 disc spaces, which are regions maximally dorsiflexed and ventroflexed, respectively, during the stance phase in this species.[5,25] It is suggested that 6% of cats suffering external trauma have SCI.[5]

CLINICAL EVALUATION OF THE PATIENT FOLLOWING SEVERE SPINAL CORD INJURY

SCI leads to a range of neurologic deficits, and a systematic approach to each case is essential to localize the origin(s) of the clinical signs and appreciate the severity of the injury. Clinically relevant concepts are presented here.

Normal Locomotion

Locomotion is achieved by sensorimotor control of the posture and gait. Limb position is perceived via ascending pathways in the spinal cord that transmit information from the limbs to sensory systems in the brain.[26] The motor response is the result of interaction between supraspinal command centers in the brain with central pattern generators (CPGs) in the spinal cord, via descending motor pathways.[27] In vertebrates, CPGs are neuronal circuits composed of groups of segmentally organized interneurons under the influence of ascending and descending pathways that produce voluntary walking movements.[28] However, when the spinal cord is transected, CPGs are still able to produce rhythmic and sequential activation of flexor and extensor motor neurons to produce walking movements independently from higher centers (ie, involuntary movements). This trait is well known in several species, including dogs, and partly explains "spinal walking" (whereby an animal with a transected spinal cord is able to ambulate on the pelvic limbs).[29] From a clinical standpoint, this observation is important because it demonstrates that severe SCI will produce loss of voluntary movements (because ascending and descending pathways are interrupted) but does not abolish movements controlled by spinal cord neurons below the lesion. Understanding the distinction between voluntary and involuntary movement also helps one to grasp the concept of upper motor neuron (UMN) and lower motor neuron (LMN), discussed later in this article.

Sequential Appearance of Neurologic Deficits After Spinal Cord Damage

Progressively more severe damage to the spinal cord causes neurologic deficits in sequence, mainly based on the diameter of fibers. Large myelinated fibers are more easily damaged than small fibers. Therefore, as injury severity increases: (1) proprioceptive deficits appear first because proprioceptive fibers (such as in the dorsal columns and spinocerebellar tracts located in the periphery of the spinal cord white matter) are large myelinated fibers; (2) loss of voluntary movement, a function controlled by medium-diameter motor fibers, occurs next; (3) loss of autonomic function (urinary and fecal continence) mediated by small myelinated fibers often occurs concomitantly; and (4) complete loss of pain sensation occurs last because fibers that mediate pain sensation are mainly small unmyelinated fibers.

Cervical injuries (C1 to T2 spinal cord segments) can cause partial loss of voluntary motor and sensory function, described as tetraparesis and ataxia of all 4 limbs.

Thoracolumbar injuries (T3 to S3 spinal cord segments) can cause partial loss of voluntary motor and sensory function, described as paraparesis and ataxia of the pelvic limbs. Complete cervical injuries cause tetraplegia, although the lesion is rarely complete because loss of autonomic function (respiration) and pain sensation remains rare in animals (most such affected animals die soon after the injury). Complete thoracolumbar injuries cause paraplegia with or without loss of urinary/fecal continence and pain sensation.

UMN Versus LMN

Clinically it is important to localize the lesion along the spinal cord to 1 of the 4 main regions: C1-C5, C6-T2 (brachial intumescence containing motor neurons to the thoracic limbs), T3-L3, and L4-S3 (lumbar intumescence containing motor neurons to the pelvic limbs) to direct subsequent diagnostics to the correct region. Tetraplegia and paraplegia indicate lesions within the C1-T2 and T3-S3 spinal cord segments, respectively. To further refine the localization of the problem, one needs to use the old but widely used concept of UMN and LMN.

Lesions of the C1-C5 and T3-L3 spinal cord segments spare the motor neurons located in the C6-T2 (ie, brachial) or L4-S3 (ie, lumbar) intumescences. Therefore, spinal reflexes mediated by these motor neurons remain intact and the muscle tone is usually normal to increased. In this instance, tetraplegia and paraplegia associated with preserved spinal reflexes is caused by a UMN lesion. When the lesion affects the C6-T2 (ie, brachial) or L4-S3 (ie, lumbar) intumescences, motor neurons in these regions are damaged, spinal reflexes become reduced or absent, and the muscle tone is often reduced. In this instance, tetraplegia and paraplegia associated with reduced or absent spinal reflexes is caused by an LMN lesion. Recently, a study questioned the utility of the thoracic limb withdrawal (flexor) reflex to distinguish a lesion of the UMN from one of the LMN.[30] In 11 of 35 cases with cervical disc herniation, the thoracic limb withdrawal reflex was considered decreased in association with a spinal cord lesion in the C1-C5 segments.[30] However, depressed flexor reflex in cranial cervical lesions might simply be caused by increased tone associated with a lesion of the UMN.

Multiple spinal cord lesions affecting both LMN and UMN may cause diagnostic difficulties because signs of LMN dysfunction mask signs of UMN dysfunction. The LMN lesion causes paralysis and loss of spinal reflexes, therefore making detection of a UMN lesion challenging. In this situation, the cutaneous trunci muscle reflex (also known as the panniculus reflex) might aid detection of the UMN lesion if a cutoff is observed along the thoracolumbar spine. The cutaneous trunci muscle reflex in normal dogs is present as far caudally as the skin overlying L5 or L6 vertebrae, as recently described in 153 of 155 normal dogs.[31] The recommendation in cases with trauma to the vertebral column is to image the entire spine to search for multiple lesions, all of which might not be clinically detectable. Five percent to 10% of cases with trauma to the vertebral column have multiple fractures or luxations.[32,33]

Spinal Shock and Schiff-Sherrington Syndrome

Sherrington originally reported that immediately after experimental thoracic spinal cord transection in dogs and cats, there is flaccid paralysis and loss of spinal reflexes in the pelvic limbs, although the lesion is created above the lumbar LMN.[34] This phenomenon, known as spinal shock, is also observed in the clinic and was reviewed by Smith and Jeffery.[35] One explanation for spinal shock is the sudden loss of synaptic control from UMN over LMN, leading to hyperpolarization of LMN and a reduction in their excitability.[36] It is long-lasting (days to weeks) in humans because LMN are under direct influence of the corticospinal tract. In dogs, this tract is poorly developed and LMN are mainly under the influence of interneurons, and the loss of UMN control over LMN is indirect. Spinal reflexes in the pelvic limbs in dogs therefore recover more quickly than in humans. In experimental thoracic spinal cord transection in dogs, the reflexes (presented in **Table 2**) reappear between 2 and 24 hours afterward, along with muscle tone from 4 to 14 days.[29,37] In the clinic, animals with spinal shock tend to have preserved patellar and perineal reflexes but a more profound depression of the withdrawal reflex (see **Table 2**).[35] Human patients sometimes exhibit the Babinski reflex (an extension of the digits in response to stimulation of the plantar surface from the heel to the toes), and is a sign of a UMN lesion (Video 1).[38] It is unknown whether spinal shock is associated with particular types of transverse myelopathy (eg, contusive/compressive).

In the Schiff-Sherrington syndrome, animals with a thoracolumbar lesion present with spasticity in the thoracic limbs (**Fig. 1**) but retain a normal gait and normal postural reactions on these limbs, whereas the pelvic limbs are paralyzed. This phenomenon is caused by sudden loss of communication with axons originating from the border cells of the L1 to L5 gray matter spinal cord segments, which normally provide inhibition to the thoracic limb extensors.[39]

Schiff-Sherrington syndrome and spinal shock are 2 separate manifestations of severe SCI but are often encountered at the same time. The clinical signs observed with spinal shock do not follow the UMN/LMN concept, which is important to remember when assessing patients with SCI. In particular, animals with severe SCI are presented increasingly commonly at early stages and repeated neurologic examination is of particular importance during the first 24 hours following trauma. Observation of a cutaneous trunci muscle reflex cutoff can help the clinician in identifying a UMN lesion in the presence of spinal shock. The Schiff-Sherrington posture is relatively characteristic, but can lead the clinician to wrongly search for a cervical lesion.

Sensory Dysfunction Following Spinal Cord Injury

Sensory dysfunction results in ataxia when the animal has retained some movement, and may cause detectable hypoesthesia and anesthesia below the lesion (eg, loss of thermal, pressure, and pain sensations). However, testing subtle sensation and pain is difficult in animals and often highly subjective. The level of force applied to test so-called deep pain sensation (often using pliers) to the nail bed, skin, or deeper

Table 2
Duration for return of recovery of spinal reflexes in the pelvic limbs following experimental spinal cord transection[37] and clinically following acute spinal cord injury (SCI)[35]

	Return of Spinal Reflexes Following Experimental SCI in Dogs	Return of Spinal Reflexes Following Clinical SCI
Anal sphincter reflex	15 min	Remained present
Patellar reflex	30 min to 2 h	Remained present
Pelvic limb withdrawal reflex	Up to 12 h	Absent after the injury and recovered over 48 h

The loss of spinal reflexes in the acute phase is caused by the spinal shock.

Data from Blauch B. Spinal reflex walking in the dog. Vet Med Small Anim Clin 1977;72:169–73; and Smith PM, Jeffery ND. Spinal shock—comparative aspects and clinical relevance. J Vet Intern Med 2005;19:788–93.

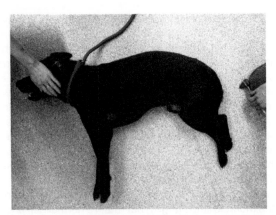

Fig. 1. Schiff-Sherrington posture in a 6-year-old male neutered Labrador retriever with acute-onset L2-L3 transverse myelopathy caused by a fibrocartilaginous embolism. Note the hyperextension of the thoracic limbs. This dog also had reduced muscle tone and withdrawal reflexes of the pelvic limbs at the time of presentation and for 48 hours following spinal cord injury (SCI), despite the lesion being in the T3-L3 region (ie, signs consistent with spinal shock).

structures has to be balanced to elicit a behavioral response but avoid tissue damage. The interpretation of the animal's response is often difficult in the acute phase of SCI, when animals may be highly anxious or in shock; therefore, new techniques are required.

Recently, an electronic von Frey esthesiometer used on the dorsal surface of the pelvic limb paw was tested in 6 normal dogs, 6 dogs with unilateral cranial cruciate ligament rupture, and 6 dogs with moderate SCI (although the exact time of testing following SCI was not specified).[40] The sensory threshold was increased for dogs with SCI, which suggests that this new method might serve as a measure in spinal cord-injured dogs.[40]

In some animals, paresthesia (one type of neuropathic pain) can occur around and below the lesion in the chronic phase of SCI (1–12 months) despite the complete lack of normal pain sensation. A recent study found that 5 dogs out of 211 cases developed neuropathic pain (~2.3%).[16] Such pain can result in self-mutilation of the pelvic limbs, tail, penis, vulva, or dorsal skin. It is difficult to recognize and even ascertain its existence in the acute phase of SCI but, given its clear description in human SCI patients postoperatively,[41] it is likely that paresthesia also occurs in animals, especially around a surgical site (Video 2).

Urinary Dysfunction Following Spinal Cord Injury

SCI disrupts sensory pathways from the bladder to the brain: (1) loss of visceral nociception mediated by sympathetic pathways when the lesion is above L1; and (2) loss of sensation of bladder stretching via the parasympathetic pathways with lesions above S1. Concomitantly, there is also loss of voluntary control of voiding. Following the acute phase of injury, neurogenic detrusor overreactivity develops within a few weeks, corresponding to involuntary detrusor contraction during the filling phase, which is mediated by lumbosacral spinal reflex pathways[42]; this causes reflex incontinence. However, this reflex activity is usually insufficient to completely empty the bladder because detrusor-sphincter dyssynergia develops, causing simultaneous contractions of the urethral sphincter when the bladder contracts. In turn this leads to urinary retention, smooth muscle tight junction disruption because of overdistention, and the need to assist bladder emptying. Urinary dysfunction often causes a range of urinary tract diseases, such as cystitis and pyelonephritis.[43] Following IVDH, urinary tract infection occurs at a frequency varying from 21% to 38% of cases,[44–46] often within 1 to 6 weeks following the injury.[45]

Do Blood Pressure Abnormalities Occur Following Spinal Cord Injury in Dogs?

Acute hypertension rapidly followed by hypotension has been demonstrated in experimental rodents after SCI but is not clearly recognized in clinically-affected dogs, as suggested by Olby.[6] This finding may reflect the delay between SCI and admission of the animal to a referral center. There is experimental evidence in dogs (using a balloon compression model developed by Griffiths and colleagues[47]) that injury and compression lead to loss of spinal cord autoregulation of blood flow. It therefore seems prudent to recommend close monitoring of blood pressure in the early stages of SCI.

In 1947, Guttman and Whitteridge[48] first described a syndrome with sudden and exaggerated onset of sympathetic activity below the lesion in response to noxious (eg, surgical intervention) or nonnoxious (eg, distended bladder or bowel) stimulation below the spinal cord lesion in human patients with lesions above the T6 spinal cord segment.[48,49] The unopposed sympathetic increase (the intact vagus nerve leads to bradycardia concomitantly) leads to vasoconstriction of the vascular beds and therefore arterial hypertension, leading to headaches, intracranial hemorrhage, retinal hemorrhage, and, less commonly, neurogenic pulmonary edema and possible death.[50] This syndrome is not reported in dogs, possibly because most spinal cord lesions are located in the lower thoracic or lumbar region. However, being aware of this syndrome might be important in cases with spinal trauma in the high thoracic region, especially when they undergo surgery for other organ damage. An elevation of 40 mm Hg over baseline systolic pressure is suggestive of autonomic dysreflexia.

Respiratory Dysfunction Following Spinal Cord Injury

In dogs and cats, the pool of motor neurons controlling the diaphragm is located between C5 and C8 spinal cord segments.[34,51,52] These neurons are under the influence of interneurons in the C1-C4 segments, themselves under bulbar control. Experimentally the C1-C4 interneurons have little influence on the activation of the phrenic motor neuron pool.[53] The high thoracic spinal cord segments T1 to T5 also contain pools of motor neurons innervating intercostal muscles and contributing to diaphragm innervation.[52] The clinical consequences are that dogs with severe SCI in the cervical region or high thoracic region are prone to neurogenic respiratory dysfunction (hypoventilation), and may need ventilatory support (**Fig. 2**, Video 3).

Hypoventilation necessitating ventilatory support has been reported in approximately 5% (13 of 263) of cases with cervical spinal cord disease undergoing surgery, although the diagnosis for these cases was not specified.[54] These dogs were commonly affected by a lesion within the C2-C4 segments (which differs from the aforementioned experimental observations) and underwent a decompressive laminectomy.[54] It is possible that clinical lesions extend over several spinal cord segments, therefore involving segments below C5 when the lesion epicenter is around C2-C4. In dogs with cervical IVDH a similar occurrence of neurogenic hypoventilation was recently found to affect 2 of 35 tetraplegic cases.[55] In one report on acute cervical hydrated nucleus pulposus extrusion between C3 and C6, 3 of 10 dogs developed respiratory dysfunction and 1 subsequently died.[56]

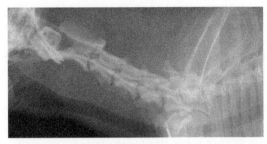

Fig. 2. Lateral radiograph of an 8-year-old female neutered Jack Russell Terrier following a road traffic accident; there is near complete luxation of the vertebral column between C5 and C6 vertebrae (also see Video 3).

The success of prolonged positive-pressure ventilation appears reasonable, although the number of reported cases is small. One case report on a dog with C3-C4 trauma had a successful outcome following 37 days of assisted ventilation.[57] In 14 other cases, the mean duration of ventilation was 4.5 days, and 9 dogs had a favorable outcome (ie, regained the ability to walk).[54] In this case series, the 2 dogs that lacked pain sensation did not recover. Hypoventilation will appear before loss of sensation; therefore, in any tetraplegic animal it is crucial to search for signs of respiratory dysfunction (poor quality of chest movements, hypo-/hyperventilation, measurements of carbon dioxide pressure and oxygen saturation). In cases with loss of pain sensation in all 4 limbs, respiratory dysfunction has to be assumed and aggressively treated. Non-neurogenic factors such as recumbency cause lung atelectasis which, combined with difficulties in clearing secretions and an impaired cough, increase the risk of pneumonia.[58]

ANCILLARY METHODS USED TO ASSESS SPINAL CORD FUNCTION
Clinical Scoring

Clinical scores are difficult to design and use in animals. The clinician scoring the animal often faces the dilemma that an observation that falls between two grades still needs to be attributed to one grade, which inevitably implies subjectivity. In animals, some neurologic functions, such as fine sensation and, to a certain extent, voluntary motor control, are omitted in clinical scores. In general, urinary and fecal incontinence are scored separately. In dogs, the severity of functional loss following SCI has been subject to clinical scoring since the 1950s, using Tarlov scales, or that implemented by Hoerlein.[59,60] Recognizing the need for more precise tools, in 2001 Olby and colleagues[61] developed a scoring scheme for use in dogs similar to the Basso, Beattie, and Bresnahan score used in rodents.[62] Although it provides more subtlety the Olby scoring scheme is not linear, which limits accurate and flexible statistical analysis over the range of possible scores. Olby and colleagues[63] have recently proposed a new gait scoring system using videos of dogs walking on treadmills without prior training. This score generates continuous data on pelvic limb function and helps to define thoracic/pelvic limb coordination in dogs walking on a treadmill. Levine and colleagues[64] also developed the Texas Spinal Cord Injury Score, an ordinal scale judging each limb and proprioceptive deficits separately, which is similar to the scheme proposed by Borgens and colleagues[65] in 1993. Overall, there is at present no consensus on the use of one particular scheme for dogs, and it is important to stress the need for blinded observations when evaluating animals. Recently, the crucial need for prospective collection of SCI clinical scores at the time of injury, as opposed to retrospective scoring, was emphasized.[66]

Kinematics

Kinematic methods using high-frequency infrared cameras have become more widely applied in dogs and have been shown to provide objective measures to quantify the gait. In SCI this mainly consists of quantifying aspects of coordination: (1) intergirdle coordination (ie, coordination between thoracic and pelvic limbs) is suggested to represent the function of short distance connections, such as propriospinal tracts, across a thoracolumbar lesion site[67]; (2) intragirdle coordination (ie, coordination between paired thoracic or pelvic limbs) represents stability of the limbs, which is a function mediated by supraspinal centers, and therefore requires long tracts from the brain.[68] Such an instrument can be exploited to assess recovery of function following SCI (**Fig. 3**).[69] However, this method requires that the dog walk on a treadmill, often while being supported by a sling. Gordon-Evans and colleagues[70] have assessed kinematic parameters such as stride time, stance time, swing time, stride length, and velocity in dogs with spinal cord dysfunction while walking freely on a walkway. These investigators proposed a multivariate model of stride length, stride time, and swing time using all limbs to provide a second objective method of assessing the gait, but its limitation is the need for patients to be ambulatory.

Advances in Magnetic Resonance Imaging

Imaging of the spinal cord parenchyma using magnetic resonance imaging (MRI), reviewed by da Costa and Samii,[13] allows identification of the lesion site, severity of compression, and characterization and extent of the lesion, therefore helping in reaching a diagnosis and guiding the surgical plan. Acute lesions usually appear hyperintense on T2-weighted images, reflecting necrosis, myelomalacia, intramedullary hemorrhage, inflammation, or edema. A variety of sequences during MRI highlight various structures associated with the vertebral column and spinal cord. MRI allows 3-dimensional examination of the spinal cord, and any examination should therefore comprise at least 2 planes of acquisition. T2-weighted sequences (usually sagittal first) allow screening and detection of a hyperintense signal, especially within the spinal cord, representing increased water content (such as with edema or mid- to long-term pathologic process). Fluid-attenuated inversion recovery sequences that suppress the signal generated by fluid, allow better differentiation of suspected edema. T1-weighted sequences provide anatomic details and are acquired before and after paramagnetic contrast injection (typically gadolinium). A variety of other MRI sequences are available, and are performed depending on initial sequence results and differential diagnoses (eg, hemorrhage can be suspected using T2* sequences, nerve root lesions might be better seen following suppression of fat signal using short-tau inversion recovery sequences, and so forth). The half-Fourier acquisition single-shot turbo spin-echo (HASTE) sequence has been found to poorly correlate with T2-weighted sequences in dogs with IVDH (ie, of 310 cases with a compression identified on T2-weighted scans, only 180 had a compression depicted by the HASTE sequence).[71]

Diffusion tensor imaging (tractography) has also recently been proposed as a means to quantify SCI, and can provide information on specific tract and white matter damage.[72–74] Diffusion tensor imaging is a form of diffusion-weighted imaging that depicts the strength and direction of movement of water molecules, allowing axonal tracts and their physical integrity to be defined.

Finally, in cases of trauma to the vertebral column, it should be kept in mind that MRI is complementary to the bony details available from computed tomography

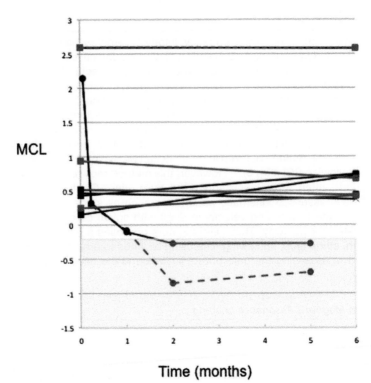

Time (months)

Fig. 3. Follow-up over 6 months (x-axis) of the thoracic/pelvic limb coordination measured using the mean cumulative lag (MCL) (y-axis). The MCL is a measure obtained following kinematic analysis of the gait of dogs with SCI. In paraplegic animals that retain involuntary movements, there is a delay between one thoracic limb step cycle and a pelvic limb step cycle (in a normal animal, each thoracic limb step cycle is almost immediately followed by a pelvic limb step cycle). The MCL corresponds to the summation of the delay between thoracic and pelvic limb steps during a large number of step cycles, and therefore quantifies thoracic/pelvic limb coordination. These data were obtained during supported treadmill walking using kinematic evaluation. The traces presented correspond to: (1) a dog with incomplete SCI (paraplegia and intact pain sensation in the pelvic limbs) following decompressive surgery (*plain black line* represents the left MCL and *dashed black line* represents the right MCL); (2) 4 dogs with complete SCI and lack of recovery at least 3 months after SCI (the 3 *red lines* and 1 *red dashed line* represent left MCL and the 4 *blue lines* represent the right MCL). The yellow shaded area represents normal values of the MCL in unaffected dogs. Note the return to normal values of the MCL in the dog with incomplete SCI, demonstrating recovery of coordination between thoracic and pelvic limbs. In this dog, pelvic limb lateral stability was also analyzed with the coefficient of variation (CV). At 7 days, 1 month, and 2 months following SCI, the CV of the pelvic limbs was 1.04, 0.44, and 0.27, respectively, approaching the normal thoracic limb value (<0.2) and demonstrating recovery of supraspinal control. The treadmill recordings were collected by Dr Lindsay Hamilton, University of Cambridge, and analyzed by Dr Nicolas Granger.

scans because it highlights the extent of SCI. Up to 60% of cases with spinal trauma have traumatic intervertebral disc herniation, of which one-third cause compression of the spinal cord, although the degree of compression does not appear to relate to probability of recovery.[75]

Utility of Electrophysiologic Measures

Electrophysiologic recordings provide quantitative data for assessing spinal cord conduction (both motor and sensory) through the damaged region of the spinal cord.[76–78]

- Magnetic motor-evoked potentials (MMEPs): Compound muscle action potentials are recorded in limb muscles below the spinal cord lesion following magnetic stimulation of the motor cortex through the skull (transcranial) or spine. Transcranial MMEP evaluation is a noninvasive and painless technique to study long-distance descending motor pathways. In humans, the latency of MMEPs is thought to reflect the speed of conduction down the corticospinal tract.[79]
- Sensory evoked potentials (SEPs): Field or ascending potentials can be recorded along and over the vertebral column. At the lumbar intumescence the impulse generated by tibial nerve stimulation is a field potential called the cord dorsum potential, which reflects the activation of neurons below the lesion. An injury potential is usually recorded at the lesion site.[76] Field potentials can be recorded over the skull (somatosensory evoked potentials [SSEPs]) following stimulation of a peripheral nerve, the spinal cord (spinal evoked potential), or the skin (dermatomal evoked potential). Evoked potentials are used to study ascending sensory pathways.
- Late waves recorded from peripheral nerves, such as the Hoffman reflex (H-reflex), reflect motor neuron excitability following SCI,[80] and can therefore detect plasticity of the lumbar spinal cord[81] and assess recovery of connection between supraspinal centers and LMN.[82]

Such electrophysiologic data available in companion animals remains extremely limited. In dogs, one study found transcranial MMEPs difficult to record in the acute phase of SCI in nonambulatory dogs,[83] but little attempt has been made so far to replicate this finding or further develop these techniques to analyze acute injury. Recent data from humans suggest that this should be pursued: recently, and for the first time in a large cohort of 255 human patients with SCI, it has been shown that recovery of motor-evoked potential amplitude closely paralleled the clinical recovery of walking function following incomplete and complete SCI.[84]

Characteristics of SSEP and spinal evoked potentials (amplitude and conduction velocity) have been shown to be clinically relevant to grade SCI in dogs.[78,85] In the acute phase of thoracolumbar disc herniation the general experience is that SSEPs are not detectable in dogs that lack pain sensation caudal to the lesion,[76,78] although Shores and colleagues[85] have shown that this was possible in some cases. It is possible to record in paraplegic animals with preserved pain sensation (**Fig. 4**). In

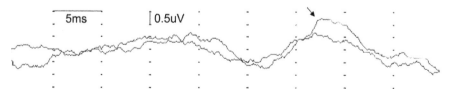

Fig. 4. Somatosensory evoked potential in the acute phase (~24 hours) of SCI in a paraplegic dog that had detectable pain sensation; the potential was obtained following submaximal electrical stimulation of the right tibial nerve at the level of the hock and recording above the left cortical hemisphere, and peaks (*black arrow*) at approximately 32 milliseconds. (*Courtesy of* Dr Milka Kwiatkowska, University of Bristol, Langford, North Somerset.)

human patients, SSEP latencies help to predict future ambulation and correlate with motor scores.[86]

STANDARD OF CARE AND TREATMENT ADVANCES FOR SPINAL CORD INJURY

The standard of care in companion animals remains to stabilize the patient physically and medically (**Fig. 5**) and decompress the spinal cord, although the evidence for early decompression in dogs has not yet been clearly demonstrated in a prospective manner. From primary reports and meta-analysis in humans, there is evidence that early decompressive surgery may reduce hospitalization time and, hence, complications, in some hospitals and improve the neurologic outcome in others.[87] In hospitals in which an effect of early decompression was not detected, there was no evidence of detrimental effects. Nevertheless, the overall level of evidence in support of early intervention remains weak.[88]

Prospects for New Pharmacologic Interventions for the Acute Phase of Spinal Cord Injury

Despite the large amount of experimental data examining neuroprotective drugs for SCI, no compound has emerged for use in clinical SCI in dogs. Recent reviews presenting novel neuroprotective drugs[4,6] and currently tested molecules in dogs include: (1) polyethylene glycol (compared with methylprednisolone sodium succinate in a phase III study, North Carolina State University), which was previously tested against historical controls[89]; (2) glial growth factor 2 (North Carolina State University) in a phase I study; and (3) matrix metalloproteinase blocker (in a large-scale randomized blinded phase II study, Texas A&M University).[90]

Selection of appropriate candidate drugs remains problematic, but it is suggested that the following should be favored in future studies: (1) drugs already in use for other related or unrelated conditions; (2) drugs that can be administered by intravenous infusion or orally; or (3) drugs for which evidence of efficacy persists if given with a delay following injury.[91]

What Is the Evidence for Cell Transplantation in the Acute Phase of Spinal Cord Injury?

A gradually increasing body of work on allogenic cell transplantation has now been conducted in either experimental or companion animals. The aim is to restore function by transplanting cells, intrathecally (ie, into the spinal cord) or intravenously, at or near the time of acute SCI, to provide neuroprotection. These data merit attention because obtaining and culturing cells (eg, mesenchymal stem cells [MSCs] from adipose tissue, umbilical cord blood, or bone marrow stromal cells[92–94]) is readily possible nowadays, and it is therefore worth examining how far veterinarians are from translating research protocols from the laboratory to pets in the clinic. Here the data on canine cell transplantation within a month of the trauma is reviewed.

One must bear in mind that injection of cells acutely into the lesion site leads to the death of most transplanted cells. In rat models of SCI, much better cell survival is achieved with acute transplantation rostral and caudal to the lesion rather than into the lesion.[95,96] This finding probably reflects the poor vascularization and oxygen supply in the lesion or the inhospitable inflammatory state of the lesion in the acute phase.[97] In one study testing the time of transplantation of allogenic canine MSCs derived from umbilical cord blood in a canine experimental model of SCI, it was suggested that transplantation 1 week after SCI gave a better motor outcome by 8 weeks, compared with transplantation at 12 hours or 2 weeks, the functional

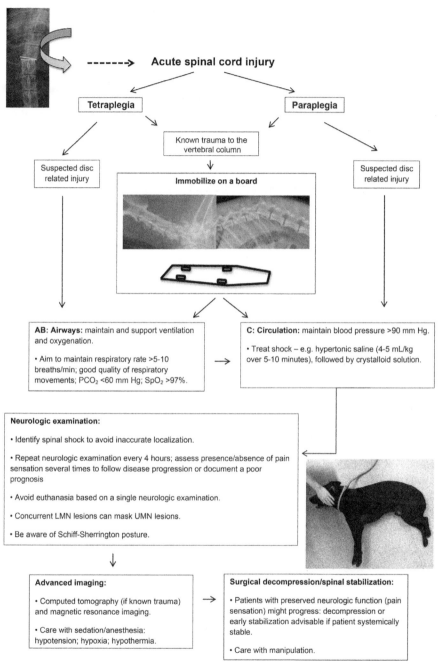

Fig. 5. Current standard of care for companion animals following acute SCI. LMN, lower motor neuron; PCO$_2$, partial pressure of carbon dioxide; SpO$_2$, oxygen saturation; UMN, upper motor neuron.

improvement being only of 1 increment of the Olby score or modified/revised Tarlov scores.[98]

Cell Transplantation in Experimental Canine Models of Spinal Cord Injury

Five studies using experimental dogs have examined the effect of cell transplantation in the acute phase of SCI. First, following the idea that inflammatory cells might help to clear debris inhibitory to axonal growth,[99,100] autologous transplants of activated macrophages were tested in a T13-L1 hemisection model.[101] This study first examined pilot data on 7 dogs (including 1 sham dog, 2 culture media–only dogs, and 4 cell transplant dogs) but found no motor or electrophysiologic benefit of the transplant over a 9-month period, and the experiment was terminated. In 4 other studies a positive effect of the transplant, composed of MSCs derived from adipose tissue, bone marrow, Wharton jelly, or umbilical cord blood, was found.[102–105] These studies, from Korea and Japan, used a ventral epidural balloon compression technique to produce a closed injury,[106] which mimics the location of the insult in clinical cases, but can be difficult to standardize in terms of severity and symmetry (the model was developed in the 1970's by the research groups of Kobrine and Griffiths.[47,107]) The study by Lim and colleagues[102] testing umbilical cord blood–derived MSCs demonstrated the biggest effect of MSCs. In the group receiving cells and a recombinant factor, the Olby score increased from 0 to 7.4 (ie, weight-bearing protraction of pelvic limb 10%–50% of the time) and there was recovery of SSEPs between L6 and T10 spinal cord segments, whereas there was no improvement in the control and media-only groups. In this study the effect could have been due to the recombinant factor, the cells, or both, because equal benefits were found in the recombinant factor–only group and the cell-only group. In one study motor benefits were not associated with recovery of evoked potentials,[105] implying that the claimed motor benefits might represent increased spinal activity below the lesion only, and not necessarily a connection across the lesion, especially because tail support was provided during clinical assessment of dogs.[102,103] Tail support is known to trigger stepping pelvic movements independently of supralesional connections.[29,108] Finally, these studies provided incomplete details of some aspects of their methodology related to: (1) blinding; (2) concealment of allocation to treatment groups before randomization; (3) prespecification of primary/secondary outcome measures; and (4) scoring systems. Therefore, their results should be interpreted with care.

Across studies, histopathologic data have suggested possible axonal regeneration, neuroprotection, and reduced inflammation in the lesion, although these findings remain observational. In the study by Ryu and colleagues,[105] transplanted cells were labeled with green fluorescent protein and identified at the termination of the experiment (9 weeks), providing direct evidence of survival of at least some transplanted cells.

Overall, the evidence of a benefit of cell transplantation in the acute phase of SCI remains limited because of the small numbers of animals and methodological flaws in published experiments. Larger studies and replication studies would help to define whether cellular transplantation forms a treatment that should be transferred to veterinary hospitals.

Cell Transplantation in Experimental Feline Models of Spinal Cord Injury

In a feline transection model, a mixed population of autologous tritium-labeled fibroblasts and Schwann cells obtained from sciatic nerve biopsies were transplanted acutely in the spinal cord of 21 cats.[109] Cells were implanted in the 0.5- to 1-mm gap and autoradiography was used to identify cells at 3 and 7 days after transplantation: ensheathment of axons by transplanted cells was observed. The functional effect of Schwann cells remains to be demonstrated.

Cell Transplantation in Clinical Cases with Spinal Cord Injury

One study examined the safety of acute spinal cord transplantation of MSCs derived from the bone marrow in clinical cases, and found no adverse reaction over a mean follow-up of 41 months.[110] Tamura and colleagues[111] reported a higher recovery proportion in paraplegic Dachshunds (32 of 36 animals) following acute spinal cord transplantation of bone marrow–derived mononuclear cells in a comparison with nontransplanted animals (26 of 46 animals). However, the group of nontransplanted animals received decompressive surgery significantly later (>24 hours) than transplanted cases, and other crucial methodological points concerning randomization and scoring were unclear. Recently, in a double-blinded and randomized clinical trial (equivalent to a phase II trial in humans), autologous spinal cord transplantation of canine olfactory ensheathing cells from the nasal mucosa had strong positive effects on thoracic/pelvic limb coordination.[69] In this trial, outcome measures were prespecified and a significant clinical effect was detected in dogs receiving olfactory ensheathing cells (1 of 24 dogs walked independently over ground, 5 others walked on a treadmill with minimal support, and 6 others had improved kinematic variables, therefore giving a response rate of 50% to the transplants), whereas none of the 12 dogs receiving only cell culture media improved. Using kinematic analysis, it was possible to tease out aspects of locomotion that are controlled by the brain and resulting from short connections between CPGs in the spinal cord (ie, independently from brain control). Results demonstrated that although olfactory ensheathing cells had positive effects on ambulation, their effects on brain-controlled locomotion were limited (eg, balance was not restored). There was also no effect on recovery of urinary continence.

Finally, there is one case report of a domestic cat transplanted with autologous MSCs derived from the bone marrow.[112] Eight months before transplantation the cat suffered from a road traffic accident, leading to lumbar spinal cord compression and loss of sensation, and incontinence (the description of the motor status of the cat is not provided in the article). Seventy-five days after surgery it is claimed that the cat showed recovery of motor function (3 minutes of weight bearing) and sensation, although the decompressive effect of the surgery is not discussed.

Standard of Care for Urinary Retention Management

There are 3 clinical techniques to empty the bladder in animals with neurogenic incontinence: intermittent urinary catheterization, indwelling urinary catheterization, and manual bladder expression. Catheterization ensures complete bladder emptying. Indwelling urinary catheterization renders management of the incontinence more comfortable for the animal and easier for the clinician, but increased duration of catheterization and hospitalization carries an increased risk of urinary tract infection.[44,113,114] Manual expression allows for early recognition of return of bladder function but can be uncomfortable for the dog and difficult in large, obese, or uncooperative dogs or cats, or if there is increased urethral tone (especially in cats). It has been suggested that manual expression may be inefficient and therefore increases the risk of urinary tract infection because of the large residual volumes of urine for prolonged periods, although there is no definitive supportive evidence.[44] The technique currently used to manage urinary retention has no clear impact on the occurrence of urinary tract infection; rather, it is the duration of required urinary bladder management that dictates the risk. It seems prudent to use the least invasive method first (ie, manual bladder expression), followed by intermittent catheterization and, finally, an indwelling catheter.

There is little available evidence in support of currently available pharmacologic interventions for bladder management. Parasympathomimetic compounds (eg, bethanechol, carbachol) used to promote detrusor contraction have not been tested in dogs or cats with SCI. An experimental study of 6 normal dogs given bethanechol for 15 days found no change in urethral or bladder pressures measured via telemetric cystometry and urethral electromyographic recordings.[115]

Sympatholytic compounds (eg, dantrolene, prazosin, acepromazine, phenoxybenzamine, diazepam) used to relax the urethral sphincter have also not been tested in the context of SCI. In healthy cats and cats with recent urethral obstructions, urethral pressure profiles in response to various medications were highly variable, with only a few recordings suggesting a minimal (2 mm Hg) drop in urethral pressures.[116–119] Prazosin and terazosin caused a reduction in urethral pressure in nonsedated healthy Beagles and in dogs with reflex dyssynergia.[120,121]

Is There a Role for Early Rehabilitation Following Spinal Cord Injury?

Conventional physiotherapy forms an integral part of the treatment of human patients with SCI, and is clearly recognized as the only available therapy to promote recovery.[122] In this respect, rehabilitation for animals lies far behind treatments provided to humans, as evidenced by the paucity of clinical data.[123]

Spinal walking, motor relearning, and postural rehabilitation

If only 5% to 10% of the spinal cord axons are spared in cats, locomotion is possible, although not normal, and this provides evidence of the robust plasticity of the nervous system to adapt to tissue loss.[124,125] In experimental animals following thoracic spinal cord transection, it has been well established that movements below the lesion, mainly in the form of stepping movements, still occur because of preservation of CPGs, and in experimental dogs recovery of the walking pattern can occur without training.[29,108] This observation was originally made by Brown,[126] who described a coordinated stepping motion in a decerebrate and spinalized cat. Later it was reported that chronically spinalized cats could be trained on a treadmill to regain near normal stepping locomotion.[127–129]

There is therefore strong experimental evidence that locomotor training leads to recovery of walking movements. However, a recent meta-analysis in human patients with SCI trained with either body-weight–supported treadmill or robotic-assisted body-weight–supported treadmill did not reveal added benefit of these treatments over conventional physiotherapy.[130] In quadrupeds, treadmill training might be easier but has not been attempted. Furthermore, the motor function would be poorly exploitable without recovery of balance. There is a range of apparatus and protocols that can be used in dogs to promote recovery of truncal posture, but none has been studied in dogs with SCI.[131]

Neuromuscular electrical stimulation

Electrical stimulation is widely used in human patients following SCI, with several therapeutic goals including increasing muscle strength and muscle mass, limiting muscular atrophy, decreasing spasticity, and reducing limb edema.[132,133] There is also evidence that neuromuscular electrical stimulation reduces muscle fatigue and improves patients' tolerance to exercise following SCI.[134,135] In dogs, this therapy has been evaluated once experimentally, following sciatic section, and was found to promote muscle metabolism.[136] The clinical effectiveness found in human patients suggests that it might also benefit dogs.

PROGNOSIS FOLLOWING SPINAL CORD INJURY
Presence or Absence of Detectable Pain Sensation

Following thoracolumbar injury, evidence of intact perception of painfully noxious stimulation in the hindquarters at the time of presentation is classically the best prognostic factor and, thus far, no other outcome measure has been shown to be equivalent. In large case series of IVDH dogs, between 60% and 80% recover ambulation following loss of detectable pain sensation,[57,136–138] compared with 86% to 96% of cases recovering function if detectable pain sensation is evident on presentation.[2,3,139] These figures show that a significant proportion of animals given a poor prognosis on examination will still go on to regain the ability to walk. In all situations, when recovery occurs the improvement begins within the first 3 weeks (usually 10 days) after injury in 92% of cases.[4,137]

Value of the Cutaneous Trunci Muscle Reflex

Recently, the utility of the cutaneous trunci muscle reflex as a predictor for recovery in a group of 36 dogs with paraplegia, loss of pain sensation, and a cutaneous trunci muscle reflex cutoff was assessed.[140] Ascension of this reflex toward the thoracic limbs (**Fig. 6**) was a sign of myelomalacia associated with a poor prognosis. Overall, 11 of 14 dogs (~78%) with caudal movement of the panniculus reflex and 6 of 8 dogs (~75%) in which the cutaneous trunci muscle reflex remained static regained the ability to walk in the long term (ie, >6 months).

Effect of Age on Prognosis

It is thought that young dogs might recover from SCI more quickly than older dogs. Only one study, which divided cases into 3 age groups, found an association between age and time to ambulation.[137] Other studies found no association between age and time to ambulation on entering the data into a linear regression model.[22,141]

Prognosis in Cats with Intervertebral Disc Disease

The prognosis for cats with IVDH treated surgically is excellent. In one series of 30 cats treated surgically, 4 either died or were lost to follow-up and the remainder had a fair to excellent outcome.[24] The prognosis is gathered from around 15 case reports or small case series.[5] Cases managed conservatively tended to have a poor outcome, but this

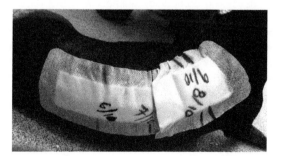

Fig. 6. Five-year-old female neutered Dachshund 72 hours following L1-L2 acute intervertebral disc herniation and decompressive spinal surgery. The dog was paraplegic and had lost pelvic limb sensation. Note the cranial progression of the cutaneous trunci muscle reflex toward the high thoracic region, evidenced by the dates recorded on the dog's dressing, consistent with ascending myelomalacia.

may reflect the willingness of owners to pursue invasive treatments. All data were collected retrospectively and were subject to the usual biases.

Biomarkers

Markers of SCI (see also the companion article by Nishida elsewhere in this issue) are investigated as prognostic factors, but also to highlight potential targets for neuroprotective drugs for SCI treatment. Biomarkers hold great promise but, again, none has been shown thus far to be able to predict recovery better than a clinician's assessment. Reported cerebrospinal fluid biomarkers include aspartate aminotransferase, calcium, glucose, nucleated cell count, protein, creatine kinase, lactate, myelin basic protein, matrix metalloproteinase 9, and tau protein.[139,142–149] Witsberger and colleagues[139] published a screening method for clinical cases of acute SCI. In this study, combined elevation of myelin basic protein and creatine kinase in dogs with no detectable pain sensation following IVDH led to the probability of a successful outcome of 10%. The probability of a successful outcome if myelin basic protein and creatine kinase were below the cutoff values was greater than 98%. Levine and colleagues[144] found that cerebrospinal fluid myelin basic protein was predictive of long-term functional outcome in dogs with thoracolumbar IVDH with sensitivity and specificity of 78% and 76%, respectively. These results are yet to be tested prospectively.

Use of MRI for Prognostication

Various groups have investigated whether spinal cord MRI changes found following injury could predict patient outcome. In a review of 67 dogs with variable degrees of SCI following thoracolumbar disc extrusion, no association was found between the severity of spinal cord compression viewed on transverse MRI scans and the preinjury neurologic grade or postsurgical outcome.[150] This finding suggests that the contusion that occurs at the time of disc herniation defines the severity of the lesion and, possibly, the prognosis, rather than the severity of compression. Ito and colleagues[151] found that in animals with loss of pain sensation (and therefore severe SCI), 31% recovered if they had an intramedullary hyperintensity identified on T2-weighted MRI images, whereas 100% recovered if no hyperintensity was seen on MRI. This finding was supported by Levine and colleagues[152] with all grades of SCI, with 76% of cases recovering with spinal cord MRI changes and 93% recovering with no spinal cord MRI changes.

SUMMARY

Basic principles for assessing companion animals with SCI remain essential in the clinic, but with the growth of clinical experience at managing these cases, detailed aspects of SCI (spinal shock, importance of autonomic dysfunction, neuropathic pain) are now recognized as equally important. The clinician's evaluation, though bearing some subjectivity, remains the most sensitive tool to assess SCI patients, and their progression or recovery. Although some new techniques to measure neurologic function are under development, they have not yet fully proved their value in the clinic. Similarly, new therapies (either pharmacologic or cellular) are still lacking in treatment of the acute phase of SCI. However, a significant number of teams around the world (United States, Europe, China, and Japan) comprising veterinary neurologists and neuroscientists have unified their efforts to test promising therapies.

SUPPLEMENTARY DATA

Supplementary data related to this article can be found online at http://dx.doi.org/10.1016/j.cvsm.2014.07.013.

REFERENCES

1. Hoerlein BF. The modern treatment of traumatic spinal compressions in the dog. Can Vet J 1960;1:216–8.
2. Brisson BA. Intervertebral disc disease in dogs. Vet Clin North Am Small Anim Pract 2010;40:829–58.
3. Jeffery ND. Vertebral fracture and luxation in small animals. Vet Clin North Am Small Anim Pract 2010;40:809–28.
4. Jeffery ND, Levine JM, Olby NJ, et al. Intervertebral disk degeneration in dogs: consequences, diagnosis, treatment, and future directions. J Vet Intern Med 2013;27(6):1318–33.
5. Marioni-Henry K. Feline spinal cord diseases. Vet Clin North Am Small Anim Pract 2010;40:1011–28.
6. Olby N. The pathogenesis and treatment of acute spinal cord injuries in dogs. Vet Clin North Am Small Anim Pract 2010;40:791–807.
7. Bray JP, Burbidge HM. The canine intervertebral disk: part one: structure and function. J Am Anim Hosp Assoc 1998;34:55–63.
8. Jeffery ND, Hamilton L, Granger N. Designing clinical trials in canine spinal cord injury as a model to translate successful laboratory interventions into clinical practice. Vet Rec 2011;168:102–7.
9. Jeffery ND, Smith PM, Lakatos A, et al. Clinical canine spinal cord injury provides an opportunity to examine the issues in translating laboratory techniques into practical therapy. Spinal Cord 2006;44:584–93.
10. Levine JM, Levine GJ, Porter BF, et al. Naturally occurring disk herniation in dogs: an opportunity for pre-clinical spinal cord injury research. J Neurotrauma 2011;28: 675–88.
11. Wewetzer K, Radtke C, Kocsis J, et al. Species-specific control of cellular proliferation and the impact of large animal models for the use of olfactory ensheathing cells and Schwann cells in spinal cord repair. Exp Neurol 2011;229:80–7.
12. Parent J. Clinical approach and lesion localization in patients with spinal diseases. Vet Clin North Am Small Anim Pract 2010;40:733–53.
13. da Costa RC, Samii VF. Advanced imaging of the spine in small animals. Vet Clin North Am Small Anim Pract 2010;40:765–90.
14. De Risio L, Platt SR. Fibrocartilaginous embolic myelopathy in small animals. Vet Clin North Am Small Anim Pract 2010;40:859–69.
15. Fluehmann G, Doherr MG, Jaggy A. Canine neurological diseases in a referral hospital population between 1989 and 2000 in Switzerland. J Small Anim Pract 2006;47:582–7.
16. Aikawa T, Fujita H, Kanazono S, et al. Long-term neurologic outcome of hemilaminectomy and disk fenestration for treatment of dogs with thoracolumbar intervertebral disk herniation: 831 cases (2000–2007). J Am Vet Med Assoc 2012; 241:1617–26.
17. Brisson BA, Holmberg DL, Parent J, et al. Comparison of the effect of single-site and multiple-site disk fenestration on the rate of recurrence of thoracolumbar intervertebral disk herniation in dogs. J Am Vet Med Assoc 2011;238:1593–600.
18. Brisson BA, Moffatt SL, Swayne SL, et al. Recurrence of thoracolumbar intervertebral disk extrusion in chondrodystrophic dogs after surgical decompression with or without prophylactic fenestration: 265 cases (1995–1999). J Am Vet Med Assoc 2004;224:1808–14.
19. Itoh H, Hara Y, Yoshimi N, et al. A retrospective study of intervertebral disc herniation in dogs in Japan: 297 cases. J Vet Med Sci 2008;70:701–6.

20. Macias C, McKee WM, May C, et al. Thoracolumbar disc disease in large dogs: a study of 99 cases. J Small Anim Pract 2002;43:439–46.

21. Necas A. Clinical aspects of surgical treatment of thoracolumbar disc disease in dogs. A retrospective study of 300 cases. Acta Vet Brno 1999;68:121–30.

22. Ruddle TL, Allen DA, Schertel ER, et al. Outcome and prognostic factors in non-ambulatory Hansen Type I intervertebral disc extrusions: 308 cases. Vet Comp Orthop Traumatol 2006;19:29–34.

23. Schulz KS, Walker M, Moon M, et al. Correlation of clinical, radiographic, and surgical localization of intervertebral disc extrusion in small-breed dogs: a prospective study of 50 cases. Vet Surg 1998;27:105–11.

24. Marioni-Henry K, Vite CH, Newton AL, et al. Prevalence of diseases of the spinal cord of cats. J Vet Intern Med 2004;18:851–8.

25. Macpherson JM, Ye Y. The cat vertebral column: stance configuration and range of motion. Exp Brain Res 1998;119:324–32.

26. Drew T, Prentice S, Schepens B. Cortical and brainstem control of locomotion. Prog Brain Res 2004;143:251–61.

27. Goulding M. Circuits controlling vertebrate locomotion: moving in a new direction. Nat Rev Neurosci 2009;10:507–18.

28. Grillner S, Wallen P. Central pattern generators for locomotion, with special reference to vertebrates. Annu Rev Neurosci 1985;8:233–61.

29. Handa Y, Naito A, Watanabe S, et al. Functional recovery of locomotive behavior in the adult spinal dog. Tohoku J Exp Med 1986;148:373–84.

30. Forterre F, Konar M, Tomek A, et al. Accuracy of the withdrawal reflex for localization of the site of cervical disk herniation in dogs: 35 cases (2004–2007). J Am Vet Med Assoc 2008;232:559–63.

31. Muguet-Chanoit AC, Olby NJ, Babb KM, et al. The sensory field and repeatability of the cutaneous trunci muscle reflex of the dog. Vet Surg 2011; 40:781–5.

32. Bali MS, Lang J, Jaggy A, et al. Comparative study of vertebral fractures and luxations in dogs and cats. Vet Comp Orthop Traumatol 2009;22:47–53.

33. Feeney DA, Oliver JE. Blunt spinal trauma in the dog and cat: insight into radiographic lesions. J Am Anim Hosp Assoc 1980;16:885–90.

34. Sherrington CS. The integrative action of the nervous system. 2nd edition. Cambridge (United Kingdom): Cambridge University Press; 1947. p. 241–50.

35. Smith PM, Jeffery ND. Spinal shock–comparative aspects and clinical relevance. J Vet Intern Med 2005;19:788–93.

36. Schadt JC, Barnes CD. Motoneuron membrane changes associated with spinal shock and the Schiff-Sherrington phenomenon. Brain Res 1980;201: 373–83.

37. Blauch B. Spinal reflex walking in the dog. Vet Med Small Anim Clin 1977;72: 169–73.

38. Marie P, Foix C. On the reflex withdrawal of the leg provoked by a toes forced flexion. Rev Neurol (Paris) 1910;20:121–3.

39. Sprague JM. Spinal border cells and their role in postural mechanism (Schiff-Sherrington phenomenon). J Neurophysiol 1953;16:464–74.

40. Moore SA, Hettlich BF, Waln A. The use of an electronic von Frey device for evaluation of sensory threshold in neurologically normal dogs and those with acute spinal cord injury. Vet J 2013;197:216–9.

41. Street JT, Lenehan BJ, DiPaola CP, et al. Morbidity and mortality of major adult spinal surgery. A prospective cohort analysis of 942 consecutive patients. Spine J 2012;12:22–34.

42. Tai C, Roppolo JR, de Groat WC. Spinal reflex control of micturition after spinal cord injury. Restor Neurol Neurosci 2006;24:69–78.
43. Lane IF. Diagnosis and management of urinary retention. Vet Clin North Am Small Anim Pract 2000;30:25–57, v.
44. Bubenik L, Hosgood G. Urinary tract infection in dogs with thoracolumbar intervertebral disc herniation and urinary bladder dysfunction managed by manual expression, indwelling catheterization or intermittent catheterization. Vet Surg 2008;37:791–800.
45. Olby NJ, MacKillop E, Cerda-Gonzalez S, et al. Prevalence of urinary tract infection in dogs after surgery for thoracolumbar intervertebral disc extrusion. J Vet Intern Med 2010;24:1106–11.
46. Stiffler KS, Stevenson MA, Sanchez S, et al. Prevalence and characterization of urinary tract infections in dogs with surgically treated type 1 thoracolumbar intervertebral disc extrusion. Vet Surg 2006;35:330–6.
47. Griffiths IR, Trench JG, Crawford RA. Spinal cord blood flow and conduction during experimental cord compression in normotensive and hypotensive dogs. J Neurosurg 1979;50:353–60.
48. Guttmann L, Whitteridge D. Effects of bladder distension on autonomic mechanisms after spinal cord injuries. Brain 1947;70:361–404.
49. Karlsson AK. Autonomic dysfunction in spinal cord injury: clinical presentation of symptoms and signs. Prog Brain Res 2006;152:1–8.
50. Assadi F, Czech K, Palmisano JL. Autonomic dysreflexia manifested by severe hypertension. Med Sci Monit 2004;10:CS77–9.
51. Bellingham MC. Synaptic inhibition of cat phrenic motoneurons by internal intercostal nerve stimulation. J Neurophysiol 1999;82:1224–32.
52. DiMarco AF, Kowalski KE. High-frequency spinal cord stimulation of inspiratory muscles in dogs: a new method of inspiratory muscle pacing. J Appl Physiol (1985) 2009;107:662–9.
53. DiMarco AF, Kowalski KE. Spinal pathways mediating phrenic activation during high frequency spinal cord stimulation. Respir Physiol Neurobiol 2013;186:1–6.
54. Beal MW, Paglia DT, Griffin GM, et al. Ventilatory failure, ventilator management, and outcome in dogs with cervical spinal disorders: 14 cases (1991–1999). J Am Vet Med Assoc 2001;218:1598–602.
55. Rossmeisl JH Jr, White C, Pancotto TE, et al. Acute adverse events associated with ventral slot decompression in 546 dogs with cervical intervertebral disc disease. Vet Surg 2013;42:795–806.
56. Beltran E, Dennis R, Doyle V, et al. Clinical and magnetic resonance imaging features of canine compressive cervical myelopathy with suspected hydrated nucleus pulposus extrusion. J Small Anim Pract 2012;53:101–7.
57. Smarick SD, Rylander H, Burkitt JM, et al. Treatment of traumatic cervical myelopathy with surgery, prolonged positive-pressure ventilation, and physical therapy in a dog. J Am Vet Med Assoc 2007;230:370–4.
58. Java MA, Drobatz KJ, Gilley RS, et al. Incidence of and risk factors for postoperative pneumonia in dogs anesthetized for diagnosis or treatment of intervertebral disk disease. J Am Vet Med Assoc 2009;235:281–7.
59. Tarlov IM, Klinger H. Spinal cord compression studies. II. Time limits for recovery after acute compression in dogs. AMA Arch Neurol Psychiatry 1954;71:271–90.
60. Hoerlein BF. Intervertebral disc protrusions in the dog. II. Symptomatology and clinical diagnosis. Am J Vet Res 1953;14:270–4.
61. Olby NJ, De Risio L, Munana KR, et al. Development of a functional scoring system in dogs with acute spinal cord injuries. Am J Vet Res 2001;62:1624–8.

62. Basso DM, Beattie MS, Bresnahan JC, et al. MASCIS evaluation of open field locomotor scores: effects of experience and teamwork on reliability. Multicenter Animal Spinal Cord Injury Study. J Neurotrauma 1996;13:343–59.

63. Olby NJ, Lim JH, Babb K, et al. Gait scoring in dogs with thoracolumbar spinal cord injuries when walking on a treadmill. BMC Vet Res 2014;10:58.

64. Levine GJ, Levine JM, Budke CM, et al. Description and repeatability of a newly developed spinal cord injury scale for dogs. Prev Vet Med 2009;89:121–7.

65. Borgens RB, Toombs JP, Blight AR, et al. Effects of applied electric fields on clinical cases of complete paraplegia in dogs. Restor Neurol Neurosci 1993;5: 305–22.

66. Van Wie EY, Fosgate GT, Mankin JM, et al. Prospectively recorded versus medical record-derived spinal cord injury scores in dogs with intervertebral disk herniation. J Vet Intern Med 2013;27:1273–7.

67. Hamilton L, Franklin RJ, Jeffery ND. Development of a universal measure of quadrupedal forelimb-hindlimb coordination using digital motion capture and computerised analysis. BMC Neurosci 2007;8:77.

68. Hamilton L, Franklin RJ, Jeffery ND. Quantification of deficits in lateral paw positioning after spinal cord injury in dogs. BMC Vet Res 2008;4:47.

69. Granger N, Blamires H, Franklin RJ, et al. Autologous olfactory mucosal cell transplants in clinical spinal cord injury: a randomized double-blinded trial in a canine translational model. Brain 2012;135:3227–37.

70. Gordon-Evans WJ, Evans RB, Conzemius MG. Accuracy of spatiotemporal variables in gait analysis of neurologic dogs. J Neurotrauma 2009;26:1055–60.

71. Mankin JM, Hecht S, Thomas WB. Agreement between T2 and haste sequences in the evaluation of thoracolumbar intervertebral disc disease in dogs. Vet Radiol Ultrasound 2012;53:162–6.

72. Griffin JF, Cohen ND, Young BD, et al. Thoracic and lumbar spinal cord diffusion tensor imaging in dogs. J Magn Reson Imaging 2013;37:632–41.

73. Hobert MK, Stein VM, Dziallas P, et al. Evaluation of normal appearing spinal cord by diffusion tensor imaging, fiber tracking, fractional anisotropy, and apparent diffusion coefficient measurement in 13 dogs. Acta Vet Scand 2013;55:36.

74. Pease A, Miller R. The use of diffusion tensor imaging to evaluate the spinal cord in normal and abnormal dogs. Vet Radiol Ultrasound 2011;52:492–7.

75. Henke D, Gorgas D, Flegel T, et al. Magnetic resonance imaging findings in dogs with traumatic intervertebral disk extrusion with or without spinal cord compression: 31 cases (2006–2010). J Am Vet Med Assoc 2013;242:217–22.

76. Holliday TA. Electrodiagnostic examination. Somatosensory evoked potentials and electromyography. Vet Clin North Am Small Anim Pract 1992;22:833–57.

77. Nollet H, Van Ham L, Deprez P, et al. Transcranial magnetic stimulation: review of the technique, basic principles and applications. Vet J 2003;166:28–42.

78. Poncelet L, Michaux C, Balligand M. Somatosensory potentials in dogs with naturally acquired thoracolumbar spinal cord disease. Am J Vet Res 1993;54: 1935–41.

79. Corthout E, Barker AT, Cowey A. Transcranial magnetic stimulation. Which part of the current waveform causes the stimulation? Exp Brain Res 2001;141:128–32.

80. Hiersemenzel LP, Curt A, Dietz V. From spinal shock to spasticity: neuronal adaptations to a spinal cord injury. Neurology 2000;54:1574–82.

81. Bianco J, Gueye Y, Marqueste T, et al. Vitamin D(3) improves respiratory adjustment to fatigue and H-reflex responses in paraplegic adult rats. Neuroscience 2011;188:182–92.

82. Xie J, Boakye M. Electrophysiological outcomes after spinal cord injury. Neurosurg Focus 2008;25:E11.

83. Sylvestre AM, Cockshutt JR, Parent JM, et al. Magnetic motor evoked potentials for assessing spinal cord integrity in dogs with intervertebral disc disease. Vet Surg 1993;22:5–10.

84. Petersen JA, Spiess M, Curt A, et al. Spinal cord injury: one-year evolution of motor-evoked potentials and recovery of leg motor function in 255 patients. Neurorehabil Neural Repair 2012;26:939–48.

85. Shores A, Redding RW, Knecht CD. Spinal-evoked potentials in dogs with acute compressive thoracolumbar spinal cord disease. Am J Vet Res 1987;48: 1525–30.

86. Curt A, Dietz V. Prognosis of traumatic spinal cord lesions. Significance of clinical and electrophysiological findings. Nervenarzt 1997;68:485–95.

87. Furlan JC, Noonan V, Cadotte DW, et al. Timing of decompressive surgery of spinal cord after traumatic spinal cord injury: an evidence-based examination of pre-clinical and clinical studies. J Neurotrauma 2011;28:1371–99.

88. van Middendorp JJ. Letter to the editor regarding: "Early versus delayed decompression for traumatic cervical spinal cord injury: results of the Surgical Timing in Acute Spinal Cord Injury Study (STASCIS)". Spine J 2012;12:540 [author reply: 541–2].

89. Laverty PH, Leskovar A, Breur GJ, et al. A preliminary study of intravenous surfactants in paraplegic dogs: polymer therapy in canine clinical SCI. J Neurotrauma 2004;21:1767–77.

90. Levine JM, Cohen ND, Heller M, et al. Efficacy of a metalloproteinase inhibitor in spinal cord injured dogs. PLoS One 2014;9:e96408.

91. Kwon BK, Okon E, Hillyer J, et al. A systematic review of non-invasive pharmacologic neuroprotective treatments for acute spinal cord injury. J Neurotrauma 2011;28:1545–88.

92. Chung CS, Fujita N, Kawahara N, et al. A comparison of neurosphere differentiation potential of canine bone marrow-derived mesenchymal stem cells and adipose-derived mesenchymal stem cells. J Vet Med Sci 2013;75:879–86.

93. Kamishina H, Cheeseman JA, Clemmons RM. Nestin-positive spheres derived from canine bone marrow stromal cells generate cells with early neuronal and glial phenotypic characteristics. In Vitro Cell Dev Biol Anim 2008;44:140–4.

94. Oda Y, Tani K, Kanei T, et al. Characterization of neuron-like cells derived from canine bone marrow stromal cells. Vet Res Commun 2013;37:133–8.

95. Pearse DD, Sanchez AR, Pereira FC, et al. Transplantation of Schwann cells and/or olfactory ensheathing glia into the contused spinal cord: survival, migration, axon association, and functional recovery. Glia 2007;55:976–1000.

96. Richter MW, Fletcher PA, Liu J, et al. Lamina propria and olfactory bulb ensheathing cells exhibit differential integration and migration and promote differential axon sprouting in the lesioned spinal cord. J Neurosci 2005;25:10700–11.

97. Deng C, Gorrie C, Hayward I, et al. Survival and migration of human and rat olfactory ensheathing cells in intact and injured spinal cord. J Neurosci Res 2006; 83:1201–12.

98. Park SS, Byeon YE, Ryu HH, et al. Comparison of canine umbilical cord blood-derived mesenchymal stem cell transplantation times: involvement of astrogliosis, inflammation, intracellular actin cytoskeleton pathways, and neurotrophin-3. Cell Transplant 2011;20:1867–80.

99. Fawcett J. Astrocytes and axon regeneration in the central nervous system. J Neurol 1994;242:S25–8.

100. Lazarov-Spiegler O, Rapalino O, Agranov G, et al. Restricted inflammatory reaction in the CNS: a key impediment to axonal regeneration? Mol Med Today 1998; 4:337–42.
101. Assina R, Sankar T, Theodore N, et al. Activated autologous macrophage implantation in a large-animal model of spinal cord injury. Neurosurg Focus 2008;25:E3.
102. Lim JH, Byeon YE, Ryu HH, et al. Transplantation of canine umbilical cord blood-derived mesenchymal stem cells in experimentally induced spinal cord injured dogs. J Vet Sci 2007;8:275–82.
103. Park SS, Lee YJ, Lee SH, et al. Functional recovery after spinal cord injury in dogs treated with a combination of Matrigel and neural-induced adipose-derived mesenchymal Stem cells. Cytotherapy 2012;14:584–97.
104. Ryu HH, Kang BJ, Park SS, et al. Comparison of mesenchymal stem cells derived from fat, bone marrow, Wharton's jelly, and umbilical cord blood for treating spinal cord injuries in dogs. J Vet Med Sci 2012;74:1617–30.
105. Ryu HH, Lim JH, Byeon YE, et al. Functional recovery and neural differentiation after transplantation of allogenic adipose-derived stem cells in a canine model of acute spinal cord injury. J Vet Sci 2009;10:273–84.
106. Lee JH, Choi CB, Chung DJ, et al. Development of an improved canine model of percutaneous spinal cord compression injury by balloon catheter. J Neurosci Methods 2008;167:310–6.
107. Kobrine AI, Evans DE, Rizzoli HV. Experimental acute balloon compression of the spinal cord. Factors affecting disappearance and return of the spinal evoked response. J Neurosurg 1979;51:841–5.
108. Naito A, Shimizu Y, Handa Y. Analyses of airstepping movement in adult spinal dogs. Tohoku J Exp Med 1990;162:41–8.
109. Wrathall JR, Kapoor V, Kao CC. Observation of cultured peripheral non-neuronal cells implanted into the transected spinal cord. Acta Neuropathol 1984; 64:203–12.
110. Nishida H, Nakayama M, Tanaka H, et al. Safety of autologous bone marrow stromal cell transplantation in dogs with acute spinal cord injury. Vet Surg 2012;41:437–42.
111. Tamura K, Harada Y, Nagashima N, et al. Autotransplanting of bone marrow-derived mononuclear cells for complete cases of canine paraplegia and loss of pain perception, secondary to intervertebral disc herniation. Exp Clin Transplant 2012;10:263–72.
112. Penha EM, Aguiar PH, Barrouin-Melo SM, et al. Clinical neurofunctional rehabilitation of a cat with spinal cord injury after hemilaminectomy and autologous stem cell transplantation. Int J Stem Cells 2012;5:146–50.
113. Barsanti JA, Blue J, Edmunds J. Urinary tract infection due to indwelling bladder catheters in dogs and cats. J Am Vet Med Assoc 1985;187:384–8.
114. Bubenik LJ, Hosgood GL, Waldron DR, et al. Frequency of urinary tract infection in catheterized dogs and comparison of bacterial culture and susceptibility testing results for catheterized and noncatheterized dogs with urinary tract infections. J Am Vet Med Assoc 2007;231:893–9.
115. Noel S, Massart L, Hamaide A. Urodynamic investigation by telemetry in Beagle dogs: validation and effects of oral administration of current urological drugs: a pilot study. BMC Vet Res 2013;9:197.
116. Frenier SL, Knowlen GG, Speth RC, et al. Urethral pressure response to alpha-adrenergic agonist and antagonist drugs in anesthetized healthy male cats. Am J Vet Res 1992;53:1161–5.

117. Marks SL, Straeter-Knowlen IM, Moore M, et al. Effects of acepromazine maleate and phenoxybenzamine on urethral pressure profiles of anesthetized, healthy, sexually intact male cats. Am J Vet Res 1996;57:1497–500.

118. Mawby DI, Meric SM, Crichlow EC, et al. Pharmacological relaxation of the urethra in male cats: a study of the effects of phenoxybenzamine, diazepam, nifedipine and xylazine. Can J Vet Res 1991;55:28–32.

119. Straeter-Knowlen IM, Marks SL, Rishniw M, et al. Urethral pressure response to smooth and skeletal muscle relaxants in anesthetized, adult male cats with naturally acquired urethral obstruction. Am J Vet Res 1995;56:919–23.

120. Fischer JR, Lane IF, Cribb AE. Urethral pressure profile and hemodynamic effects of phenoxybenzamine and prazosin in non-sedated male beagle dogs. Can J Vet Res 2003;67:30–8.

121. Haagsman AN, Kummeling A, Moes ME, et al. Comparison of terazosin and prazosin for treatment of vesico-urethral reflex dyssynergia in dogs. Vet Rec 2013;173:41.

122. Wolfe DL, Hsieh JT, Metha S. Rehabilitation practices and associated outcomes following spinal cord injury. In: Eng JJ, Teasell WC, Miller DL, et al, editors. Spinal cord injury rehabilitation evidence. 3rd edition. Harish Pai K; 2006. p. 3.1–3.44.

123. Drum MG. Physical rehabilitation of the canine neurologic patient. Vet Clin North Am Small Anim Pract 2010;40:181–93.

124. Blight AR. Cellular morphology of chronic spinal cord injury in the cat: analysis of myelinated axons by line-sampling. Neuroscience 1983;10:521–43.

125. Kloos AD, Fisher LC, Detloff MR, et al. Stepwise motor and all-or-none sensory recovery is associated with nonlinear sparing after incremental spinal cord injury in rats. Exp Neurol 2005;191:251–65.

126. Brown TG. The intrinsic factors in the progression of the mammal. Proc Roy Soc Lond 1911;84:308–19.

127. Barbeau H, Rossignol S. Recovery of locomotion after chronic spinalization in the adult cat. Brain Res 1987;412:84–95.

128. Eidelberg E, Story JL, Meyer BL, et al. Stepping by chronic spinal cats. Exp Brain Res 1980;40:241–6.

129. Lovely RG, Gregor RJ, Roy RR, et al. Effects of training on the recovery of full-weight-bearing stepping in the adult spinal cat. Exp Neurol 1986;92:421–35.

130. Morawietz C, Moffat F. Effects of locomotor training after incomplete spinal cord injury: a systematic review. Arch Phys Med Rehabil 2013;94:2297–308.

131. Vallani C, Carcano C, Piccolo G, et al. Postural pattern alterations in orthopaedics and neurological canine patients: postural evaluation and postural rehabilitation techniques. Vet Res Commun 2004;28(Suppl 1):389–91.

132. de Abreu DC, Cliquet A Jr, Rondina JM, et al. Electrical stimulation during gait promotes increase of muscle cross-sectional area in quadriplegics: a preliminary study. Clin Orthop Relat Res 2009;467:553–7.

133. Doucet BM, Lam A, Griffin L. Neuromuscular electrical stimulation for skeletal muscle function. Yale J Biol Med 2012;85:201–15.

134. Dean JC, Yates LM, Collins DF. Turning on the central contribution to contractions evoked by neuromuscular electrical stimulation. J Appl Physiol (1985) 2007;103:170–6.

135. Lagerquist O, Collins DF. Stimulus pulse-width influences H-reflex recruitment but not H(max)/M(max) ratio. Muscle Nerve 2008;37:483–9.

136. David E, Jayasree V, Ramakrishna O, et al. Effect of in vivo electrical stimulation on the carbohydrate metabolism of control and denervation atrophied muscle of dog, *Canis domesticus*. Indian J Physiol Pharmacol 1983;27:289–97.

137. Olby N, Levine J, Harris T, et al. Long-term functional outcome of dogs with severe injuries of the thoracolumbar spinal cord: 87 cases (1996–2001). J Am Vet Med Assoc 2003;222:762–9.
138. Scott HW, McKee WM. Laminectomy for 34 dogs with thoracolumbar intervertebral disc disease and loss of deep pain perception. J Small Anim Pract 1999;40:417–22.
139. Witsberger TH, Levine JM, Fosgate GT, et al. Associations between cerebrospinal fluid biomarkers and long-term neurologic outcome in dogs with acute intervertebral disk herniation. J Am Vet Med Assoc 2012;240:555–62.
140. Muguet-Chanoit AC, Olby NJ, Lim JH, et al. The cutaneous trunci muscle reflex: a predictor of recovery in dogs with acute thoracolumbar myelopathies caused by intervertebral disc extrusions. Vet Surg 2012;41:200–6.
141. Davis GJ, Brown DC. Prognostic indicators for time to ambulation after surgical decompression in nonambulatory dogs with acute thoracolumbar disk extrusions: 112 cases. Vet Surg 2002;31:513–8.
142. Anderson DK, Prockop LD, Means ED, et al. Cerebrospinal fluid lactate and electrolyte levels following experimental spinal cord injury. J Neurosurg 1976;44:715–22.
143. Bock P, Spitzbarth I, Haist V, et al. Spatio-temporal development of axonopathy in canine intervertebral disc disease as a translational large animal model for nonexperimental spinal cord injury. Brain Pathol 2013;23:82–99.
144. Levine GJ, Levine JM, Witsberger TH, et al. Cerebrospinal fluid myelin basic protein as a prognostic biomarker in dogs with thoracolumbar intervertebral disk herniation. J Vet Intern Med 2010;24:890–6.
145. Levine JM, Ruaux CG, Bergman RL, et al. Matrix metalloproteinase-9 activity in the cerebrospinal fluid and serum of dogs with acute spinal cord trauma from intervertebral disk disease. Am J Vet Res 2006;67:283–7.
146. Nagano S, Kim SH, Tokunaga S, et al. Matrix metalloprotease-9 activity in the cerebrospinal fluid and spinal injury severity in dogs with intervertebral disc herniation. Res Vet Sci 2011;91:482–5.
147. Nečas A, Sedláková D. Changes in the creatine kinase and lactate dehydrogenase activities in cerebrospinal fluid of dogs with thoracolumbar disc disease. Acta Vet Brno 1999;68:111–20.
148. Olby NJ, Sharp NJ, Munana KR, et al. Chronic and acute compressive spinal cord lesions in dogs due to intervertebral disc herniation are associated with elevation in lumbar cerebrospinal fluid glutamate concentration. J Neurotrauma 1999;16:1215–24.
149. Roerig A, Carlson R, Tipold A, et al. Cerebrospinal fluid tau protein as a biomarker for severity of spinal cord injury in dogs with intervertebral disc herniation. Vet J 2013;197:253–8.
150. Penning V, Platt SR, Dennis R, et al. Association of spinal cord compression seen on magnetic resonance imaging with clinical outcome in 67 dogs with thoracolumbar intervertebral disc extrusion. J Small Anim Pract 2006;47:644–50.
151. Ito D, Matsunaga S, Jeffery ND, et al. Prognostic value of magnetic resonance imaging in dogs with paraplegia caused by thoracolumbar intervertebral disk extrusion: 77 cases (2000–2003). J Am Vet Med Assoc 2005;227:1454–60.
152. Levine JM, Fosgate GT, Chen AV, et al. Magnetic resonance imaging in dogs with neurologic impairment due to acute thoracic and lumbar intervertebral disk herniation. J Vet Intern Med 2009;23:1220–6.

Perspectives on Meningoencephalomyelitis of Unknown Origin

Joan R. Coates, DVM, MS[a],*,
Nicholas D. Jeffery, BVSc, PhD, MSc, FRCVS[b]

KEYWORDS

- Necrotizing meningoencephalitis • Necrotizing leukoencephalitis
- Granulomatous meningoencephalomyelitis • Central nervous system
- Immune-mediated • Inflammatory • Immunomodulation

KEY POINTS

- Meningoencephalomyelitis of unknown origin (MUO) is a syndrome of idiopathic noninfectious central nervous system inflammatory diseases defined by their clinical presentation, advanced imaging characteristics, and cerebrospinal fluid analysis.
- Genetic and immune-mediated processes underlie the disease, but it likely has a multifactorial pathogenesis.
- Management is focused on remission of clinical signs through judicious use of immunosuppressive therapies, including glucocorticoids.
- Future studies on the therapeutic efficacy of different strategies using a more targeted approach may depend on identification of prognostic indicators and case stratification using molecular genetic discoveries.

INTRODUCTION

Recent advances in the understanding of noninfectious inflammatory diseases of the central nervous system (CNS) have resulted in an increasing subdivision of this parent category, each with its own specific name. The recognition that specific histologic subtypes cannot be identified on routine antemortem clinical tests has led to the use of an umbrella term: meningoencephalomyelitis of unknown origin (MUO). Because each of the subtype conditions has an extremely unwieldy name, there is

The authors have nothing to disclose.
[a] Department of Veterinary Medicine and Surgery, Veterinary Medical Teaching Hospital, College of Veterinary Medicine, University of Missouri, 900 East Campus Drive, Clydesdale Hall, Columbia, MO 65211, USA; [b] Department of Veterinary Clinical Sciences, Lloyd Veterinary Medical Center, College of Veterinary Medicine, Iowa State University, 1600 South 16th Street, Ames, IA 50011, USA
* Corresponding author.
E-mail address: Coatesj@missouri.edu

Vet Clin Small Anim 44 (2014) 1157–1185
http://dx.doi.org/10.1016/j.cvsm.2014.07.009   **vetsmall.theclinics.com**

a plethora of acronyms, and the resulting alphabet soup (which has even been exacerbated though differences in United States and United Kingdom spellings; explaining why this article uses the term "meningoencephalomyelitis of unknown origin" throughout) can be very confusing to navigate.

It is uncertain whether the various breed-specific idiopathic encephalitides of dogs that constitute the cases known as MUO are variations on a common etiologic theme or are truly distinct pathologic entities.[1–3] This review primarily focuses on providing an overview of the subtypes, illustrating how the differences in histopathologic classification and underlying neuroinflammatory responses may have relevance to the therapeutic approach and prognosis.

Clinical signs of noninfectious CNS inflammatory disorders are frequently very similar to those of infectious CNS diseases and even those of neoplasia. Diagnosis in the clinic therefore rests predominantly on advanced imaging, cerebrospinal fluid (CSF) analysis, and serologic tests designed to rule in or rule out infectious disease. In most cases, neoplastic lesions, which are generally unifocal, are easily differentiated from inflammatory disease, which are usually multifocal. Therefore, the major diagnostic decision is between infectious and noninfectious disease. Nowadays in the developed world, noninfectious inflammatory diseases of the CNS, which can affect the brain, spinal cord, and/or the meninges, are much more common.

MUO has long been assumed to have an autoimmune and genetic pathogenesis.[4] In general, major factors that contribute to the development of autoimmunity are genetic susceptibility and environmental factors (eg, infections, tissue injury). Nevertheless, a trigger factor is assumed to initiate signs of disease in each specific dog at a specific time.[5–8] Suspected agents include environmental or infectious antigenic triggers that might activate autoreactive cells in the CNS, although no such agent has yet been incriminated in the development of MUO.[9–12] Susceptibility genes may confer susceptibility or protection for autoimmunity by influencing the maintenance of self-tolerance. Data from inbred rodent studies have identified a strong influence of genetic background as a competing influence in the variability of lymphocyte responses in clearing pathogens from the CNS and promoting neuroprotection.[13–15]

Categorization of Noninfectious Inflammatory Disease of the CNS

Noninfectious inflammatory disease of the CNS can be divided into several subtypes, based mainly on the specific regions of the CNS that are affected and the specific histopathology (**Fig. 1**). These subtypes include steroid-responsive meningitis-arteritis (SRMA), eosinophilic meningoencephalitis, granulomatous meningoencephalomyelitis (GME), and necrotizing encephalitis (NE). SRMA, which affects the meninges only, and eosinophilic meningoencephalitis have fairly distinct disease signatures based on clinical presentation, CSF abnormalities, and histopathology,[16] and are not considered further here.

Recently, the term MUO has been introduced to encompass all clinically diagnosed (ie, dependent on advanced imaging and CSF analysis) cases of noninfectious inflammatory CNS disease.[4,17] MUO thus includes all the specific subtypes of noninfectious inflammatory disease that can be identified through histopathology, including GME, necrotizing meningoencephalitis (NME), necrotizing leukoencephalitis (NLE), and so forth, but does not include the diseases without evidence of overt CNS involvement (such as SRMA). NME and NLE are inflammatory disorders described with neuropathologic nomenclature reflective of the affected region of the brain. However, there is much overlap in clinical signs, signalment, and neuropathology for these conditions and, therefore, the more inclusive term NE, incorporating NME and NLE, is preferred for antemortem diagnosis.[4,18]

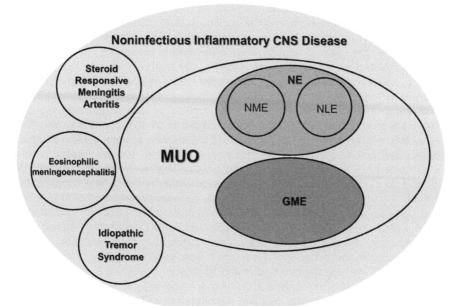

Fig. 1. Various noninfectious inflammatory central nervous system (CNS) diseases. Meningoencephalomyelitis of unknown origin (MUO) includes the necrotizing encephalidites, necrotizing leukoencephalitis (NLE) and necrotizing meningoencephalitis (NME), and granulomatous meningoencephalomyelitis (GME). Note that the noninfectious inflammatory CNS diseases, steroid-responsive meningitis arteritis, idiopathic tremor syndrome, and eosinophilic meningoencephalitis stand apart, with the distinctive disease signatures based on cerebrospinal fluid analysis or clinical signs.

AN OVERVIEW OF NEUROINFLAMMATION

Although many of the general features of CNS inflammation are similar to those affecting other body systems, an important feature of the CNS is its relative isolation from the peripheral immune system, which has important implications regarding the pathogenesis, diagnostic criteria, and therapy for inflammatory CNS diseases. The blood-brain barrier (BBB), usually understood to also include the blood–spinal cord barrier, implies that there is "gating" of the flow of cells and macromolecules from the systemic circulation to the CNS.[19] This selectively permeable barrier is formed through the influence of the endothelial cells and basement membrane, and the neighboring perivascular pericytes, glial cells (astrocytes, microglia), and neurons, and tends to temper the intensity of inflammatory responses within the CNS.[19–21] However, although the CNS traditionally has been considered immunologically privileged, current data confirm that the CNS is immunocompetent and actively interacts with the peripheral immune system.[22] In fact, peripheral inflammation can trigger a neuroinflammatory response involving BBB endothelia, glia, and neurons. Neuroinflammation is characterized by a broad range of immune responses, differing from peripheral inflammation primarily in the principal cells involved, most notably the astrocytes and microglia.[23]

Immune-Mediated CNS Disease

Autoimmune diseases arise from dysregulation of either or both of the innate and adaptive immune systems to produce inflammatory responses leading to cellular dysfunction and tissue destruction.[24,25] Innate immunity comprises immediate, nonspecific, short-term responses of the immune system usually triggered by distinctive pathogen-derived molecules, known as pathogen-associated molecular patterns (PAMPs) or, in the case of noninfectious inflammatory responses, by damage or danger-associated molecular patterns (DAMPs). By contrast the adaptive immune response, which involves humoral (antibody production) and cell-mediated immunity, is delayed but highly specific, and capable of memory responses.

CNS autoimmune disease responses are targeted at cellular components that are normally shielded, in part by the BBB. Infections or other antigens may also alter the way in which self-antigens are displayed to the immune system, leading to failure of self-tolerance and activation of self-reactive lymphocytes. Antigen-presenting cells may present CNS self-antigen (or foreign antigen that is similar to self-antigen) fragments to CNS-reactive T cells in peripheral lymph nodes where lymphocytes that traffic through the brain will ultimately arrive. Activated T cells then exit the lymph nodes, upregulate molecules that facilitate migration across the BBB,[26,27] and participate in a proinflammatory sequence of events within the CNS. Signals arising from injured neurons and surrounding glia create a milieu of cytokines that activate resident microglia and subsets of T cells.[23,28] Polarization of the response toward neurotoxicity or neuroprotection is dictated by altered activation states of 2 arms of the immune system: (1) T cells and (2) the microglia and infiltrating macrophages (**Fig. 2**). Once an autoimmune reaction develops, amplification mechanisms (eg, cytokines) promote activation of autoreactive lymphocytes, and release of self-antigens from damaged cells leads to epitope spreading and exacerbation of the disease.[24]

T-cell responses

Intra-CNS inflammatory responses tend to be dominated by mononuclear cells. All T cells express surface receptor cluster of differentiation (CD) 3 (CD3) antigen. CD4 surface receptor is found only on T-helper (Th) cells that can recognize and process antigens. CD8 surface receptor is only expressed on cytotoxic T cells that attack and kill abnormal cells. Classic major histocompatibility complex (MHC) class I molecules are required for $CD8^+$ T cells to recognize antigen, whereas CD4 is the receptor for MHC class II molecules on antigen-presenting cells. Cytotoxic and helper T-cell subsets and T-regulatory (Treg) cells are divergent in promotion of protective or deleterious responses to neuroinflammation, and are orchestrated through cytokine release.[29] Th-cell subsets modulate cytotoxicity and dictate anti-inflammatory (eg, Th2, Treg) or proinflammatory (eg, Th1, Th17) phenotypes.[30] Cytokine expression includes the interleukins (IL), interferons (IFN), and members of the tumor necrosis factor (TNF) family.

During disease, cytokines in the CNS exert proinflammatory and anti-inflammatory actions, and cause oxidative stress, neurotoxicity, apoptosis, astrogliosis and microglial activation.[22,29,31] For example, Th1 cells that secrete high levels of IFN-γ and TNF-α activate M1 microglia. Th2 and Treg cells tend to contribute to neuroprotection through cytokine mediators (eg, IL-4, IL-10, IL-13 via Th2) that drive M2 microglia and suppress cytotoxic T-cell function. Chemokines are small chemotactic cytokines that guide the migration of immune cells throughout the body, and are key molecules in promoting entry of immune cells into the CNS. Typically chemokines, such as monocyte chemoattractant protein 1 (MCP-1; CCL-2) or fractalkine (CX3CL), have very low physiologic concentrations within the CNS but are strongly upregulated in chronic neuroinflammation.[32,33] Such increased chemokine expression then attracts myeloid dendritic cells, monocytes, and activated T cells.[34,35]

Microglial responses

Microglia, the resident macrophages of the CNS, play a crucial role in the process of neuroinflammation. Microglia are derived from a specific embryonic myeloid cell population and invade the CNS during development,[36] where they exhibit regional variation. Microglia display functional plasticity during activation, which involves changes in cell number, morphology, and surface receptor expression, and production of growth factors and cytokines.[37–39] Microglia are the most prominent MHC-expressing cells in the CNS and are capable of processing and presenting antigen by expression of MHC classes I and II, and thereby have a bidirectional interaction with neurons and other microglia.[40] As with macrophages, the cytokine-mediated phenotype switch of microglia directs development of either a proinflammatory (M1) or anti-inflammatory phenotype (M2).[37,41–43] In response to cytokines (eg, high levels of IFN-γ) and other signaling molecules resulting from acute inflammation or injury, microglia are transformed from an inactivated to an activated phagocytic state, releasing proinflammatory mediators in the process.[28,39,44] M1 microglia increase secretion of proinflammatory cytokines such as TNF-α, IL-6, and IL-1β, reactive oxygen species (ROS), and nitric oxide (NO), and reduce the production of neurotrophic factors, all of which lead to cytotoxicity, astrocyte activation, and neurodegeneration. When induced by a variety of cytokines (eg, IL-4, IL-10) or immune complexes, M2 microglia reduce proinflammatory responses, and produce high levels of anti-inflammatory cytokines (eg, IL-10, transforming growth factor β) and neurotrophic factors.[41,45] The balance between M2 neuroprotective microglia and M1 neurotoxic microglia fluctuate according to the physiologic conditions they encounter during disease.[37,39,46] Despite advances in the understanding of microglia in the healthy dog, it remains unclear as to whether these cells respond to various disease states stereotypically or if they adapt their responses to the underlying pathologic conditions.[47] In many canine diseases, microglial markers are upregulated to varying degrees and the cells show enhanced phagocytosis.[48,49]

Histopathology of Neuroinflammation

Immunophenotyping for a variety of cellular markers in the MUOs can assist in determining the inflammatory signatures that influence perivascular and parenchymal hypercellularity, disease distribution between white and gray matter, and disease progression. Canine microglial cells share antigenic markers with macrophages, which has complicated identification of these cells, but the combined analysis of antigenicity, cell size, and cell complexity allows them to be distinguished. In dogs, several differences between resident microglia and infiltrating macrophages have been noted, along with topographic differences within the CNS.[49–51] Although both express CD18+, CD11b/c+, and CD45, microglia have lower levels of expression of CD45.[50] Moreover, stimulated microglia in healthy dogs generate lower levels of ROS.[49,51]

Neuroinflammation in MUO

Although neuroinflammation has been investigated in several spontaneous canine CNS diseases,[48,49,52–54] mechanisms still remain enigmatic for the MUOs. When the normal immune regulatory mechanisms of the CNS are rendered dysfunctional, for instance by age, pathogen exposure, or neurodegeneration, the threshold to initiate CNS inflammation and the ability of the CNS to direct immune effector functions will change.[22] Such alteration may also decrease neuroprotective responses and support controlled proinflammatory responses against pathogens and other insults. Knowledge of what dictates the predominance of neurotoxic or neuroprotective

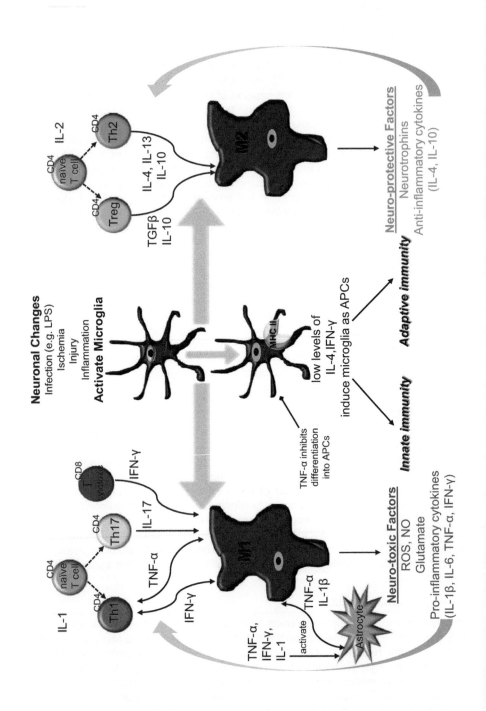

immunomodulation through cross-talk between the periphery (extraneural) and the CNS,[29,55] and how to limit cytotoxicity and enhance neuroprotection, would help identify appropriate targets for immune-based therapy.[56] Immunohistochemistry studies of the MUOs are summarized in **Table 1**.

SIGNALMENT, NEUROLOGIC SIGNS, AND HISTOPATHOLOGIC FEATURES

Clinical signs associated with GME and NE simply reflect the region of CNS involved; common presenting syndromes include meningoencephalitis, although signs vary widely, even including myelopathy alone.[57] Although the syndrome can affect any dog, small, female dogs aged between approximately 3 and 7 years are most commonly affected by all subtypes of MUO. Although there are some apparent breed predispositions for specific subtypes, those between GME and NE (for example) are indistinct; similar breeds are commonly affected and there are no differences in age or sex predilection between the 2 groups.[58] It is thought that the spectrum of pathologic lesions for the MUOs may represent combinations of genetic influences on the cascade of neuroinflammatory responses.[16]

Granulomatous Meningoencephalomyelitis

GME may represent up to 25% of all canine inflammatory CNS diseases.[16] Neurologic signs of GME are nonspecific and can be localized to forebrain, brainstem, or spinal cord, or appear as a multifocal syndrome.[58] The clinical presentation correlates with 3 pathologic distributions: multifocal (disseminated), focal, and ocular.[59,60] Multifocal GME typically is characterized clinically by acute onset and rapid progression of multifocal neurologic signs.[60–62] In the acute phase, dogs may have fever and exhibit paraspinal hyperesthesia, especially localizing to the cervical region.[59] By contrast, focal GME tends to have a more insidious or slower progression of neurologic signs that may suggest a space-occupying lesion,[59,60] with differential diagnoses including intracranial neoplasia. Forebrain and brainstem signs are reported most frequently with multifocal GME, whereas forebrain signs alone are more frequent with focal GME.[59,62] The third form, ocular GME, clinically manifests with acute signs of visual dysfunction attributable to optic neuritis and is sometimes considered one aspect of disseminated GME.[17,63–67] Anterior and posterior uveitis also can occur.[68]

GME is a distinct pathologic entity in which neuropathologic lesions consist of whorling, perivascular, disseminated, or focal infiltrates of mononuclear cells in the white matter and meninges of the brain and spinal cord (**Fig. 3**).[59,69,70] Originally GME was referred to as inflammatory or neoplastic reticulosis,[71,72] and reclassification as CNS lymphosarcoma or malignant histiocytosis is a viable alternative for some cases.[73] It appears that in acute progressive disease the gray and white matter is equally affected, whereas in more chronic GME white matter is predominantly

---

Fig. 2. A mechanism by which cytokines activate microglia, in response to neuronal changes that thereby promote neurotoxicity (*red*) or neuroprotection (*green*). Low levels of both IFN-γ and IL-4 can induce microglia to express MHC to function as APCs that mediate innate and adaptive immunity. This figure is a simplification of the neuroinflammatory processes based on interpretation of the current literature. The types of cellular responses to the milieu of cytokines/chemokines and cellular contact mechanisms are influenced by other environmental factors and differences between species. APCs, antigen-presenting cells; CD, cluster of differentiation; IFN, interferon; IL, interleukin; LPS, lipopolysaccharide; MHC, major histocompatibility complex; NO, nitric oxide; ROS, reactive oxygen species; TGF, transforming growth factor; Th, helper T cell; TNF, tumor necrosis factor; Treg, regulatory T cell.

Table 1
Summary of clinical and histologic characteristics of the meningoencephalitides of unknown origin

	GME	NME	NLE
Clinical signs	Multifocal (disseminated), focal and ocular; forebrain, hindbrain, spinal cord	Focal or multifocal forebrain; seizures most common	Focal or multifocal; forebrain and hindbrain signs
MR imaging characteristics	Multifocal or diffuse lesion hyperintensity on T2W and FLAIR sequences; variable T1W contrast enhancement; gray and white matter lesions; minimal meningeal enhancement; mass effect	Asymmetric, multifocal cerebrocortical gray and white matter lesions; lesions appear iso- to hypointense on T1W and hyperintense on T2W and FLAIR sequences; variable T1W contrast enhancement of parenchymal lesions; meningeal enhancement; mass effect; varying ventriculomegaly	Asymmetric cerebral white matter and brainstem lesions. Lesions appear iso- to hypointense on T1W and hyperintense on T2W and FLAIR sequences; minimal contrast enhancement of parenchymal lesions; lack of meningeal enhancement and mass effect; varying ventriculomegaly
Histologic characteristics	Whorling perivascular mononuclear cell infiltrates; white matter, meninges, spinal cord; acute lesions in gray and white matter; chronic lesions in white matter	Asymmetric extensive necrosis and cavitation; mononuclear infiltrates involve cerebral cortex, corona radiata, subcortical white matter; prominent reactive astrogliosis effacing areas of cavitation; inflammation can occur in brainstem and cerebellum; extensive leptomeningeal inflammation	Asymmetric extensive necrosis and cavitation; mononuclear infiltrate and prominent reactive astrogliosis effacing areas of cavitation; predominantly white matter; meninges minimally affected

| Immunohistochemistry characteristics | CD3 lymphocytes in perivascular cuffs, parenchymal granulomas, and leptomeninges; CD43 and CD45R$^+$ expression were low; expressions for B cells and plasma cells were low; strong MHC class II antigen expression observed in resting and activated T and B lymphocytes; MAC-387$^+$ common; CD163$^+$ macrophages, epithelioid cells more frequent in perivascular cuffs than in parenchymal lesions; CCR2 and highest in GME compared with NME and NLE; lysozyme$^+$ histiocytes[6,76,77] | GFAP$^+$ astrocytes distributed widely over cerebrum; CD3$^+$ lymphocytes scattered in meninges, perivascular cuffs, and brain lesions but less compared with GME; MAC-387$^+$ cells limited in NME but mainly in meninges and perivascular cuffs; lysozyme$^+$ cells faint compared with GME; expression of IFN-γ and CXCR3 highest in NME compared with NLE and GME. CD163+ macrophages localized in active inflammatory lesions perivascular cuffs and brain parenchyma[1,76,77] | Intralesional GFAP expression; CD3$^+$ T cells dominate in perivascular cuffing and in diffuse histiocytic and lymphocytic infiltrates; rare B cells; MAC-387$^+$ histiocytic cells were detected in lesions of Yorkshire terrier but few in French bulldog; IgG deposits in white matter associated with inflammation; faint labeling IgM and IgA; CD163$^+$ cells diffusely infiltrated the cerebral white matter[77,96,98] |

Abbreviations: CD, cluster of differentiation; FLAIR, fluid-attenuated inversion-recovery; GFAP, glial fibrillary acidic protein; GME, granulomatous meningoencephalomyelitis; IFN, interferon; IgA, -G, -M, immunoglobulin A, G, M; MHC, major histocompatibility complex; NLE, necrotizing leukoencephalitis; NME, necrotizing meningoencephalitis; T1W, T1-weighted; T2W, T2-weighted.

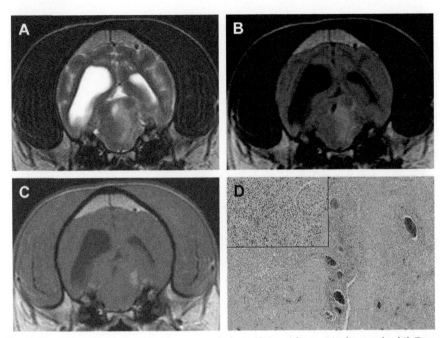

Fig. 3. Focal granulomatous meningoencephalomyelitis with ventriculomegaly. (*A*) Transverse T2-weighted magnetic resonance (MR) image at the level of the midbrain, caudal colliculi, and cerebral cortex. Diffuse and right-sided hyperintensity involving the central gray substance, brachium of caudal colliculus, reticular formation, medial lemniscus, and mass effect of the mesencephalic aqueduct. (*B*) Transverse, T2-weighted fluid-attenuated inversion-recovery (FLAIR) image at the same level as in *A*. Edema in the right midbrain is more conspicuous as a result of suppression of signal intensity in the mesencephalic aqueduct. (*C*) Transverse T1-weighted image at the same level as in *A* after intravenous administration of a gadolinium-based contrast medium. The lesion displays variable contrast enhancement. (*D*) Hematoxylin and eosin staining of multifocal perivascular infiltrates consisting of macrophages, histiocytes, plasma cells, and lymphocytes. There is whorling of mixed cell infiltrates around blood vessels (see inset). Original magnification 100×; inset 400× (*Courtesy of* Gayle C. Johnson, DVM, PhD, Columbia, MO.)

involved.[59] Multifocal granuloma can predominate in the cerebellum and brainstem with epithelioid cells in advanced stages,[6,69,74] and tryptase-positive mast cells have been found in the perivascular cuffs, meninges, and CNS parenchyma of dogs with acute forms of GME.[75] Focal lesions represent a coalescence of a large number of perivascular lesions, which commonly involve the pontomedullary region and cerebral white matter.[61,62,66,73] Kipar and colleagues[6] have suggested, based on a predominance of MHC class II and CD3+ T cells, that GME is a result of delayed type hypersensitivity. However, CD3+ immunoreactivity varies little between GME and NME or between GME and CNS histiocytosis.[74,76] Park and colleagues[77] also reported a tendency toward higher numbers of CD163+ macrophages in GME than in NME and NLE.

Necrotizing Encephalitis

NE is a subtype of MUO that appears histopathologically distinct from GME because of characteristic necrotic lesions in cerebral white or gray matter. The onset of neurologic signs of NE ranges from 6 months to 7 years of age but most commonly occurs in younger dogs with a mean age of 2.5 years.[58] In general, signs associated with NE are rapidly progressive and commonly include seizures, abnormal mentation, vestibulocerebellar dysfunction, central visual deficits, and death. Histology typical of the NEs includes nonsuppurative meningoencephalitis and bilaterally asymmetric cerebral necrosis (see **Fig. 4**). There are 2 subtypes of this category of lesion, namely NME and NLE, which appear to have considerable overlap in breed association and lesion distributions.

Necrotizing meningoencephalitis

NME was originally reported as a breed-specific disease in Pug dogs (Pug dog encephalitis),[78] and many other reports have followed.[76,79–84] NME has now also been reported in the Maltese,[76,84,85] Chihuahua,[1] Pekingese,[86] West Highland White Terrier,[87] Papillon,[3,76] Shih Tzu,[3,76] Coton de Tulear,[3] Brussels Griffon,[3] and other

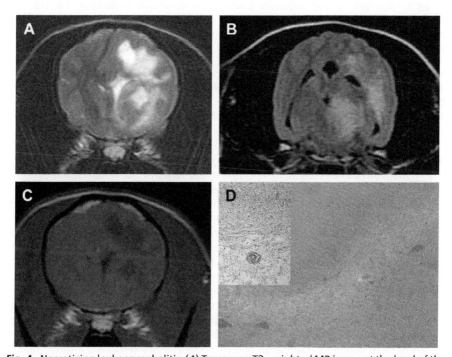

Fig. 4. Necrotizing leukoencephalitis. (*A*) Transverse T2-weighted MR image at the level of the caudate nucleus and cerebral cortex. Note the hyperintensity of the white matter (internal capsule, centrum semiovale, and corona radiate) of the right cerebrum. (*B*) Transverse T2-weighted FLAIR image at the level of the thalamus. Edema in the right centrum semiovale and internal capsule is more conspicuous as a result of suppression of signal intensity in the lateral ventricle. Edema is also noted in the region of the right thalamus. (*C*) Transverse T1-weighted image at the same level as in *A* after intravenous administration of a gadolinium-based contrast medium. The lesion displays mild peripheral contrast enhancement and hypointensity, suggestive of necrosis. (*D*) Hematoxylin and eosin staining of internal capsule with edema, dissolution of white matter, and multifocal perivascular cuffing of mostly lymphocytes. Multifocal small areas of white matter surrounding affected vessels are effaced and replaced by foamy macrophages, glial cells, and gemistocytic astrocytes (see inset). Original magnification 100×; inset 400× (*Courtesy of* Gayle C. Johnson, DVM, PhD, Columbia, MO.)

breeds.[4] Dogs with NME commonly manifest forebrain signs, especially seizures, because of lesions in the cerebral cortex.[3,58,80,82] Other forebrain signs include lethargy, anorexia, central blindness, circling, and head-pressing.[78,80] Cervical spinal hyperesthesia may be evident depending on the extent of leptomeningitis.[78]

The hallmark of NME is extensive necrosis, which varies in severity from neuronal necrosis and gliosis in the early stage to gross cavitation of parenchyma in advanced disease.[1,78,84] Lesions, dominated by plasma cells, lymphocytes, and histiocytes, commonly involve the leptomeninges, cerebral cortex, corona radiata, and subcortical white matter, and lead to loss of demarcation between gray and white matter.[78,84] Lesions are most common in the cerebrum, but have also been identified in the brainstem and cerebellum of Pugs and other breeds.[3,80] A distinctive segmental, multifocal pattern of intense meningitis and encephalitis is a consistent finding in Chihuahuas,[1] Maltese,[85] and Pug dogs.[78,83] Park and colleagues[88] divided the histopathologic lesions of NME dogs into 3 phases: mild inflammatory cell infiltration in the acute phase; moderate malacic changes and intense inflammatory reactions, especially in the leptomeninges, in the subacute phase; and extensive malacia in the chronic phase. Lesion topography also includes extensive leptomeningeal inflammation.[3,78,84] Immunohistochemistry studies of lesions in a small cohort of dogs with NME suggest that IFN-γ plays a major role in NME.[88]

Necrotizing leukoencephalitis

NLE has been described in Yorkshire terriers[89–94] and French Bulldogs[95,96] with differing clinical and topographic features. Clinically most dogs with NLE have presented with visual loss, seizures, and central vestibular signs reflecting forebrain and brainstem involvement.[89–91,93,95,96]

Histopathology of NLE is characterized by nonsuppurative leukoencephalitis with multiple necrotizing foci affecting the white matter of the forebrain and brainstem, with subsequent cavitary necrosis and prominent reactive gemistocytic astrogliosis (**Fig. 4**).[91,93,95–98] It is noteworthy that leptomeningeal involvement usually is minimal, in contrast to NME (see previous section). Neurons within gray matter appear to be unaffected despite parenchymal inflammation.[90,97] Areas of necrosis and cavitation with NLE are more extensive in comparison with NME, although the cavitation is less prominent in the brainstem and cerebellum. A recent report of NLE in the French Bulldog described inflammatory changes in the optic nerves and retina,[96] and one case report describes similar lesions in the spinal cord.[91] Spitzbarth and colleagues[96] demonstrated that a dominant T-cell response was associated with a marked upregulation of MHC class II expression, and that resident activated microglial cells rather than blood-derived macrophages play a central role as antigen-presenting and phagocytic cells in NLE of French Bulldogs. Similarly to GME, these findings are suggestive of local antigen presentation and possible immune-mediated inflammation.[6] However, these findings differ from those of GME, in which macrophages represent the dominant cell type of infiltrating lesions.[76,77,88]

DIAGNOSTIC EVALUATION

MUO is a clinical diagnosis based on neurologic examination, cross-sectional imaging findings, and CSF abnormalities, supplemented by exclusion of infectious diseases.[4,99] For this reason there is no specific noninvasive antemortem diagnostic test, and many other diseases can mimic the MUOs; definitive diagnosis of noninfectious inflammatory CNS disease requires histopathology.[16,100,101] However, Granger and colleagues[58] used a meta-analysis to formulate guidelines for establishing a presumptive diagnosis of MUO in the absence of histopathologic diagnosis (**Table 2**): In summary, most cases

Table 2
Proposed guidelines for diagnosis of meningoencephalomyelitis of unknown origin

Diagnostic Variables	Descriptions
Signalment	Dogs older than 6 mo
Magnetic resonance (MR) imaging findings	Multiple, single, or diffuse intra-axial hyperintense lesions on T2W MR images
Cerebrospinal fluid analysis	Pleocytosis with >50% mononuclear (monocytes/lymphocytes) cells and increased protein concentration
Infectious disease testing	Infectious diseases based on geographic area should be ruled out
Image-guided biopsy and histopathology	Stereotactic systems, ultrasound-guided, endoscopic-guided, free-hand computed tomography–guided

Adapted from Granger N, Smith PM, Jeffery ND. Clinical findings and treatment of noninfectious meningoencephalomyelitis in dogs: a systematic review of 457 published cases from 1962 to 2008. Vet J 2010;184:290–7; with permission.

diagnosed with MUO have multifocal neurologic signs, CSF mononuclear pleocytosis, and hyperintense lesions on T2-weighted (T2W) magnetic resonance (MR) imaging.[58]

Although some MR imaging features are common to the NEs and GME, none are considered specific for the diagnosis of any disease process. Moreover, the diagnostic efficiency of both CSF analysis and MR imaging is incomplete because some cases lack abnormalities in one or the other test.[1,58] Lamb and colleagues[102] determined that approximately 25% of brain MR images of dogs with an inflammatory CSF revealed no abnormalities, emphasizing that a normal brain MR image does not rule out CNS inflammatory disease.

Cross-Sectional Imaging

Before MR imaging became widely available, computed tomography (CT) provided some help in the diagnosis of inflammatory CNS disease, especially when combined with CSF analysis.[103] CT imaging characteristics of NE include multifocal areas of hypoattenuation, absence of mass effect, and lack of contrast enhancement.[89] CT abnormalities in GME consist of multifocal or focal distributions, mass effect associated with edema and granuloma, and ventricular asymmetry.[103,104] However, lesions may be difficult to detect using CT if they are located in the caudal fossa or lack contrast enhancement.

MR imaging is a recommended diagnostic tool for all dogs with possible CNS inflammatory disease. Compared with cerebral parenchyma, inflammatory lesions are hyperintense on T2W and fluid-attenuated inversion-recovery (FLAIR) sequences, variably hypointense to isointense on T1-weighted (T1W) sequences without contrast, and have variable degrees of contrast enhancement. Although T2W sequences are sensitive in detecting MUOs, MR imaging does not identify all MUO lesions and lacks specificity in distinguishing the different subtypes of MUO.[58,105] Use of a gadolinium-based paramagnetic contrast agent increases the sensitivity of T1W MR imaging for inflammatory parenchymal or meningeal lesions.[102,106] However, the FLAIR sequence has been reported to have higher sensitivity when compared with T2W and precontrast and postcontrast T1W sequences in detecting brain lesions in dogs with multifocal localization and abnormal CSF analysis.[107] The presence or absence of contrast enhancement with inflammatory CNS disease depends on the degree of BBB disruption or presence of vasodilation or neovascularization, and as such is a nonspecific finding associated with a variety of CNS diseases[102] and does not distinguish between specific infectious and noninfectious inflammatory diseases.[108] Moreover, lack of meningeal (ie, leptomeningeal) enhancement does not rule out meningeal disease that still can be evident on histopathology.[106,107] None the less, within the subtypes of MUO leptomeningeal enhancement is characteristic in Pug dogs[79,82] and other breeds[3] with NME, but is not a typical imaging feature of GME[107] or NLE.

The histologic characteristics that form the basis of the diagnosis of CNS disease cannot be determined using MR imaging, but a clinical diagnosis may be based on the pattern and number of lesions detected on MR images,[109] which can aid differentiation of intracranial neoplasia and meningoencephalitis.[102,104,107,110,111] Differential diagnoses for multifocal intracranial lesions include infectious meningoencephalitis, cerebrovascular lesions, CNS lymphosarcoma, and glial and metastatic neoplasms. A recent study determined that MR imaging is highly sensitive and specific for identifying brain lesions and classifying disease as inflammatory, but very poorly sensitive for diagnosing cerebrovascular disease.[104]

The most common MR imaging findings in GME include regions of multifocal or diffuse hyperintensity with irregular margins on T2W and FLAIR sequences in any part of the CNS, with variable enhancement after intravenous contrast is administered (see **Fig. 3**).[107,112] Although histopathologic lesions of GME typically are distributed primarily in the white matter, lesions on MR imaging are distributed throughout both gray and white matter[107]; mass effect with a suggestion of increased intracranial pressure also may be observed.[112]

NME is typically associated with asymmetric, multifocal cortical gray and white matter lesions with loss of gray/white matter demarcation and variable contrast enhancement; forebrain predilection, perilesional edema, mass effect, and irregular lesion margins are common.[1,79,82] Lesions appear isointense to hypointense on T1W images and hyperintense on T2W and FLAIR images,[3,79,113] and the mass effect may be sufficient to cause herniation.[1,3,79,82,113] However, although meningeal enhancement, mass effect, and ventricular dilation are frequent in Pugs with NME, NME and GME cannot be differentiated according to these features alone.[79,82] MR imaging characteristics of mass effect and contrast enhancement in NME also share similarities to those of neoplastic lesions; therefore, MR imaging findings common to NME lack specificity.[82,114,115] Increased lesion burden as evidenced on imaging in Pugs with NME has been correlated with increased disease time but not with prognosis.[82,116,117]

NLE lesions on MR imaging predominantly affect the subcortical white matter and brainstem.[91,94,96] Multifocal distribution of lesions and cavitation with mild to absent contrast enhancement in the brainstem are highly suggestive of NLE.[92,95,97] Affected areas appear hypointense on T1W images and hyperintense on T2W and FLAIR images (see **Fig. 4**).[90,97] The hyperintensity on FLAIR sequences within lesions likely reflects higher protein content in comparison with CSF. Varying degrees of ventriculomegaly also can be apparent.[90–92,95]

Especially for necrosis in the NEs, MR imaging can identify lesion topography reflective of the gross types of lesion associated with the different disorders.[1,82] It has been suggested that cavitary lesions, characterized by sharply demarcated T1W hypointensity and T2W and FLAIR hyperintensity without contrast enhancement, may be highly indicative of NE.[91,92,95] However, there was no such correlation in a study of Pug dogs with NME.[82] Brain MR imaging of dogs with chronic NE and necrosis showed widened sulci and dilation of the adjacent ventricle reflective of loss of tissue volume,[90,113] and there is a suggestion that necrotic lesions may imply disease chronicity.[91,116,118]

Cerebrospinal Fluid Analysis

Typically CSF analysis of MUOs reveals mononuclear pleocytosis and elevated protein concentration, both of which may vary considerably in severity. Increased protein concentration is a nonspecific indicator of CNS disease, typically caused by either BBB disruption or increased intrathecal immunoglobulin production. The CSF in GME has been described as containing a mild to moderate lymphocytic, neutrophilic, or mixed cell pleocytosis.[62,119] In dogs with NE, CSF analysis similarly typically consists of a moderate to marked lymphocytic pleocytosis with greater than 80% lymphocytes, but a mixed cell pleocytosis may occasionally be seen.[58,69,80,93] Although CSF analysis is more sensitive than MR imaging in identifying abnormalities consistent with inflammatory disease, normal CSF analysis has been described in cases with histopathologically confirmed inflammatory CNS disease.[5,16,58,75,80,107] Overall, CSF analysis is highly variable in the various types of MUOs but with little difference between these groups.[58,120]

Other analyses of CSF have been studied for CNS inflammatory diseases, but lack disease specificity. CSF protein composition can be further defined by semiquantitative electrophoretic techniques, and abnormalities have been reported to be useful in the identification of inflammatory, neoplastic, and degenerative disease.[121-123] For instance, CSF electrophoresis of dogs with GME may reveal an increase in β- and γ-globulins.[59,122] The lesser degree of BBB disturbance and increased intrathecal production of (autoreactive) immunoglobulins in dogs with chronic GME reflect the immune-mediated nature of the condition.[59] Antiastrocytic autoantibodies in canine CSF were suggested to be specific for NME and GME,[81,124,125] but this seems unlikely because antiastrocytic autoantibodies have also been detected in cases of brain tumors and in clinically normal dogs.[11,124] Flow cytometry and immunophenotyping has been used to identify mononuclear cells in the CSF of inflammatory disorders[126] and identification of lineages of neoplastic cells, but its practical use for CNS inflammatory disease is hindered by the need for large volumes (4–5 mL) of CSF unless the cell count is very high.

Brain Biopsy

A definitive diagnosis of CNS inflammatory disease is based on histopathology. Antemortem brain biopsy may yield a more definite diagnosis by which to guide treatment approaches, although such procedures depend on obtaining biopsy material from representative portions of the lesion. Minimally invasive techniques such as CT-guided[127-131] or MR-guided[132] stereotactic systems, free-handed techniques that use ultrasound,[133] CT,[134] or MR imaging,[101] and endoscopic-guided biopsy[135] have recently been developed for brain biopsy in dogs. Diagnostic accuracy of brain biopsy in canine CNS inflammatory disease ranges from 82% to 100%, based on the limited available data, and such information highly depends on the population disease types from which the biopsies were obtained.[101,127] Diagnostic yield for biopsy of inflammatory lesions may be influenced by sample size and difficulty in distinguishing between changes in the primary and secondary lesions such as edema and necrosis. Intraoperative cytologic evaluation of the biopsy sample may aid in diagnostic accuracy.[127,136] In addition to limitations in accuracy of diagnosis from biopsy, there are also risks that cannot be easily overlooked; a recent study suggested mortality and morbidity rates of 6% and 29%, respectively.[101]

Infectious Disease Testing

Infectious causes of meningoencephalomyelitis should also be investigated to help differentiate infectious meningoencephalomyelitis from the MUOs and neoplastic diseases.[99] Microbial culture of CSF has low yield, and culture of blood and urine may also be considered in cases of suspected bacterial infection.[137] More usefully, CSF, serum, or both can conveniently be analyzed for antibodies to infectious diseases, most notably *Neospora caninum*, *Ehrlichia* spp, *Anaplasma* spp, *Rickettsia rickettsia*, and *Coccidioides immitis*, although prevalent diseases vary with global location. Infection by *Cryptococcus* spp is usually detected by antigen testing, and other microbial DNA or RNA can also be detected by polymerase chain reaction (PCR) assays, which have high sensitivity and specificity.[8–10,99] Results should still be interpreted carefully to avoid false positives, and rigorous negative controls must be evaluated in parallel with the clinical sample. A negative PCR result needs to take into account that the nucleic acid may be present but at undetectable levels, the agent may be in the neural tissue but not in CSF, and the disorder may have been triggered by an agent that is no longer present.[99] Nonetheless, specific pathogens in CSF and diseased tissues have not been identified as being associated with the MUOs.[4,8–10]

Genetic Testing

Many autoimmune diseases are complex polygenic traits whereby affected individuals inherit multiple genetic polymorphisms that contribute to disease susceptibility, and consequently act with environmental factors to cause disease.[24] Although strong familial inheritance was reported in Pugs with NME, a simple Mendelian inheritance pattern could not be demonstrated.[138] Along with the wide range of age of onset and variable clinical course, this finding suggested the possibility of genetic modifiers or other influences contributing to the disease phenotype.[80,138] Genome-wide association studies identified CFA 12 near the dog leukocyte antigen (DLA) complex with the development of NME,[12,139] and this region was subsequently focused on the region containing *DLA- DRB1*, *-DQA1*, and *-DQB1* genes.[12] Although the causative mutation had not been identified, fine mapping and candidate gene sequencing implicated linked-allelic homozygosity in the risk of developing NME.[12] Furthermore, it is possible to attain risk assessments for NME by sequencing only the *DQB1* gene that is now being used as a susceptibility haplotype when in the homozygous state.[140] Such findings strongly support the role of the immune system in NME. The strong DLA class II association of NME in Pugs resembles that of atypical variant/fulminant forms in the disease spectrum of human multiple sclerosis (MS).[12] A widely held concept is that MS occurs when certain environmental exposures (eg, viruses), or lack thereof (eg, sunlight and vitamin D), trigger the activation of CNS autoreactive T cells in genetically susceptible individuals, which leads to a CNS inflammatory disease[141,142]; therefore a similar pathogenesis is suspected for NME in Pugs.

TREATMENT

Once infectious causes have been ruled out, the primary treatment of the MUOs is immunosuppression with corticosteroids or other agents. Initial treatment begins with patient stabilization based on severity of neurologic dysfunction followed by maintenance therapy. If there are seizures, anticonvulsant therapy is also required. Stabilization may necessitate supplementary oxygen for hypoxemia, crystalloid/colloid support to maintain cerebral perfusion and control hypotension, and osmotic therapy (eg, mannitol, hypertonic saline) to reduce elevated intracranial pressure.

Immunosuppression is central to the therapeutic management of MUO, despite the incompletely understood pathogenic mechanisms or triggers. The rationale of immunosuppression for autoimmune diseases is to induce disease remission through the inhibition of inflammation and modulation of lymphocyte function.[143] The ultimate goal is to achieve disease remission while minimizing adverse effects. Corticosteroids historically have been the first-line therapy for the treatment of MUO. Often anti-inflammatory to immunosuppressive doses of corticosteroids (eg, prednisone, 0.25–0.5 mg/kg by mouth daily) are initiated until review of negative infectious disease testing, and then increased to immunosuppressive doses (2–4 mg/kg by mouth daily) for 2 to 4 weeks; after which the dose is gradually reduced or tapered every 4 weeks when clinical signs stabilize or improve. The ultimate goal is alternate-day therapy at the lowest effective dose to maintain remission of clinical signs or discontinuation of the drug.[144] Animals often will respond initially, but relapses are common; sustaining remission thus may require long-term high-dose corticosteroids, or administration of alternative immunosuppressive agents whereby the undesirable side effects of high-dose corticosteroid therapy can be avoided. Adverse effects of high-dose corticosteroids include gastric ulceration, steroid hepatopathy, alopecia, urinary tract infection, muscle weakness, and iatrogenic hyperadrenocorticism (see the article on corticosteroid therapy elsewhere in this issue by Jeffery).

Reported second-line immunosuppressive drug therapies for MUO include leflunomide,[145] procarbazine,[146] cytosine arabinoside,[17,147–152] lomustine,[144,153] mycophenolate mofetil,[154] azathioprine[155]; COP[149] (cyclophosphamide, vincristine, prednisone), and cyclosporine (**Table 3**).[118,155–159] Radiation therapy has also proved to be effective for focal GME lesions.[62] Not uncommonly, second-line therapies may be introduced early in the disease process in response to severe neurologic signs or rapid neurologic deterioration. Many of these secondary immunosuppressive agents have potential risks for myelosuppression, hepatotoxicity, gastrointestinal disturbances, and other drug-specific systemic effects; therefore, regular monitoring of complete blood count and serum biochemistry is recommended. A systematic review suggested a benefit, based on median survival, of prednisone combined with other immunosuppressive agents.[58] Overall median survival for dogs treated with corticosteroids plus a second-line immunosuppressive protocol ranged from 240 to 590 days. By comparison, survival in dogs treated with corticosteroids alone ranged from 28 to 357 days. However, in dogs with GME and NE, oral administration of lomustine and prednisolone or prednisolone alone had similar efficacy.[144]

Selection of a specific immunosuppressive protocol depends on the clinician's decision, the patient's clinical status, and the pet owner's financial considerations. In accordance with guidelines from other studies,[17,147,148,151] a common protocol is daily administration of prednisone at an immunosuppressive dose combined with cytosine arabinoside administered at 50 mg/m^2 every 12 hours as a subcutaneous bolus for 2 consecutive days, or by intravenous infusion at 200 mg/m^2 over 8 hours. The treatment cycle is repeated every 3 to 4 weeks for 3 cycles. Subsequently the interval between treatment cycles is increased by 1 week for 3 cycles at the new treatment interval. The treatment cycles are gradually extended to every 6 weeks. Concurrently the dose of prednisone is gradually tapered to a low-dose administration every other day. Intravenous administration of cytosine arabinoside has been described at higher doses (up to 600 mg/m^2) in severe cases of MUO.[152,160] The route of cytosine arabinoside administration and protocol likely to be most effective has been controversial. A pharmacokinetic study comparing subcutaneous bolus administration versus intravenous infusion revealed that based on Fick's first law of diffusion, intravenous infusion may produce a more prolonged exposure of cytosine arabinoside at cytotoxic levels in plasma in comparison with the concentrations after subcutaneous administration.[161] However, further study in dogs with MUO is needed to identify whether the sustained concentrations produced by intravenous infusion would improve penetration of cytosine arabinoside across the BBB and produce higher

Table 3
Summary of immunomodulatory therapies for meningoencephalomyelitis of unknown origin

Drug[a]	Mechanisms of Action	Dosages
Azathioprine[155]	Alters purine metabolism by inhibiting DNA synthesis and mitosis; chromosome breaks; interferes with lymphocyte proliferation, reduces lymphocyte numbers, decreased T-cell–dependent antibody synthesis	2 mg/kg PO, every 24 h for 2 wk, then decrease to 2 mg/kg every 48 h indefinitely; goal is to achieve alternate-day therapy with prednisone
Cyclosporine[155–159]	Inhibits T-cell activation through intracellular target calcineurin; decreases IL-2 and other cytokines preventing proliferation of T-cell and B lymphocytes; also decreases IL-3, IL-4, and TNF-α	3–15 mg/kg PO every 12 h; or 5–12 mg/kg PO every 24 h when used in combination with ketoconazole 8 mg/kg PO every 24 h. Therapeutic target: trough levels between 200 and 400 ng/mL
Cyclophosphamide, vincristine, prednisone (COP)[149]	Cyclophosphamide is alkylating agent; introduces alkyl radicals into DNA strands of cells Vincristine inhibits microtubule function and leads to a disruption in the mitotic spindle causing metaphase arrest and cytotoxicity	Cyclophosphamide: 50 mg/m^2 PO, every 48 h for 8 wk, then given in alternate weeks Vincristine: 0.5 mg/m^2 IV, every 7 d for 8 wk, then every 14 d Prednisone: 40 mg/m^2 PO, every 24 h for 7 d, then 20 mg/m^2 every 48 h for 7 wk, then same dose given in alternate weeks
Cytosine arabinoside[17,147–152]	Inhibits DNA polymerase; causes topoisomerase dysfunction and prevents DNA repair; cell cycle (S phase)	50 mg/m^2 SC, every 12 h for 2 consecutive days, then repeat every 3 wk for 4 cycles; treatment interval is lengthened by 1 wk every 4 cycles with a maximum interval of 6–8 wk Alternatively dose at same interval using IV infusion at 200 mg/m^2 over 8 h
Leflunomide[145]	Pyrimidine synthesis inhibitor; tyrosine kinase inhibition; targets B and T lymphocytes	1.5–4.0 mg/kg PO every 24 h and adjusted based on blood levels (20–40 μg/mL)
Lomustine[144,153]	Alkylating agent; induction of intrastrand and interstrand DNA cross-linking; suppresses B- and T-cell proliferation	60 mg/m^2 PO every 6 wk
Mycophenolate mofetil[154]	Purine synthesis inhibitor; selective to lymphocytes (B and T) via depletion of guanosine and deoxyguanosine nucleotides; suppresses dendritic cell maturation and reduces monocyte recruitment	Initial dose of 10–20 mg/kg PO every 12 h (lower dose, eg, 5 mg/kg, may be administered if concern for gastrointestinal side effects); after 1 mo reduce to 5–10 mg/kg every 12 h

(continued on next page)

Table 3 *(continued)*		
Drug[a]	**Mechanisms of Action**	**Dosages**
Prednisone[151]	Targets macrophages via downregulating Fc receptor expression, decreases responsiveness to antibody-sensitized cells and decreases antigen processing; suppresses T-cell function and induces apoptosis of T cells; inhibits B-cell antibody production	1 to 2 mg/kg PO, every 12 h for 3–4 wk; 0.5–1 mg/kg every 12 h for 6 wk, then 0.25–0.5 mg/kg every 12 h for 3 wk, then 0.25–0.5 mg/kg every 24 h for 3 wk, then 0.25–0.5 mg/kg every 48 h indefinitely
Procarbazine[146]	T-cell specific; monoamine oxidase inhibitor; cell cycle nonspecific with cytotoxicity in the S and G2 phases, DNA methylation, and free radical production	25–50 mg/m^2 PO every 24 h

Abbreviations: IL, interleukin; IV, intravenously; PO, by mouth; SC, subcutaneously; TNF, tumor necrosis factor.
[a] Immunomodulatory drugs are administered in combination with prednisone, which is gradually tapered.
Data from Refs.[17,144–159]

efficacy for the treatment of MUO. Alternative approaches include prolonged use of oral leflunomide or cyclosporine in combination with prednisone tapered over approximately 6 to 12 weeks.

Treatment effect often is monitored by clinical response and resolution of neurologic deficits, and occasional repeated CSF analysis and MR imaging. Serial MR imaging has been used to monitor resolution of clinical signs or evolution of lesions in dogs with meningoencephalitis.[91,102,116,117] In a small cohort of dogs presumptively diagnosed with MUO, Lowrie and colleagues[151] suggested that a combination of MR imaging and CSF analysis provided greater sensitivity for predicting relapse than one modality alone, although an abnormal CSF analysis at the 3-month reexamination, despite normal MR imaging findings, was associated with an increased risk of relapse. However, discontinuing treatment before MR-identified lesions resolved always resulted in relapse, suggesting that treatment can be tapered according to MR imaging or CSF findings.

PROGNOSIS

Prognostic indicators and effects of the treatment of MUO have not been well characterized, but typically focus on the underlying disease process and severity of clinical signs. Focal forebrain lesions have been associated with a significantly longer survival time than those with multifocal/disseminated or brainstem lesions,[62] although subsequent studies have been unable to corroborate this finding.[146,151] Dogs presenting specifically with seizures have been found to have a significantly reduced survival time.[162] However, selection bias for (poor) prognosis also exists for series of dogs that must include a postmortem diagnosis, and may account for some reports of poor prognosis.[62,146] None the less, approximately 15% of dogs with GME die even before being treated.[58]

MR imaging may offer a broader assessment by which to guide therapy in dogs with MUO. MR imaging abnormalities of foramen magnum herniation, loss of cerebral sulci, or mass effect attributable to MUO have been associated with reduced survival time.[151] By contrast, postcontrast hyperintense lesions, rostral fossa involvement, caudal fossa involvement, and transtentorial herniation were not associated with mortality.[151] Lowrie and colleagues[151] also determined that none of the described MR imaging findings was associated with relapse or was predictive of long-term outcome. Others investigating MR imaging findings also report that contrast enhancement or lesion burden was not predictive of survival time.[82,94] Familiarity with MR imaging and CSF abnormalities indicating a poorer prognosis may facilitate more aggressive therapy and follow-up in these patients to improve survival.[151] However, these prognostic variables need further validation in the context of more tightly controlled prospective studies.

Determining prognosis based on the treatment effect for recovery in dogs with MUOs is challenging because of the difficulty in making definitive diagnoses, disease heterogeneity, treatment variability, and low sample size.[57,58] Outcomes described in dogs treated for MUO by various treatment regimens often are based on survival time, and the probability of long-term survival increases with increased disease duration.[149] Of note, Pugs with NE only receiving an anticonvulsant had mean survival intervals similar to those for dogs with other subsets of MUO.[58,80] Described risk factors in determining outcome or relapse are often based on post hoc analyses with multiple comparisons of low case numbers, which increases the potential for type I error, low power, and inability to take into account other confounding influences (eg, pet owner's decision, concurrent medical problems, financial considerations, indications to treat). Validated outcome measures (eg, neurodisability score) specific for the MUOs are needed to allow novel treatments to be tested objectively over a relatively short time scale.[149] There is still a need for a gold-standard treatment against which a new treatment can be tested. Although the criterion-referenced standard for a clinical trial is a randomized, placebo-controlled, double-blinded, prospective study, it is generally accepted that use of a placebo control treatment group is unethical because dogs with MUO have a poor outcome without treatment.[62,146] Nevertheless, treatment trials comparing 1 or more protocols would be simple to establish, although they would require multicenter collaboration. The lack of data acquisition using well-designed clinical trials means that treatment recommendations for MUO still remain empiric. It will be important to expand our understanding of the pathogenesis of MUO to enable the development of more targeted therapies for improved survival times and sustained remission.

REFERENCES

1. Higgins RJ, Dickinson PJ, Kube SA, et al. Necrotizing meningoencephalitis in five chihuahua dogs. Vet Pathol 2008;45:336–46.
2. Higgins RJ, LeCouteur RA. GME, NME, and breed specific encephalitis and allied disorders: Variations of the same theme or different diseases? A clinical and pathological perspective. 20th Annual Symposium of the European College of Veterinary Neurology. Bern (Switzerland), September 27–29, 2007. p. 35–7.
3. Cooper JJ, Schatzberg SJ, Vernau KM, et al. Necrotizing meningoencephalo-myelitis in atypical dog breeds: a case series and literature review. J Vet Intern Med 2014;28:198–203.
4. Talarico LR, Schatzberg SJ. Idiopathic granulomatous and necrotising inflammatory disorders of the canine central nervous system: a review and future perspectives. J Small Anim Pract 2010;51:138–49.

5. Thomas JB, Eger C. Granulomatous meningoencephalomyelitis in 21 dogs. J Small Anim Pract 1989;30:287–93.
6. Kipar A, Baumgartner W, Vogl C, et al. Immunohistochemical characterization of inflammatory cells in brains of dogs with granulomatous meningoencephalitis. Vet Pathol 1998;35:43–52.
7. Schwab S, Herden C, Seeliger F, et al. Non-suppurative meningoencephalitis of unknown origin in cats and dogs: an immunohistochemical study. J Comp Pathol 2007;136:96–110.
8. Schatzberg SJ, Haley NJ, Barr SC, et al. Polymerase chain reaction screening for DNA viruses in paraffin-embedded brains from dogs with necrotizing meningoencephalitis, necrotizing leukoencephalitis, and granulomatous meningoencephalitis. J Vet Intern Med 2005;19:553–9.
9. Barber RM, Li Q, Diniz PP, et al. Evaluation of brain tissue or cerebrospinal fluid with broadly reactive polymerase chain reaction for *Ehrlichia, Anaplasma*, spotted fever group *Rickettsia, Bartonella*, and *Borrelia* species in canine neurological diseases (109 cases). J Vet Intern Med 2010;24:372–8.
10. Barber RM, Porter BF, Li Q, et al. Broadly reactive polymerase chain reaction for pathogen detection in canine granulomatous meningoencephalomyelitis and necrotizing meningoencephalitis. J Vet Intern Med 2012;26:962–8.
11. Matsuki N, Fujiwara K, Tamahara S, et al. Prevalence of autoantibody in cerebrospinal fluids from dogs with various CNS diseases. J Vet Med Sci 2004;66: 295–7.
12. Greer KA, Wong AK, Liu H, et al. Necrotizing meningoencephalitis of pug dogs associates with dog leukocyte antigen class II and resembles acute variant forms of multiple sclerosis. Tissue Antigens 2010;76:110–8.
13. Tsunoda I, Kuang LQ, Theil DJ, et al. Antibody association with a novel model for primary progressive multiple sclerosis: induction of relapsing-remitting and progressive forms of EAE in H2s mouse strains. Brain Pathol 2000;10:402–18.
14. Kipnis J, Yoles E, Schori H, et al. Neuronal survival after CNS insult is determined by a genetically encoded autoimmune response. J Neurosci 2001;21: 4564–71.
15. Kipnis J, Mizrahi T, Hauben E, et al. Neuroprotective autoimmunity: naturally occurring CD4+CD25+ regulatory T cells suppress the ability to withstand injury to the central nervous system. Proc Natl Acad Sci U S A 2002;99:15620–5.
16. Tipold A. Diagnosis of inflammatory and infectious diseases of the central nervous system in dogs: a retrospective study. J Vet Intern Med 1995;9:304–14.
17. Zarfoss M, Schatzberg S, Venator K, et al. Combined cytosine arabinoside and prednisone therapy for meningoencephalitis of unknown aetiology in 10 dogs. J Small Anim Pract 2006;47:588–95.
18. Tipold A, Vandevelde M, Schatzberg SJ. Necrotizing encephalitis. In: Greene CE, editor. Infectious diseases of the dog and cat. 4th edition. St Louis (MO): Elsevier; 2012. p. 856–8.
19. Cardoso R, Brites D, Brito MA. Looking at the blood-brain barrier: molecular anatomy and possible investigation approaches. Brain Res Rev 2010;64: 328–64.
20. Engelhardt B, Sorokin L. The blood-brain and the blood-CSF barriers: function and dysfunction. Semin Immunopathol 2009;31:497–511.
21. Abbott NJ, Ronnback L, Hansson E, et al. Astrocyte–endothelial interactions at the blood–brain barrier. Nat Rev Neurosci 2006;7:41–53.
22. Carson MJ, Doose JM, Melchior B, et al. CNS immune privilege: hiding in plain sight. Immunol Rev 2006;213:48–65.

23. Lyman M, Lloyd DG, Sunming J, et al. Neuroinflammation: the role and consequences. Neurosci Res 2014;79:1–12.

24. Abbas AK, Lichtman AH, Pillai S. Cellular and molecular immunology. St Louis (MO): Elsevier; 2012.

25. Gershwin LJ. Autoimmune diseases in small animals. Vet Clin North Am Small Anim Pract 2010;40(3):439–57.

26. Ransohoff RM, Kivisakk P, Kidd G. Three or more routes for leukocyte migration into the central nervous system. Nat Rev Immunol 2003;3:569–81.

27. Lyck R, Engelhardt B. Going against the tide – how encephalitogenic T cells breach the blood-brain barrier. J Vasc Res 2012;49:497–509.

28. Smith JA, Das A, Ray SK, et al. Role of pro-inflammatory cytokines released from microglia in neurodegenerative diseases. Brain Res Bull 2012;87:10–20.

29. Kierschensteiner M, Meinl E, Holfeld R. Neuro-immune crosstalk in CNS diseases. Neuroscience 2009;158:1122–32.

30. Hendrix S, Nitsch R. The role of T helper cells in neuroprotection and regeneration. J Neuroimmunol 2007;184:100–12.

31. Wang CX, Shuaib A. Involvement of inflammatory cytokines in central nervous system injury. Prog Neurobiol 2002;67:161–72.

32. Sokolova A, Hill MD, Rahimi F, et al. Monocyte chemoattractant protein-1 plays a dominant role in the chronic inflammation observed in Alzheimer's disease. Brain Pathol 2009;19:392–8.

33. Cardona AE, Pioro EP, Sasse ME, et al. Control of microglial neurotoxicity by the fractalkine receptor. Nat Neurosci 2006;9:917–24.

34. Carr MW, Roth SJ, Luther E, et al. Monocyte chemoattractant protein 1 acts as a T-lymphocyte chemoattractant. Proc Natl Acad Sci U S A 1994;91:3652–6.

35. Taub DD, Proost P, Murphy WJ, et al. Monocyte chemotactic protein-1 (MCP-1), -2, and -3 are chemotactic for human T lymphocytes. J Clin Invest 1995;95:1370–6.

36. Neumann H, Wekerle H. Brain microglia: watchdogs with pedigree. Nat Neurosci 2013;16:253–5.

37. Ransohoff RM, Perry VH. Microglial physiology: unique stimuli, specialized responses. Annu Rev Immunol 2009;27:119–45.

38. Biber K, Owens T, Boddeke E. What is microglia neurotoxicity (not?). Glia 2014;62:841–54.

39. Carson MJ, Bilousova TV, Puntambekar SS, et al. A rose by any other name? The potential consequences of microglial heterogeneity during CNS health and disease. Neurotherapeutics 2007;4:571–9.

40. Suzumura A. Neuron-microglia interaction in neuroinflammation. Curr Protein Pept Sci 2013;14:16–20.

41. Michelucci A, Heurtaux T, Grandbarbe L, et al. Characterization of the microglial phenotype under specific pro-inflammatory and anti-inflammatory conditions: effects of oligomeric and fibrillar amyloid-beta. J Neuroimmunol 2009;210:3–12.

42. Geissmann F, Auffray C, Palframan R, et al. Blood monocytes: distinct subsets, how they relate to dendritic cells, and their possible roles in the regulation of T cell responses. Immunol Cell Biol 2008;86:398–408.

43. Martinez FO, Sica A, Mantovani A, et al. Macrophage activation and polarization. Front Biosci 2008;13:453–61.

44. Dheen ST, Kaur C, Ling EA. Microglial activation and its implications in the brain diseases. Curr Med Chem 2007;14:1189–97.

45. Benoit M, Benoit D, Mege JL. Macrophage polarization in bacterial infections. J Immunol 2008;181:3733–9.

46. Schwartz M, Butovsky O, Bruck W, et al. Microglial phenotype: is the commitment reversible. Trends Neurosci 2006;29:68–74.
47. Stein VM, Puff C, Genini S, et al. Variations on brain microglial gene expression of MMPs, RECK and TIMPs in inflammatory and non-inflammatory diseases in dogs. Vet Immunol Immunopathol 2011;144:17–26.
48. Stein VM, Baumgartner W, Kreienbrock L, et al. Canine microglial cells: stereotypy in immunophenotype and specificity in function? Vet Immunol Immunopathol 2006;113:277–87.
49. Boekhoff TM, Ensinger EM, Calrson R, et al. Microglial contribution to secondary injury evaluated in a large animal model of human spinal cord trauma. J Neurotrauma 2012;29:1000–11.
50. Stein VM, Czub M, Hansen R, et al. Characterization of canine microglial cells isolated ex vivo. Vet Immunol Immunopathol 2004;99:73–85.
51. Ensinger EM, Boekhoff TM, Carlson R, et al. Regional topographical differences of canine microglial immunophenotype and function in the healthy spinal cord. J Neuroimmunol 2010;227:144–52.
52. Spitzbarth I, Baumgartner W, Beineke A. The role of pro- and anti-inflammatory cytokines in the pathogenesis of spontaneous canine diseases. Vet Immunol Immunopathol 2012;147:6–24.
53. Beineke A, Markus S, Borlak J, et al. Increase of pro-inflammatory cytokine expression in non-demyelinating early cerebral lesions in nervous canine distemper. Viral Immunol 2008;21:401–10.
54. Beineke A, Puff C, Seehusen F, et al. Pathogenesis and immunopathology of systemic and nervous canine distemper. Vet Immunol Immunopathol 2009; 127:1–18.
55. Appel SH, Beers DR, Henkel JS. T cell-microglial dialogue in Parkinson's disease and amyotrophic lateral sclerosis: are we listening? Trends Immunol 2009;31:7–17.
56. Schwartz M, Kipnis J. Protective autoimmunity and neuroprotection in inflammatory and noninflammatory neurodegenerative diseases. J Neurol Sci 2005;233: 163–6.
57. Griffin JF, Levine JM, Levine GJ, et al. Meningomyelitis in dogs: a retrospective review of 28 cases (1999-2007). J Small Anim Pract 2008;49:509–17.
58. Granger N, Smith PM, Jeffery ND. Clinical findings and treatment of non-infectious meningoencephalomyelitis in dogs: a systematic review of 457 published cases from 1962 to 2008. Vet J 2010;184:290–7.
59. Sorjonen DC. Clinical and histopathological features of granulomatous meningoencephalomyelitis in dogs. J Am Anim Hosp Assoc 1990;26:141–7.
60. Braund KG. Granulomatous meningoencephalitis. J Am Vet Med Assoc 1985; 186:138–41.
61. Russo ME. Primary reticulosis of the central nervous system in dogs. J Am Vet Med Assoc 1979;174:492–500.
62. Munana KR, Luttgen PJ. Prognostic factors for dogs with granulomatous meningoencephalomyelitis: 42 cases (1982–1996). J Am Vet Med Assoc 1998;212: 1902–6.
63. Fischer CA, Liu SK. Neuro-ophthalmologic manifestations of primary reticulosis of the central nervous system in a dog. J Am Vet Med Assoc 1971;158:1240–8.
64. Smith J, DeLahunta A, Riss R. Reticulosis of the visual system in a dog. J Small Anim Pract 1977;18:643–52.
65. Garmer N, Naeser P, Bergman A. Reticulosis of the eyes and the central nervous system in a dog. J Small Anim Pract 1981;22:39–45.

66. Cuddon PA, Smith-Maxie L. Reticulosis of the central nervous system in the dog. Compend Contin Educ Vet Prac 1984;6:23–32.

67. Kitagawa M, Okada M, Toshihiro W, et al. Ocular granulomatous meningoencephalomyelitis in a dog: magnetic resonance images and clinical findings. J Vet Med Sci 2009;71:233–7.

68. Smith R. A case of ocular granulomatous meningoencephalitis in a German Shepherd dog presenting as bilateral uveitis. Aust Vet Pract 1995;25:76–8.

69. Cordy DR. Canine granulomatous meningoencephalomyelitis. Vet Pathol 1979; 16:325–33.

70. Braund KG, Vandevelde M, Walker TL. Granulomatous meningoencephalomyelitis in six dogs. J Am Vet Med Assoc 1978;172:1195–200.

71. Fankhauser R, Fatzer R, Luginbuhl H. Reticulosis of the central nervous system (CNS) in dogs. Adv Vet Sci Comp Med 1972;16:35–72.

72. Koestner A. Primary lymphoreticuloses of the nervous system in animals. Acta Neuropathol Suppl 1975;6:85–9.

73. Vandevelde M, Fatzer R, Fankhauser R. Immunohistological studies on primary reticulosis of the canine brain. Vet Pathol 1981;18:577–88.

74. Suzuki M, Uchida K, Morozumi M, et al. A comparative pathological study on granulomatous meningoencephalomyelitis and central malignant histiocytosis in dogs. J Vet Med Sci 2003;65:1319–24.

75. Demierre S, Tipold A, Griot-Wenk ME, et al. Correlation between the clinical course of granulomatous meningoencephalomyelitis in dogs and the extent of mast cell infiltration. Vet Rec 2001;148:467–72.

76. Suzuki M, Uchida K, Morozumi M, et al. A comparative pathological study on canine necrotizing meningoencephalitis and granulomatous meningoencephalomyelitis. J Vet Med Sci 2003;65:1233–9.

77. Park ES, Uchida K, Nakayama H. Comprehensive immunohistochemical studies on canine necrotizing meningoencephalitis (NME), necrotizing leukoencephalitis (NLE), and granulomatous meningoencephalomyelitis (GME). Vet Pathol 2012; 49:682–92.

78. Cordy DR, Holliday TA. A necrotizing meningoencephalitis of pug dogs. Vet Pathol 1989;26:191–4.

79. Flegel T, Henke D, Boettcher IC, et al. Magnetic resonance imaging findings in histologically confirmed pug dog encephalitis. Vet Radiol Ultrasound 2008;49: 419–24.

80. Levine JM, Fosgate GT, Porter B, et al. Epidemiology of necrotizing meningoencephalitis in pug dogs. J Vet Intern Med 2008;22:961–8.

81. Uchida K, Hasegawa T, Ikeda M, et al. Detection of an autoantibody from Pug dogs with necrotizing encephalitis (pug dog encephalitis). Vet Pathol 1999;36:301–7.

82. Young B, Levine JL, Fosgate A, et al. Magnetic resonance imaging characteristics of necrotizing meningoencephalitis in pug dogs. J Vet Intern Med 2009;23(3):527–35.

83. Kobayashi Y, Ochiai K, Umemura T, et al. Necrotizing meningoencephalitis in pug dogs in Japan. J Comp Pathol 1994;110:129–36.

84. Summers BA, Cummings JF, de Lahunta A. Veterinary neuropathology. St Louis (MO): Mosby; 1995.

85. Stalis IH, Chadwick B, Dayrell-Hart B, et al. Necrotizing meningoencephalitis of Maltese dogs. Vet Pathol 1995;32:230–5.

86. Cantile C, Chianini F, Arispici M, et al. Necrotizing meningoencephalitis associated with cortical hippocampal hamartia in a Pekingese dog. Vet Pathol 2001;38:119–22.

87. Aresu L, D'Angelo A, Zanatta R, et al. Canine necrotizing encephalitis associated with antiglomerular basement membrane glomerulonephritis. J Comp Pathol 2007;136:279–82.
88. Park ES, Uchida K, Nakayama H. Th1-, Th2-, and Th17-related cytokine and chemokine receptor mRNA and protein expression in the brain tissues, T cells, and macrophages of dogs with necrotizing and granulomatous meningoencephalitis. Vet Pathol 2013;50:1127–34.
89. Ducote JM, Johnson KE, Dewey CW, et al. Computed tomography of necrotizing meningoencephalitis in 3 Yorkshire terriers. Vet Radiol Ultrasound 1999;40: 617–21.
90. Jull BA, Merryman JI, Thomas WB, et al. Necrotizing encephalitis in a Yorkshire terrier. J Am Vet Med Assoc 1997;211:1005–7.
91. Kuwamura M, Adachi T, Yamate J, et al. Necrotising encephalitis in the Yorkshire terrier: a case report and literature review. J Small Anim Pract 2002;43: 459–63.
92. Sawashima Y, Sawashima K, Aura Y, et al. Clinical and pathological findings of a Yorkshire terrier affected with necrotizing encephalitis. J Vet Med Sci 1996;58: 659–61.
93. Tipold A, Fatzer R, Jaggy A, et al. Necrotizing encephalitis in Yorkshire terriers. J Small Anim Pract 1993;34:623–8.
94. von Praun F, Matiasek K, Grevel V, et al. Magnetic resonance imaging and pathologic findings associated with necrotizing encephalitis in two Yorkshire terriers. Vet Radiol Ultrasound 2006;47:260–4.
95. Timmann D, Konar M, Howard J, et al. Necrotising encephalitis in a French bulldog. J Small Anim Pract 2007;48:339–42.
96. Spitzbarth I, Schenk HC, Tipold A, et al. Immunohistochemical characterization of inflammatory and glial responses in a case of necrotizing leucoencephalitis in a French bulldog. J Comp Pathol 2010;142:235–41.
97. Lotti D, Capucchio T, Gaidolfi E, et al. Necrotizing encephalitis in a Yorkshire terrier: clinical imaging, and pathological findings. Vet Radiol Ultrasound 1999;40:622–6.
98. Lezmi S, Toussaint Y, Prata D, et al. Severe necrotizing encephalitis in a Yorkshire terrier: topographic and immunohistochemical study. J Vet Med A Physiol Pathol Clin Med 2007;54:186–90.
99. Nghiem PP, Schatzberg SJ. Conventional and molecular diagnostic testing for the acute neurologic patient. J Vet Emerg Crit Care (San Antonio) 2010;20: 46–61.
100. Thomas WB. Inflammatory diseases of the central nervous system in dogs. Clin Tech Small Anim Pract 1998;13:167–78.
101. Flegel T, Oevermann A, Oechtering G, et al. Diagnostic yield and adverse effects of MRI-guided free-hand brain biopsies through a mini-burr hole in dogs with encephalitis. J Vet Intern Med 2012;26:969–76.
102. Lamb CR, Croson PJ, Cappellow R, et al. Magnetic resonance imaging findings in 25 dogs with inflammatory cerebrospinal fluid. Vet Radiol Ultrasound 2005;46: 17–22.
103. Plummer SB, Wheeler SJ, Thrall DE, et al. Computed tomography of primary inflammatory brain disorders in dogs and cats. Vet Radiol Ultrasound 1992; 33:307–12.
104. Speciale J, Van Winkle TJ, Steinberg SA, et al. Computed tomography in the diagnosis of focal granulomatous meningoencephalitis: retrospective evaluation of three cases. J Am Anim Hosp Assoc 1992;28:327–32.

105. Wolff CA, Holmes SP, Young BD, et al. Magnetic resonance imaging for the differentiation of neoplastic, inflammatory, and cerebrovascular brain disease in dogs. J Vet Intern Med 2012;26:589–97.

106. Keenihan EK, Summers BA, David FH, et al. Canine meningeal disease: associations between magnetic resonance imaging signs and histologic findings. Vet Radiol Ultrasound 2013;54:504–15.

107. Cherubini GB, Platt SR, Anderson TJ, et al. Characteristics of magnetic resonance images of granulomatous meningoencephalomyelitis in 11 dogs. Vet Rec 2006;159:110–5.

108. Mellema LM, Samii VF, Vernau KM, et al. Meningeal enhancement on magnetic resonance imaging in 15 dogs and 3 cats. Vet Radiol Ultrasound 2002;43:10–5.

109. Vite CH, Cross JR. Correlating magnetic resonance findings with neuropathology and clinical signs in dogs and cats. Vet Radiol Ultrasound 2011; 52(Suppl 1):S23–31.

110. Lobetti RG, Pearson J. Magnetic resonance imaging in the diagnosis of focal granulomatous meningoencephalitis in two dogs. Vet Radiol Ultrasound 1996; 37:424–7.

111. Kitagawa M, Kanayama K, Satoh T, et al. Cerebellar focal granulomatous meningoencephalitis in a dog: clinical findings and MR imaging. J Vet Med A Physiol Pathol Clin Med 2004;51:277–9.

112. Cherubini GB, Platt SR, Howson S, et al. Comparison of magnetic resonance imaging sequences in dogs with multi-focal intracranial disease. J Small Anim Pract 2008;49(12):634–40.

113. Kuwabara M, Tanaka S, Fujiwara K. Magnetic resonance imaging and histopathology of encephalitis in a Pug. J Vet Med Sci 1998;60:1353–5.

114. Cherubini GB, Mantis P, Martinez TA, et al. Utility of magnetic resonance imaging for distinguishing neoplastic from non-neoplastic brain lesions in dogs and cats. Vet Radiol Ultrasound 2005;46:384–7.

115. Rodenas S, Pumarola M, Gaitero L, et al. Magnetic resonance imaging findings in 40 dogs with histologically confirmed intracranial tumours. Vet J 2011;187: 85–91.

116. Kitagawa M, Okada M, Kanayama K, et al. A canine case of necrotizing meningoencephalitis for long-term observation: clinical and MRI findings. J Vet Med Sci 2007;69:1195–8.

117. Hasegawa T. Long-term management of necrotizing meningoencephalitis in a Pug dog. Canine Pract 2000;25:20–2.

118. Jung DI, Kang BT, Park C, et al. A comparison of combination therapy (cyclosporine plus prednisolone) with sole prednisolone therapy in 7 dogs with necrotizing meningoencephalitis. J Vet Med Sci 2007;69:1303–6.

119. Bailey C, Higgins R. Characteristics of cerebrospinal fluid associated with canine meningoencephalomyelitis: a retrospective study. J Am Vet Med Assoc 1986;188:418–21.

120. Bohn AA, Wills TB, West CL, et al. Cerebrospinal fluid analysis and magnetic resonance imaging in the diagnosis of neurologic disease in dogs: a retrospective study. Vet Clin Pathol 2006;35:315–20.

121. Tipold A, Pfister H, Zurbriggen A, et al. Intrathecal synthesis of major immunoglobulin classes in inflammatory diseases of the canine CNS. Vet Immunol Immunopathol 1994;42:149–59.

122. Sorjonen DC. Cerebrospinal fluid electrophoresis. Use in canine granulomatous meningoencephalomyelitis. Veterinary Medicine Report 1989;1:399–403.

123. Sorjonen DC. Total protein, albumin quota, and electrophoretic patterns in cerebrospinal fluid of dogs with central nervous system disorders. Am J Vet Res 1987;48:301–5.
124. Shibuya M, Matsuki N, Fujiwara K, et al. Autoantibodies against glial fibrillary acidic protein (GFAP) in cerebrospinal fluids from Pug dogs with necrotizing meningoencephalitis. J Vet Med Sci 2007;69:241–5.
125. Toda Y, Matsuki N, Shibuya M, et al. Glial fibrillary acidic protein (GFAP) and anti-GFAP autoantibody in canine necrotising meningoencephalitis. Vet Rec 2007;161:261–4.
126. Duque C, Parent J, Bienzle D. The immunophenotype of blood and cerebrospinal fluid mononuclear cells in dogs. J Vet Intern Med 2002;16:714–9.
127. Koblik PD, LeCouteur RA, Higgins RJ, et al. CT-guided brain biopsy using a modified Pelorus Mark III stereotactic system: experience with 50 dogs. Vet Radiol Ultrasound 1999;40:434–40.
128. Moissonnier P, Bordeau W, Delisle F, et al. Accuracy testing of a new stereotactic CT-guided brain biopsy device in the dog. Res Vet Sci 2000;68:243–7.
129. Flegel T, Podell M, March PA, et al. Use of a disposable real-time CT stereotactic navigator device for minimally invasive dog brain biopsy through a mini-burr hole. AJNR Am J Neuroradiol 2002;23:1160–3.
130. Giroux A, Jones JC, Bøhn JH, et al. A new device for stereotactic CT-guided biopsy of the canine brain: design, construction, and needle placement accuracy. Vet Radiol Ultrasound 2002;43:229–36.
131. Troxel MT, Vite CH. CT-guided stereotactic brain biopsy using the Kopf stereotactic system. Vet Radiol Ultrasound 2008;49:438–43.
132. Chen AV, Wininger FA, Frey S, et al. Description and validation of a magnetic resonance imaging-guided stereotactic brain biopsy device in the dog. Vet Radiol Ultrasound 2012;53:150–6.
133. Thomas WB, Sorjonen DC, Hudson JA, et al. Ultrasound-guided brain biopsy in dogs. Am J Vet Res 1993;54:1942–7.
134. Harari J, Moore MM, Leathers CW, et al. Computed tomographic-guided free-hand needle biopsy of brain tumors in dogs. Progress Vet Neurology 1994;4:41–4.
135. Klopp LS, Ridgway M. Use of an endoscope in minimally invasive lesion biopsy and removal within the skull and cranial vault in two dogs and one cat. J Am Vet Med Assoc 2009;234:1573–7.
136. Vernau KM, Higgins RJ, Bollen AW, et al. Primary canine and feline nervous system tumors: Intraoperative diagnosis using the smear technique. Vet Pathol 2001;38:47–57.
137. Radaelli ST, Platt SR. Bacterial meningoencephalomyelitis in dogs: a retrospective study. J Vet Intern Med 2002;16:159–63.
138. Greer KA, Schatzberg SJ, Porter BF, et al. Heritability and transmission analysis of necrotizing meningoencephalitis in the pug. Res Vet Sci 2009;86(3):438–42.
139. Barber RM, Schatzberg SJ, Corneveaux JJ, et al. Identification of risk loci for necrotizing meningoencephalitis in pug dogs. J Hered 2011;102(S1): S40–46.
140. Pedersen N, Liu H, Millon L, et al. Dog leukocyte antigen class II-associated genetic risk testing for immune disorders of dogs: simplified approaches using Pug dog necrotizing meningoencephalitis as a model. J Vet Diagn Invest 2011; 23:68–76.
141. Storch MK, Bauer J, Linington C, et al. Cortical demyelination can be modeled in specific rat models of autoimmune encephalomyelitis and is major

histocompatibility complex (MHC) haplotype-related. J Neuropathol Exp Neurol 2006;65:1137–42.

142. Bar-Or A. The immunology of multiple sclerosis. Semin Neurol 2008;28:29–45.

143. Viviano KR. Update on immunosuppressive therapies for dogs and cats. Vet Clin Small Anim 2013;43:1149–70.

144. Flegel T, Boettcher IC, Matiasek K, et al. Comparison of oral administration of lomustine and prednisolone or prednisolone alone as treatment for granulomatous meningoencephalomyelitis or necrotizing encephalitis in dogs. J Am Vet Med Assoc 2011;238:337–45.

145. Gregor CR, Stewar A, Sturges B, et al. Leflunomide effectively treats naturally occurring immune-mediated and inflammatory diseases of dogs that are unresponsive to conventional therapy. Transplan Proceed 1998;30:4143–8.

146. Coates JR, Barone G, Dewey CW, et al. Procarbazine as adjunctive therapy for treatment of dogs with presumptive antemortem diagnosis of granulomatous meningoencephalomyelitis: 21 cases (1998–2004). J Vet Intern Med 2007;21:100–6.

147. Nuhsbaum MT, Powell CC, Gionfriddo JR, et al. Treatment of granulomatous meningoencephalomyelitis in a dog. Vet Ophthalmol 2002;5:29–33.

148. Menaut P, Landart J, Behr S, et al. Treatment of 11 dogs with meningoencephalomyelitis of unknown origin with a combination of prednisolone and cytosine arabinoside. Vet Rec 2008;162:241–5.

149. Smith PM, Stalin CE, Shaw D, et al. Comparison of two regimens for the treatment of meningoencephalomyelitis of unknown etiology. J Vet Intern Med 2009;23:520–6.

150. Behr S, Llabres-Dias FJ, Radaelli ST. Treatment of meningoencephalitis of unknown origin in a dog. Vet Rec 2009;164:627–9.

151. Lowrie M, Smith PM, Garosi L. Meningoencephalitis of unknown origin: investigation of prognostic factors and outcome using a standard treatment protocol. Vet Rec 2013;172:527–34.

152. de Stefani A, De Risio L, Matiasek K. Intravenous cytosine arabinoside in the emergency treatment of 9 dogs with central nervous system inflammatory disease of unknown etiology. In: 20th Annual Symposium of the European College of Veterinary Neurology. Bern (Switzerland), 2007. p. 508.

153. Uriarte JL, Thibaud K, Gnirs S. Lomustine treatment in noninfectious meningoencephalitis in 8 dogs. In: 20th Annual Symposium of the European College of Veterinary Neurology. Bern (Switzerland), 2007. p. 508.

154. Feliu-Pascual AL, Matiasek K, de Stefani A, et al. Efficacy of mycophenolate mofetil for the treatment of presumptive granulomatous meningoencephalomyelitis: preliminary results. In: 20th Annual Symposium of the European College of Veterinary Neurology. Bern (Switzerland), 2007. p. 509.

155. Wong MA, Hopkins AL, Meeks JC, et al. Evaluation of treatment with a combination of azathioprine and prednisone in dogs with meningoencephalomyelitis of undetermined etiology: 40 cases (2000-2007). J Am Vet Med Assoc 2010;237:929–35.

156. Gnirs K. Ciclosporin treatment of suspected granulomatous meningoencephalitis in three dogs. J Small Anim Pract 2006;47:201–6.

157. Adamo PF, Rylander H, Adams WM. Cyclosporin use in multidrug therapy for meningoencephalomyelitis of unknown aetiology in dogs. J Small Anim Pract 2007;48(9):486–96.

158. Adamo FP, O'Brien RT. Use of cyclosporine to treat granulomatous meningoencephalitis in three dogs. J Am Vet Med Assoc 2004;225:1211–6.

159. Pakozdy A, Leschnik M, Kneissl S, et al. Improved survival time in dogs with suspected GME treated with ciclosporin. Vet Rec 2009;164:89–91.
160. Scott-Moncrieff JC, Chan TC, Samuels ML, et al. Plasma and cerebrospinal fluid pharmacokinetics of cytosine arabinoside in dogs. Cancer Chemother Pharmacol 1991;29:13–8.
161. Crook KI, Early PJ, Messenger KM, et al. The pharmacokinetics of cytarabine in dogs when administered via subcutaneous and continuous intravenous infusion rates. J Vet Pharmacol Ther 2013;36:408–11.
162. Bateman SW, Parent JM. Clinical findings, treatment, and outcome of dogs with status epilepticus or cluster seizures: 156 cases (1990-1995). J Am Vet Med Assoc 1999;215:1463–8.

Biomarkers for Neural Injury and Infection in Small Animals

Hidetaka Nishida, DVM, PhD

KEYWORDS

- Biomarker • Diagnosis • Infectious disease testing • Neural injury • Prognosis
- Small animals

KEY POINTS

- Biomarkers can assist in understanding the cause, diagnosis, severity, and prognosis for neural injury.
- Integration of conventional testing and new diagnostic techniques will overcome current shortcomings in understanding CNS infectious diseases.
- Diagnostic tests may be limited because of poor positive and negative predictive values, which must be recognized when interpreting test results.

NEURAL INJURY MARKERS

Introduction

Cross-sectional imaging techniques such as computed tomography (CT) and magnetic resonance imaging (MRI) have become more widely available to veterinarians during the past quarter of a century and have facilitated diagnosis of central nervous system (CNS) diseases. However, there is still frequently a lack of definition of the cause of neurologic lesions, because tissue sampling from the pathologic site is often difficult and there are few clinical diagnostic tools to assist diagnosis. A biomarker is a potential option to improve current shortcomings.

A biomarker is a characteristic that can be objectively measured as an indicator of a physiologic or pathologic process or a response to a therapeutic intervention.[1] Biomarkers can be associated with each step of gene-to-protein processing or metabolites that are produced during subsequent intracellular reactions and can be expected to aid in understanding the cause, diagnosis, severity, prediction, or outcome of treatments. Molecular biological techniques have advanced rapidly in

The author reports no financial or other conflicts relevant to this article.
Institute for Regenerative Medicine, Texas A&M Health Science Center, College of Medicine at Scott & White, 5701 Airport Road, Module C, Temple, TX 76502, USA
E-mail address: nishida@medicine.tamhsc.edu

recent years allowing emergence of the so-called omics technologies of genomics, proteomics, and metabolomics, which has increased the opportunities for developing efficient biomarkers. The omics techniques allow the simultaneous analysis of many candidate molecules and allow selection of disease-specific biomarkers through comparison between groups of healthy and disease-affected animals. Candidates can subsequently be further investigated to determine whether they are clinically useful.

Blood, urine, cerebrospinal fluid (CSF), and tissue samples from the pathologic site have been the main source of biomarkers for CNS disease. Blood and urine are easily collected but CNS tissues and CSF sampling are more difficult and can incur the risk of significant morbidity. However, the blood-brain barrier (BBB) presents a highly selective barrier, which means that pathologic processes in the CNS are not necessarily reflected in the blood, unless its permeability is increased.

Diagnostic Testing

Diagnostic accuracy depends on 2 parameters (**Fig. 1**): sensitivity and specificity. Sensitivity is the identification of true-positives, and specificity indicates true-negatives; both are conventionally expressed as proportions or percentages. The relationship between sensitivity and specificity can be shown using the receiver-operating characteristic (ROC) curve. Poor to fair biomarkers have area under the curve (AUC) values ranging between 0.5 and 0.8, good markers have AUC values between 0.8 and 0.9, and excellent markers have AUC values between 0.9 and 1.0. Positive predictive value (PPV) is the percentage of patients with a positive test that have the disease and negative predictive value (NPV) is the percentage of patients with a negative test that do not have the disease (**Box 1**).

Limitations of Biomarkers

An ideal biomarker specifically and sensitively reflects a disease state and can be used for diagnosing, determining prognosis, and monitoring disease progression during therapy. Although a large number of studies have reported new biomarkers for predicting prognosis with spinal cord injury (SCI) and brain tumors, none are ideal in terms of accuracy and availability. The transfer of biomarkers from discovery to clinical practice encounters many obstacles.

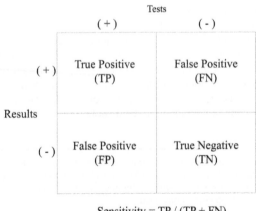

$$\text{Sensitivity} = \text{TP} / (\text{TP} + \text{FN})$$
$$\text{Specificity} = \text{TN} / (\text{FP} + \text{TN})$$

Fig. 1. Diagnostic accuracy depends on 2 parameters: sensitivity and specificity.

Box 1
Key points regarding biomarkers

- Biomarkers can provide an indication of physiologic and pathologic changes in the CNS.
- Diagnostic accuracy depends on sensitivity and specificity.

One of the limitations of biomarkers is that they may detect the physiologic and pathologic changes in the body resulting from a disease process but they do not detect the disease itself. For example, CSF matrix metalloproteinase (MMP)-9 activity is increased in the CSF of dogs with thoracolumbar intervertebral disc herniation (IVDH)[2] but is also increased in the CSF of dogs with visceral leishmaniasis[3] or meningiomas.[4] Increased MMP-9 in the CSF suggests an inflammatory state within the CNS but does not provide specific evidence that the process is the result of any specific lesion. It is therefore useless as a diagnostic test, but potentially extremely useful as a prognostic biomarker.

Although diagnostic accuracy depends on sensitivity and specificity, they do not directly apply to many clinical situations, because they do not predict the certainty with which a diagnosis will be made.[5] These parameters are determined in research that uses a reference standard to confirm the true disease status,[6] and sensitivity and specificity calculated against a poor reference standard may be inaccurate. The common way to recruit patients for biomarker studies is to use case-control sampling, in which a group of diseased patients is compared with a group of nondiseased patients. However, this method does not eliminate uncertainty regarding the rate of false-positive results. For rare diseases, erroneous results may be obtained because it is not known how often false-positives occur because the number of true-positives is small. PPV provides information about the likelihood of the diseases, but it cannot be derived from 1 population sample alone.[7]

Variability is a major concern. Biomarker studies are normally conducted on body fluid or tissue samples collected from patients and healthy subjects of a range of ages, sexes, and breeds. It is also important that difference in types and locations of the lesions can affect the results.

The timing for sampling and measuring biomarkers is crucial to accurate interpretation. For example, the serum ubiquitin C-terminal hydrolase-L1 level is most reliably associated with traumatic brain injury (TBI) of human patients when measured within the first 6 hours after injury, but accuracy decreases markedly thereafter.[8] For use in prognostication, useful biomarkers should accurately track the likely course of disease in patients that are not treated (**Box 2**).[9]

There are 2 major ways to discover useful biomarkers in small animal practice. First, candidate biomarkers already investigated in other species can be applied to small animals. Second, comprehensive analysis such as genomics, proteomics, and

---

Box 2
Key points regarding limitations of biomarkers

- Sensitivity and specificity do not always generalize to all clinical situations.
- Signalment and characteristics of lesions (eg, locations and types of lesions) can affect the results of biomarkers.
- The timing for sampling is crucial for accurate interpretation.

---

metabolomics can allow selection of disease-specific biomarkers. A summary of biomarkers that have been investigated in a range of canine CNS diseases is given later. They are largely being investigated for their use as prognostic tools, but many are still in the developmental stage.

Neuron-specific enolase

Neuron-specific enolase (NSE) was initially found in the cytoplasm of neurons, but it is also localized in neuroendocrine cells, oligodendrocytes, thrombocytes, and erythrocytes. It is released from damaged neurons as a result of ischemia, multiple sclerosis, SCI, and TBI, in rodent models and human patients.[10–13] Therefore, an increase of the CSF NSE might be useful for detecting evidence of neuronal damage in the CNS.

CSF NSE concentrations are increased in dogs with GM1 gangliosidosis[14] and in dogs with meningoencephalitis.[15] However, at present there is not sufficient evidence to use it as a diagnostic test in practice because it does not aid in differentiating different causes of neuronal injury.

Myelin basic protein

Myelin basic protein (MBP) is produced by oligodendrocytes and is a major constituent of the axonal myelin sheath, and is therefore predicted to be a marker of white matter injury. It has been detected in the CSF of humans with multiple sclerosis, SCI, and TBI.[12,13,16]

In dogs, a potential use for this marker is in defining important differences in severity of SCI, especially within the thoracolumbar region (where white matter injury is of predominant importance in determining prognosis). In accordance with that notion, CSF MBP concentration was higher in dogs with thoracolumbar IVDH that had an unsuccessful long-term outcome than in those with a successful long-term outcome.[17] Furthermore, a CSF MBP concentration of 3 ng/mL had a sensitivity of 78% and specificity of 76% for predicting a successful outcome after thoracolumbar IVDH (although values of 50% can be achieved through a coin flip). The area under the ROC curve was estimated as 0.688, which is rated as reasonable. The CSF MBP concentration did not correlate with the T2-weighted (T2W) hyperintensity with the SCI, which is also known to be associated with functional outcome in dogs with thoracolumbar IVDH.[18,19]

In an effort to improve the value of this test, an investigation was made into combining these results with those available from CSF creatine kinase (CK) measurements. Successful long-term functional recovery occurred in 98% of cases when CSF CK activity was less than or equal to 38 U/L and MBP concentration was less than or equal to 3 ng/mL.[20] Therefore, combined use of CK and MBP might have value in predicting outcome after the SCI caused by thoracolumbar IVDH. However, to be clinically useful they need to show either greater diagnostic accuracy than simple physical assessment (eg, deep pain testing) or show that they could add value to the discrimination already available via physical examination. Furthermore, developments in testing technology to allow kennel-side testing will eventually be required.

It is also feasible that estimation of CSF MBP levels might aid in antemortem diagnosis of degenerative myelopathy, because affected animals have increased levels compared with controls.[21] Nevertheless, the same caveats apply: increases in MBP occur in any white matter disease, and so they may not aid in discrimination between degenerative myelopathy and other lesions, such as chronic cord compression.

Glial fibrillary acidic protein

Glial fibrillary acidic protein (GFAP) is a monomeric intermediate filament protein found in astrocytes that forms an important cellular component in maintaining the BBB. In humans, GFAP levels in blood and CSF increase with CNS diseases such as Alzheimer disease, multiple sclerosis, SCI, stroke, and TBI.[10–13,22]

Serum GFAP was investigated for potential diagnosis of progressive myelomalacia[23]; 8 of 51 dogs had clinical signs suggesting progressive myelomalacia, of which 6 were positive and 2 were negative for GFAP in the serum. The sensitivity and specificity of serum GFAP for progressive myelomalacia were 75% and 97.7%, respectively. Therefore, this report suggested that the clinical assessment was more sensitive than serum GFAP; the question remains as to whether serum GFAP may increase before the onset of clinical signs.

Dogs with necrotizing meningoencephalitis (NME) have been shown to have increased levels of GFAP compared with naive controls and those affected by miscellaneous CNS diseases including idiopathic epilepsy, malignant lymphoma, meningioma, and glioma.[24] However, there was no significant difference between dogs with NME and dogs with other inflammatory CNS diseases, which would be the major reason for wishing to use the test. In pugs, which are commonly affected by NME (see the article elsewhere in this issue by Coates and colleagues), serum GFAP concentration of 0.1 ng/mL had a sensitivity of 67% and specificity of 100% for diagnosing this disease.[25]

Cleaved tau

Cleaved tau (c-tau) protein has a microtubule structure and is localized in axons where it binds to axonal microtubules and forms axonal microtubule bundles, which are important structural elements in the axonal cytoskeleton. c-Tau protein can be detected in the serum and CSF after neural damage. Increased c-tau protein levels in the CSF have been detected in human patients with neurodegenerative disorders such as Alzheimer disease, multiple sclerosis, SCI, and TBI.[12,13,26,27]

CSF c-tau concentration was significantly higher in paraplegic or tetraplegic dogs with IVDH than in healthy dogs or dogs with paresis.[28] More importantly, dogs with IVDH that improved by 1 neurologic grade within a week had significantly lower CSF tau levels than dogs that needed more time for neurologic improvement or dogs that did not show any improvement. In dogs with IVDH, ROC analysis showed a moderate correlation between the CSF c-tau concentration and prognosis (AUC, 0.887). The CSF c-tau concentration of 41.3 pg/mL had a sensitivity of 86% and specificity of 83%. These results, although promising, need to be replicated in further groups of patients, because cutoff values derived from initial exploratory studies are optimized based on the available data, whereas clinical tests need to rely on previously defined reference intervals. The CSF tau concentration was not associated with T2W spinal cord hyperintensity on MRI.

Phosphorylated neurofilament heavy chain

Neurofilaments form a major cytoskeletal component in axons; they consist of light chain (NF-L), medium chain (NF-M), and heavy chain (NF-H). NF-H is one of the most abundant protein components of neurons, and contains many repeated lysine-proline-serine sequences in which essentially all of the serine residues are phosphorylated. This feature makes it resistant to proteases, so that it remains as an undegraded form in the CSF and serum after release from damaged axons. In humans, the phosphorylated NF-H (pNF-H) level in blood has been reported to be increased in amyotrophic lateral sclerosis, SCI, and TBI.[12,13,29]

Blood pNF-H values in dogs that were paraplegic with absent deep pain perception (DPP) were significantly increased compared with those in dogs with paraplegia and intact DPP and control dogs.[30] In paraplegic dogs with absence of DPP, ROC analysis revealed a weak correlation between the serum pNF-H concentration and prognosis (AUC, 0.613). Using a cutoff value of 1590 pg/mL, the serum pNF-H value was 34.8% sensitive and 100% specific for predicting recovery of ambulation. Again, this biomarker may have value in prognostication, but needs to be tested again in further groups of patients.

MMPs

MMPs are zinc-dependent endopeptidases that degrade various components of the extracellular matrix. They are released in an inactive state, requiring proteolytic activation after interaction with other proteinases, and are thought to play a major role in tissue remodeling and development, tumorigenesis, and tumor invasion. MMP-9 has recently emerged as a novel regulator of physiologic processes in the healthy adult CNS.[31]

Increased CSF MMP-9 activity was detected in 6 of 35 dogs with thoracolumbar IVDH, whereas it was detected in 1 of 8 control dogs.[2] Dogs that were paraplegic at admission had a significantly greater likelihood of expressing MMP-9 in the CSF than those that had voluntary motor activity (5 of 13 dogs, compared with 1 of 22 dogs). Serum MMP-9 was detected more frequently in dogs with IVDH than in the control dogs (27 of 31 dogs, compared with 1 of 8 dogs). However, the correlation with functional recovery has not been investigated and MMP-9 was also detected in dogs with different diseases, such as leishmaniasis.[4]

MMP-9 has been detected in dogs with intracranial tumors such as meningiomas, gliomas, pituitary tumors, choroid plexus tumors, and lymphoma.[3] Dogs with intracranial tumors were significantly more likely than those without tumors to have detectable MMP-9 in the CSF. In one study the level of MMP-2 and MMP-9 expression were correlated with recurrence of meningiomas or with higher meningioma grade in human patients,[32] although another study did not show this correlation.[33] The data collected from a small number of canine and feline meningiomas suggested that MMP is not correlated with morphologic malignancy patterns.[34]

Growth factors

Growth factors are naturally occurring substances capable of stimulating cell growth, differentiation, and proliferation. Growth factors such as vascular endothelial growth factor (VEGF) and transforming growth factor beta are involved in recurrence and progression of tumors. In human brain tumors, VEGF expression is positively correlated with tumor grade and degree of malignancy.[35] VEGF was strongly expressed in canine meningiomas, and the degree of VEGF expression is associated with survival times.[36] Intratumoral VEGF expression may be a useful marker for predicting prognosis of meningiomas.

Summary

Biomarkers show a great deal of potential for detecting, and perhaps for prognostication, in CNS injury, but much further work is required to define suitable cutoff values to permit reliable differentiation of varying severities of damage. Many studies compare groups of nondiseased patients with results derived from animals carrying specific diseases of interest, but differentiation of these two groups is not usually a relevant clinical question. Furthermore, it is important to take into account the stage of disease, heterogeneity of patients, and the possible effects of treatment interventions such as surgery, antiinflammatory medications, and nutritional supplements.

Even if a single biomarker does not have sufficient sensitivity and specificity to diagnose and determine prognosis, a combination may prove valuable (eg, the combination of CSF CK and CSF MBP in dogs with an acute thoracolumbar IVDH).[20]

Interpretation of mechanisms by which combinations of biomarkers are affected by disease and intervention may assist the development of novel therapeutic approaches for CNS diseases.

INFECTIOUS DISEASE TESTING
Introduction

Infectious CNS diseases may be caused by bacterial, viral, protozoan, rickettsial, or fungal agents. CNS infections, unlike most infections affecting other organ systems, are often not associated with systemic signs such as fever and increased white blood cell counts. Therefore diagnostic testing to identify causes becomes more critical. There are multiple options: cytologic/histologic examination, microbial culture, antibody titer testing, and detection of microorganism-specific molecules, especially nucleic acids (**Table 1**).

Cytologic or histologic examination and microbial culture of the CSF or tissue samples may reveal infectious agents in the CNS, thus achieving a definitive diagnosis. However, such tests are often falsely negative, which may be the consequence of a low concentration of the agent in the CSF or tissue samples. In addition, some agents may take several weeks to grow, or may be difficult to isolate in culture media.[37] Therefore, evidence of a systemic response to infection (ie, antibody titers) are also helpful in establishing diagnosis. Nevertheless, increase in CSF antibody titer is supportive but not diagnostic because, for instance, previous exposure, vaccination, or leakage of antibodies from serum to CSF also cause increased levels.

Advances in molecular biology over the past 10 years have revolutionized microbial identification and characterization. This article provides general principles, diagnostic values, and limitations of current molecular biology techniques.

Polymerase Chain Reaction–based Techniques

Polymerase chain reaction (PCR) is a molecular biological test developed by Kary Mullis, who was awarded the Nobel Prize for chemistry in 1993. It generally has higher sensitivity than conventional methods because it can detect even fragments of infectious agent in the CNS. The basic techniques of PCR include repeated cycles of 3 steps (denaturation, primer annealing, and DNA synthesis). In the

Table 1		
Advantages and disadvantages of infectious CNS disease testing		
	Advantages	**Disadvantages**
Cytology/histology Microbial culture	Easily accessible, cheap	Low sensitivity Takes several days to weeks
Antibody titer testing	Quick turnaround time, cheap	Low specificity High chance of false-negative during acute phase of infection
PCR	High sensitivity	Low specificity because of contamination
Nested PCR	Specificity is higher than standard PCR	Needs technical expertise
Multiplex PCR	Two or more agents can be detected at once	Difficult to design experimental conditions
Broad-range PCR	Can identify a class of agents	Higher chance of false-positive than standard PCR

Abbreviation: PCR, polymerase chain reaction.

denaturation step, the double strands of DNA are separated by heating. Second, primers anneal to their complementary target sequences. In the last step, DNA polymerase extends the sequences between the primers. Repeating for 30 to 50 thermal cycles exponentially increases the total amount of the copied DNA. Reverse transcriptase PCR (RT-PCR) was developed to amplify RNA targets, such as RNA virus infections. This technique clones the expressed gene by reversely transcribing the RNA of interest into complementary DNA (cDNA) through the use of reverse transcriptase.

To increase specificity, a double amplification step using nested primers may help. The first round of amplification consists of 15 to 30 cycles and the products are subjected to a second round of amplification with other primers. The second primers are specific for an internal sequence amplified by the first primers.[38] Nested PCR is intended to reduce nonspecific binding resulting from amplification of unexpected primer binding sites.

Multiplex PCR is a modification of PCR in which 2 or more primer pairs specific for different targets are introduced in the same tube,[39] allowing more than 1 target DNA sequence to be amplified simultaneously. The primers must be carefully designed to have similar annealing temperatures, which often requires extensive empirical testing.

Another important technique is broad-range PCR.[40] This technique identifies agents by using a single pair of primers targeting conserved sequences within phylogenetically informative genes and therefore recognizes a class of agents. Research has focused on identifying sequences of the ribosome RNA genes, which are conserved in many bacterial species.

Limitations of PCR

Although PCR analysis is useful in assessing infectious CNS diseases in dogs and cats, there are many limitations of these techniques (see **Table 1**). DNA strands are exponentially amplified by PCR, therefore false-positive outcomes can easily occur because of exogenous DNA sources,[41] such as contamination from normal skin flora. Carryover contamination can also be derived from reagents, pipetting devices, or laboratory surfaces. Nested PCR has a higher probability of contamination during transfer of the first amplification products to the second tubes. Furthermore, false-positive results may occur if the patients received modified live vaccines. PCR techniques can also provide false-negative results. Clinical specimens may contain PCR inhibitors that bind to polymerase and inhibit its activity; such inhibitors are detected frequently in CSF.[42,43]

The application of PCR in small animal practice has many potential pitfalls because of its susceptibility to experimental conditions. The choice of target genes and the design of primers are important to determine sensitivity and a 100-fold to 1000-fold sensitivity difference between primers has been reported even when the same target gene is selected.[44] There are several different detection methods for PCR products, such as traditional electrophoresis methods using an ethidium bromide–containing agarose gel. Southern hybridization has recently been developed, in which DNA fragments separated by the agar gel are transferred to a membrane and a specific probe is used to PCR amplicons. The membrane is probed with a radioprobe or nonradioprobe that hybridizes to 1 or more of the separated fragments. This detection method can provide a higher sensitivity than the ethidium bromide detection method (**Box 3**).[41]

Microbial Agents

Bacteria
Bacterial infections of the CNS are uncommon. CSF culture may be useful in detecting bacterial CNS infections but the sensitivity is low because of low concentrations of

---

Box 3
Key points regarding testing for CNS infectious disease

- Multiple types of diagnostic tests can be used to diagnose CNS infectious diseases: cytologic or histologic examination, microbial culture, antibody titer testing, and PCR assays.
- PCR techniques have higher sensitivity than conventional methods, but clinicians should understand the limitations and pitfalls of this technique.

---

bacteria in the CSF and tissue samples, and can be falsely negative because of improper sample preparation or culture technique. Broad-range PCR has higher sensitivity and may detect almost all bacterial infectious agents in the CSF.[45] Broad-range PCR detected meningitis pathogens in 65% of CSF samples from human patients with suspected CNS infection compared with a 35% detection rate by culture and microscopy.[46] However, it has low specificity because of difficulty in differentiating contaminants, such as skin flora.

Virus

Increased CSF antibody titer against canine distemper virus (CDV) with normal serum titer is supportive but not definitive evidence of CNS infection with CDV.[47] In contrast, serum CDV RNA detection using RT-PCR was 86% sensitive and 100% specific, and whole-blood and CSF CDV RNA was 88% sensitive and 100% specific.[48] Nested PCR allows characterization of various CDV lineages and differentiates the field strains from vaccine-related CDV strains.[49]

Feline infectious peritonitis (FIP) is the most commonly detected infectious cause of CNS diseases in cats. Definitive antemortem diagnosis can be difficult because conventional methods, such as CSF antibody titer, have low specificity and sensitivity.[50] In 1 previous study, blood FIP RNA was 93% sensitive and 100% specific compared with diagnosis confirmed by necropsy.[51] Achieving definitive diagnosis of CNS viral infections is difficult but can be accomplished by combining cytology or histology, antibody titer testing, and PCR analysis.

Protozoa

Toxoplasma gondii and *Neospora caninum* are commonly detected protozoan agents that can infect any area of the CNS in dogs and cats. Definitive diagnosis can be confirmed by identification of protozoan agents by cytologic examination, but they are rarely found in the CNS even in active infection. For toxoplasmosis, immunoglobulin (Ig) M antibody or increasing convalescent IgG titers in the serum and CSF is supportive of toxoplasma infection. IgM antibodies for *T gondii* usually appear in serum 1 to 2 weeks following infection and generally are undetectable within 16 weeks.[52] IgG antibodies appear by the fourth week of infection, increase over 2 to 3 weeks, and may persist for months or even years. However, false-negative and false-positive results can occur with these antibody titer tests. In one study in cats previously infected with *T gondii*, inoculation with adjuvant alone increased IgG titers in the serum and CSF, suggesting that increasing IgG titers should be interpreted with care.[53]

As an alternative, multiplex PCR has been used to detect *T gondii* and *N caninum*.[39] The combination of CSF-specific antibody detection and detection of agents by PCR is the most accurate way to diagnose protozoiasis in the CNS in animals with a clinical picture suggesting protozoal infection.[54,55] Even so, identification of Protozoa, or evidence of their antigen, does not necessarily indicate that they are responsible for clinical signs. Evidence of inflammation or tissue destruction in the vicinity of protozoan structures within the CNS is required confirm their pathologic importance.

Rickettsia

Isolation of rickettsial agents requires living cells for propagation and considerable expertise,[56] therefore culture is rarely used as a diagnostic technique. Although it is possible to observe *Rickettsia* microscopically in blood and CSF, the sensitivity is low because of the low concentration of infectious agent. Detection of antibodies for *Rickettsia rickettsii* and *Ehrlichia canis* can support the diagnosis of rickettsial infections. A 4-fold increase or decrease of the immunofluorescence antibody titer within 4 weeks is considered to indicate active infection.[57] However, these tests take time and the results are often available only after the disease has progressed or the patient has recovered. Furthermore, antibody titer results should be interpreted cautiously because they are often detected in clinically normal patients as a result of past infection or recent infection with other closely related *Rickettsia* spp, many of which are not known to be pathogenic.[58] PCR-based assays are helpful in diagnosing rickettsial infections if the results are positive.[56] An accurate diagnosis of rickettsial infection is based on the combination of history of tick exposure, thrombocytopenia, microscopic examination of CSF, serum or CSF antibody titer, and PCR assay.

Fungus

Diagnosis of CNS fungal infections is often made by cytologic or histologic examination of CSF or biopsy samples. The sensitivity of fungal culture alone is low so additional tests are usually necessary; in particular, molecular analysis and antibody and antigen (in the case of cryptococcal infections) titer measurement can be helpful. Although antigen titers are sensitive and specific if available, it is difficult to interpret the results of antibody titer tests because no large veterinary epidemiologic studies have been performed to determine the true sensitivity of these tests.[59] A panfungal PCR is usually performed when conventional diagnostic tests have not diagnosed the disease, but it is not regarded as a routinely useful clinical tool. The combination of cytologic/histologic examination, fungal culture, antibody titer testing, and molecular analysis can help detect specific infectious agents. The urine blastomyces/coccidioides antigen test is most useful and is highly sensitive and specific.[60]

REFERENCES

1. Jain KK. Introduction. In: The handbook of biomarkers. New York: Springer; 2010. p. 1–20.
2. Levine JM, Ruaux CG, Bergman RL, et al. Matrix metalloproteinase-9 activity in the cerebrospinal fluid and serum of dogs with acute spinal cord trauma from intervertebral disk disease. Am J Vet Res 2006;67:283–7.
3. Mariani CL, Boozer LB, Braxton AM, et al. Evaluation of matrix metalloproteinase-2 and -9 in the cerebrospinal fluid of dogs with intracranial tumors. Am J Vet Res 2013;74:122–9.
4. Marangoni NR, Melo GD, Moraes OC, et al. Levels of matrix metalloproteinase-2 and metalloproteinase-9 in the cerebrospinal fluid of dogs with visceral leishmaniasis. Parasite Immunol 2011;33:330–4.
5. Mayeux R. Biomarkers: potential uses and limitations. NeuroRx 2004;1:182–8.
6. Naeger DM, Kohi MP, Webb EM, et al. Correctly using sensitivity, specificity, and predictive values in clinical practice: how to avoid three common pitfalls. AJR Am J Roentgenol 2013;200:W566–70.
7. Jeffery ND, Levine JM, Olby NJ, et al. Intervertebral disk degeneration in dogs: consequences, diagnosis, treatment, and future directions. J Vet Intern Med 2013;27:1318–33.

8. Mondello S, Linnet A, Buki A, et al. Clinical utility of serum levels of ubiquitin C-terminal hydrolase as a biomarker for severe traumatic brain injury. Neurosurgery 2012;70:666–75.

9. Bruenner N. What is the difference between "predictive and prognostic biomarkers"? Can you give some examples? Connection 2009;13:18.

10. Herrmann M, Ehrenreich H. Brain derived proteins as markers of acute stroke: their relation to pathophysiology, outcome prediction and neuroprotective drug monitoring. Restor Neurol Neurosci 2003;21:177–90.

11. Giovannoni G. Multiple sclerosis cerebrospinal fluid biomarkers. Dis Markers 2006;22:187–96.

12. Yokobori S, Zhang Z, Moghieb A, et al. Acute diagnostic biomarkers for spinal cord injury: review of the literature and preliminary research report. World Neurosurg 2013;19. pii:S1878-8750(13)00459-2.

13. Yokobori S, Hosein K, Burks S, et al. Biomarkers for the clinical differential diagnosis in traumatic brain injury-a systematic review. CNS Neurosci Ther 2013;19: 556–65.

14. Satoh H, Yamato O, Asano T, et al. Cerebrospinal fluid biomarkers showing neurodegeneration in dogs with GM1 gangliosidosis: possible use for assessment of a therapeutic regimen. Brain Res 2007;1133:200–8.

15. Nakamura K, Miyasho T, Nomura S, et al. Proteome analysis of cerebrospinal fluid in healthy beagles and canine encephalitis. J Vet Med Sci 2012;74:751–6.

16. Barkhof F, Frequin ST, Hommes OR, et al. A correlative triad of gadolinium-DTPA MRI, EDSS, and CSF-MBP in relapsing multiple sclerosis patients treated with high-dose intravenous methylprednisolone. Neurology 1992;42:63–7.

17. Levine GJ, Levine JM, Witsberger TH, et al. Cerebrospinal fluid myelin basic protein as a prognostic biomarker in dogs with thoracolumbar intervertebral disk herniation. J Vet Intern Med 2010;24:890–6.

18. Ito D, Matsunaga S, Jeffrey ND, et al. Prognostic value of magnetic resonance imaging in dogs with paraplegia caused by thoracolumbar intervertebral disk extrusion: 77 cases (2000–2003). J Am Vet Med Assoc 2005;227:1454–60.

19. Levine JM, Fosgate GT, Chen AV, et al. Magnetic resonance imaging findings associated with neurologic impairment in dogs with acute thoracic and lumbar intervertebral disk herniation. J Vet Intern Med 2009;23:1220–6.

20. Witsberger TH, Levine JM, Fosgate GT, et al. Associations between cerebrospinal fluid biomarkers and long-term neurologic outcome in dogs with acute intervertebral disk herniation. J Am Vet Med Assoc 2012;240:555–62.

21. Oji T, Kamishina H, Cheeseman JA, et al. Measurement of myelin basic protein in the cerebrospinal fluid of dogs with degenerative myelopathy. Vet Clin Pathol 2007;36:281–4.

22. Fukuyama R, Izumoto T, Fushiki S. The cerebrospinal fluid level of glial fibrillary acidic protein is increased in cerebrospinal fluid from Alzheimer's disease patients and correlates with severity of dementia. Eur Neurol 2001;46:35–8.

23. Sato Y, Shimamura S, Mashita T, et al. Serum glial fibrillary acidic protein as a diagnostic biomarker in dogs with progressive myelomalacia. J Vet Med Sci 2013;75:949–53.

24. Toda Y, Matsuki N, Shibuya M, et al. Glial fibrillary acidic protein (GFAP) and anti-GFAP autoantibody in canine necrotising meningoencephalitis. Vet Rec 2007;161:261–4.

25. Miyake H, Inoue A, Tanaka M, et al. Serum glial fibrillary acidic protein as a specific marker for necrotizing meningoencephalitis in Pug dogs. J Vet Med Sci 2013;75:1543–5.

26. Blennow K, Wallin A, Agren H, et al. Tau protein in cerebrospinal fluid: a biochemical marker for axonal degeneration in Alzheimer disease? Mol Chem Neuropathol 1995;26:231–45.

27. Kapaki E, Paraskevas GP, Michalopoulou M, et al. Increased cerebrospinal fluid tau protein in multiple sclerosis. Eur Neurol 2000;43:228–32.

28. Roerig A, Carlson R, Tipold A, et al. Cerebrospinal fluid tau protein as a biomarker for severity of spinal cord injury in dogs with intervertebral disc herniation. Vet J 2013;197:253–8.

29. Boylan K, Yang C, Crook J, et al. Immunoreactivity of the phosphorylated axonal neurofilament H subunit (pNF-H) in blood of ALS model rodents and ALS patients: evaluation of blood pNF-H as a potential ALS biomarker. J Neurochem 2009;111:1182–91.

30. Nishida H, Nakayama M, Tanaka H, et al. Evaluation of serum phosphorylated neurofilament subunit NF-H as a prognostic biomarker in dogs with thoracolumbar intervertebral disc herniation. Vet Surg 2014;43:289–93.

31. Rivera S, Khrestchatisky M, Kaczmarek L, et al. Metzincin proteases and their inhibitors: foes or friends in nervous system physiology. J Neurosci 2010;30: 15337–57.

32. Nordqvist AC, Smurawa H, Mathiesen T. Expression of matrix metalloproteinase 2 and 9 in meningiomas associated with different degrees of brain invasiveness and edema. J Neurosurg 2001;95:839–44.

33. von Randow AJ, Schindler S, Tews DS. Expression of extracellular matrix-metalloproteinase protein in classic, atypical, and anaplastic menigiomas. Pathol Res Pract 2006;202:365–72.

34. Mandara MT, Pavone S, Mandrioli L, et al. Matrix metalloproteinase-2 and metalloproteinase-9 expression in canine and feline meningioma. Vet Pathol 2009;46:836–45.

35. Pietsch T, Valter MM, Wolf HK, et al. Expression and distribution of vascular endothelial growth factor protein in human brain tumors. Acta Neuropathol 1997;93:109–17.

36. Platt SR, Scase TJ, Adams V, et al. Vascular endothelial growth factor expression in canine intracranial meningiomas and association with patients survival. J Vet Intern Med 2006;20:663–8.

37. Lappin MR. Infectious disease diagnostic assays. Top Companion Anim Med 2009;24:199–208.

38. Tang YW, Procop GW, Persing DH. Molecular diagnostics of infectious diseases. Clin Chem 1997;43:2021–38.

39. Schatzberg SJ, Haley NJ, Barr SC, et al. Use of a multiplex polymerase chain reaction assay in the antemortem diagnosis of toxoplasmosis and neosporosis in the central nervous system of cats and dogs. Am J Vet Res 2003;64:1507–13.

40. Messner JH, Wagner SO, Baumwart RD, et al. A case of canine streptococcal meningoencephalitis diagnosed using universal bacterial polymerase chain reaction assays. J Am Anim Hosp Assoc 2008;44:205–9.

41. Yamamoto Y. PCR in diagnosis of infection: detection of bacteria in cerebrospinal fluids. Clin Diagn Lab Immunol 2002;9:508–14.

42. Dennett C, Klapper PE, Cleator GM, et al. CSF pretreatment and the diagnosis of herpes encephalitis using the polymerase chain reaction. J Virol Methods 1991;34:101–4.

43. Bouquillon C, Dewilde A, Andreoletti L, et al. Simultaneous detection of 6 human herpesviruses in cerebrospinal fluid and aqueous fluid by a single PCR using stair primers. J Med Virol 2000;62:349–53.

44. He Q, Marjamäki M, Soini H, et al. Primers are decisive for sensitivity of PCR. Biotechniques 1994;17:82, 84, 86–7.

45. Lu JJ, Perng CL, Lee SY, et al. Use of PCR with universal primers and restriction endonuclease digestions for detection and identification of common bacterial pathogens in cerebrospinal fluid. J Clin Microbiol 2000;38:2076–80.

46. Meyer T, Franke G, Polywka SK, et al. Improved detection of bacterial central nervous system infections by use of a broad-range PCR assay. J Clin Microbiol 2014;52:1751–3.

47. Soma T, Uemura T, Nakamoto Y, et al. Canine distemper virus antibody test alone increases misdiagnosis of distemper encephalitis. Vet Rec 2013;173:477.

48. Frisk AL, Konig M, Moritz A, et al. Detection of canine distemper virus nucleo-protein RNA by reverse transcription-PCR using serum, whole blood, and cere-brospinal fluid from dogs with distemper. J Clin Microbiol 1999;37:3634–43.

49. Martella V, Elia G, Lucente MS, et al. Genotyping canine distemper virus (CDV) by a hemi-nested multiplex PCR provides a rapid approach for investigation of CDV outbreaks. Vet Microbiol 2007;122:32–42.

50. Boettcher IC, Steinberg T, Matiasek K, et al. Use of anti-coronavirus antibody testing of cerebrospinal fluid for diagnosis of feline infectious peritonitis involving the central nervous system in cats. J Am Vet Med Assoc 2007;230:199–205.

51. Simons FA, Vennema H, Rofina JE, et al. A mRNA PCR for the diagnosis of feline infectious peritonitis. J Virol Methods 2005;124:111–6.

52. Lappin MR, Chavkin MJ, Munana KR, et al. Feline ocular and cerebrospinal fluid *Toxoplasma gondii*-specific humoral immune responses following specific and nonspecific immune stimulation. Vet Immunol Immunopathol 1996;55:23–31.

53. Lappin MR, Greene CE, Prestwood AK, et al. Diagnosis of recent *Toxoplasma gondii* infection in cats by use of an enzyme-linked immunosorbent assay for immunoglobulin M. Am J Vet Res 1989;50:1580–5.

54. Powell CC, McInnis C, Fontenelle J, et al. *Bartonella* species, feline herpesvirus 1, and *Toxoplasma gondii* PCR assay results from blood and aqueous humor samples from 104 cats with naturally occurring endogenous uveitis. J Feline Med Surg 2010;12:923–8.

55. Lappin MR, Burney DP, Dow SW, et al. Polymerase chain reaction for the detec-tion of *Toxoplasma gondii* in aqueous humor of cats. Am J Vet Res 1996;57:1589–93.

56. Allison RW, Little SE. Diagnosis of rickettsial diseases in dogs and cats. Vet Clin Pathol 2013;42:127–44.

57. Carrade DD, Foley JE, Borjesson DL, et al. Canine granulocytic anaplasmosis: a review. J Vet Intern Med 2009;23:1129–41.

58. Apperson CS, Engber B, Nicholson WL, et al. Tick-borne diseases in North Car-olina: is "*Rickettsia amblyommii*" a possible cause of rickettsiosis reported as Rocky Mountain spotted fever? Vector Borne Zoonotic Dis 2008;8:597–606.

59. Dial SM. Fungal diagnostics: current techniques and future trends. Vet Clin North Am Small Anim Pract 2007;37:373–92.

60. Foy DS, Trepanier LA, Kirsch EJ, et al. Serum and urine blastomyces antigen concentration as markers of clinical remission in dogs treated for systemic blas-tomycosis. J Vet Intern Med 2014;28:305–10.

Acute Lower Motor Neuron Tetraparesis

Sònia Añor, DVM, PhD

KEYWORDS

- Flaccid tetraparesis • Polyradiculoneuritis • Botulism • Tick paralysis
- Fulminant myasthenia gravis

KEY POINTS

- Acute flaccid nonambulatory tetraparesis is a neurologic emergency in dogs and cats that may need intensive care unit treatment in some cases because of respiratory muscle involvement.
- The 4 major disease conditions causing acute flaccid tetraparesis in dogs and cats are idiopathic polyradiculoneuritis, botulism, tick paralysis, and acquired acute fulminating myasthenia gravis.
- A careful and complete neurologic examination on presentation is essential and might be very helpful in differentiating between these diseases.

INTRODUCTION

Flaccid nonambulatory tetraparesis or tetraplegia is an infrequent neurological presentation, but is characteristic of neuromuscular disease (lower motor neuron [LMN] disease), rather than spinal cord disease. Paresis that begins in the pelvic limbs and progresses to involve the thoracic limbs, resulting in flaccid tetraparesis or tetraplegia within 24 to 72 hours, is actually a common presentation of peripheral nerve or neuromuscular junction disease.[1] The thoracic limbs rarely may be involved first. Often, complete body flaccidity develops with severe decrease or complete loss of spinal reflexes in pelvic and thoracic limbs. Animals with acute generalized LMN tetraparesis commonly show severe motor dysfunction in all 4 limbs, and severe generalized weakness in all muscles of the body. Flaccidity is evident in the limb muscles, but also in the neck and sometimes in muscles of the head. Thus, affected dogs and cats often show inability to walk and support weight in any limb, and inability to hold their heads up in a normal position. In addition, some of the diseases affecting the LMN system might affect cranial nerves, causing difficulties in swallowing, prehending, or chewing food; changes in phonation (bark or meow); or other cranial nerve signs. Finally,

Facultat de Veterinària, Department of Animal Medicine and Surgery, Veterinary School, Autonomous University of Barcelona, Bellaterra, Barcelona 08193, Spain
E-mail address: sonia.anor@uab.es

Vet Clin Small Anim 44 (2014) 1201–1222
http://dx.doi.org/10.1016/j.cvsm.2014.07.010
0195-5616/14/$ – see front matter © 2014 Elsevier Inc. All rights reserved.

respiratory paresis or paralysis may develop in some of these animals as a result of intercostal and/or phrenic nerve involvement.

The 4 major causes of acute LMN tetraparesis are acute idiopathic polyradiculoneuritis (AIP) (coonhound paralysis [CHP]), botulism, tick paralysis, and acute fulminating myasthenia gravis (MG). Less common causes include coral snake envenomation, blue and green algae intoxications, black widow spider envenomation (latter stages), and other rare toxicities (lasalocid). Other diseases causing LMN tetraparesis most often cause chronic progressive clinical signs (ie, endocrinopathies, neoplasia, toxicities and drugs, infectious and inflammatory diseases, hereditary and idiopathic neuropathies), although acute exacerbations may occur.

Clinical differentiation of the 4 major causes of acute LMN tetraparesis should be based on presenting clinical signs, routine diagnostic tests (complete blood cell count, serum biochemistry panel, urinalysis), and complementary diagnostic procedures (cerebrospinal fluid analysis and electrophysiological examination). More specific confirmatory tests (eg, determination of serum anti-acetylcholine receptor antibody titers, muscle and fascicular nerve biopsies) can be performed eventually to reach a definitive diagnosis in some cases.[2] However, the initial emergency approach of an animal with severe, nonambulatory LMN tetraparesis should be the same in all cases, regardless of the underlying cause (**Fig. 1**), and should be centered on assessing respiration.

ACUTE IDIOPATHIC POLYRADICULONEURITIS (COONHOUND PARALYSIS)

Acute idiopathic polyradiculoneuritis (AIP) or coonhound paralysis (CHP) is the most common form of acute polyneuropathy in dogs.[1-3] The syndrome was first described in 1954 as an ascending flaccid paralysis that developed in dogs 7 to 10 days after they had been bitten by a raccoon.[4] Although contact with raccoon saliva seems to have an etiologic role in some cases in America, an identical syndrome has been

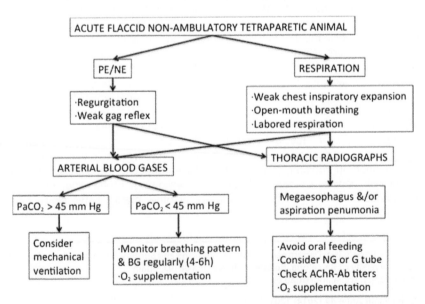

Fig. 1. Emergency approach of an animal with acute nonambulatory lower motor neuron tetraparesis. O_2, oxygen.

described in dogs that did not have contact with raccoons and in many countries around the world without a raccoon population.[5–11] Following the observation of the disease in animals without contact with raccoons, the disease has been subclassified according to cause as CHP, idiopathic polyradiculoneuritis, and postvaccinal polyradiculoneuritis (rare).[12] Regardless of the cause, however, the clinical signs are identical in all cases described.

Pathophysiology

AIP has been historically regarded as the canine equivalent of the acute human polyneuropathy Guillain-Barré syndrome (GBS).[2,3,8,12,13] Both diseases seem to be immune-mediated disorders affecting peripheral myelin, axons, or both. GBS is most commonly a postinfectious disorder that occurs in otherwise healthy people.[14] About two-thirds of patients with GBS have symptoms of an infection in the 3 weeks before the onset of weakness, and most studies state that symptoms of a preceding upper respiratory tract or gastrointestinal tract infection predominate. The most frequently identified cause of infection is *Campylobacter jejuni*, but other types of infection have also been related to GBS (cytomegalovirus, Epstein-Barr virus, *Mycoplasma pneumoniae*, and *Haemophilus influenzae*).[15,16] In addition, there are many reports of people developing GBS after vaccinations (influenza, hepatitis, and tetanus vaccinations), operations, or stressful events.[14,17–20] Studies in humans and animals provide evidence that in many cases GBS is caused by an infection-induced aberrant immune response that damages nerve roots and spinal and peripheral nerves[21] and that antiganglioside antibodies (Abs) are important mediators of the disorder.[22,23] Gangliosides are found in high concentrations in membranes of neural tissue. When antiganglioside Abs bind to gangliosides, the complement cascade is activated resulting in an attack to membrane complexes, pathologic changes, and dysfunction of the structures targeted.[24,25] A wide spectrum of antiganglioside Abs has been described in human patients with GBS: anti-GM1, anti-GM2, anti-GD1a, anti-GD1b, anti-GQ1b, and Abs against ganglioside complexes.[26,27] A recent study in dogs has demonstrated the presence of anti-GM2 ganglioside Abs in sera from a high percentage of dogs with AIP, which very strongly suggests that the disease is the canine equivalent to GBS.[28] Another potential triggering factor recently described for dogs with AIP is Toxoplasma gondii infection.[29]

In both AIP and GBS, in addition to humoral mechanisms, there is also evidence for cell-mediated immune responses involving autoreactive CD4+ T cells, interferon-γ, proliferating B cells, and macrophages that directly or indirectly damage myelin and axons.[2]

The immune-mediated reaction in AIP seems to target ventral (motor) nerve roots and spinal nerves primarily, with variable but always minor involvement of dorsal nerve roots. Pathologic changes in ventral roots and spinal and peripheral nerves consist of leukocytic infiltration of variable intensity and composition, paranodal and segmental demyelination, and axonal degeneration.[3,30,31] The lumbosacral nerve roots seem to be affected more severely than the thoracic or cervical nerve roots.[30]

Clinical Signs

The disease has been described in dogs of different ages and breeds. Affected animals start showing clinical signs 7 to 14 days after the antecedent event, if present. A stilted, stiff, short-stride gait may be seen in the initial period and progresses rapidly (2–4 days) to a flaccid, generalized lower motor neuron (LMN) tetraparesis or tetraplegia. Typically, signs are first evident in the pelvic limbs, but the thoracic limbs can be occasionally affected first.[2,32] The disease has a progressive phase that lasts between 5 and 10 days. During this period, clinical signs worsen rapidly but variably in different dogs. Some dogs remain ambulatory tetraparetic, whereas others experience a rapid deterioration and develop a flaccid, nonambulatory tetraparesis or tetraplegia, are unable to hold their heads up, and might develop respiratory paresis or paralysis caused by intercostal or phrenic nerve involvement. Most affected dogs display dysphonia or aphonia as a result of cranial nerve involvement, and some may show facial paresis.[33] Although there is no sensory loss, some animals demonstrate hyperesthesia on palpation or manipulation of the lumbar spine or limbs. Mental status and autonomic functions are normal; thus, affected animals are bright and alert, able to eat and drink normally if their heads are supported, and can voluntarily urinate and defecate. A surprising finding is that most dogs can keep wagging their tails during the whole process.

The neurologic examination shows flaccid tetraparesis or tetraplegia with severely decreased to absent spinal reflexes in all limbs, with the exception of the perineal reflex, which is normal. Because the disease affects mostly the ventral nerve roots, proprioception is not affected in AIP. Thus, affected animals attempt to reposition their feet when testing proprioceptive positioning if given enough support and provided they maintain some degree of motor function to perform the efferent pathway of the test. All dogs rapidly develop severe and generalized neurogenic muscle atrophy.

After the progressive phase of the disease, neurologic signs stabilize for a period of time; most dogs recover within 3 to 6 weeks. However, prolonged courses (up to 3–4 months) and incomplete recoveries are possible.[34] Usually, the more severe the clinical signs are, the longer the recovery time is.[2] Several repeated bouts of AIP have been described in raccoon hunting dogs.[2]

Acute onset of areflexic flaccid tetraparesis or tetraplegia similar to AIP in dogs and GBS in people has been described in cats.[35,36] The age of onset varied from 3 months to 4 years of age. Affected cats developed a rapidly ascending flaccid tetraparesis with severely decreased to absent spinal reflexes within 72 hours from the onset of clinical signs. Some cats (2 of 9) in one of the studies developed respiratory paralysis that led to euthanasia, whereas the others recovered uneventfully in 4 to 6 weeks.[36] This author has seen 2 cats with rapidly progressive, flaccid nonambulatory tetraparesis following vaccination against rabies. In both cases, recovery was complete in 2 to 4 weeks after the onset of signs.

Diagnosis

The first step in the diagnosis of AIP is to obtain an accurate history from the owner, especially concerning potential antecedent events (signs of upper respiratory or gastrointestinal tract infection, vaccinations) that may have occurred 1 to 2 weeks before the onset of neurologic signs. It is also essential to perform complete and accurate physical and neurologic examinations in order to identify other possible systemic abnormalities as well as to clinically differentiate the disease from the 3 other main causes of acute LMN tetraparesis (botulism, tick paralysis, acute fulminating myasthenia gravis [MG]) (**Table 1**). Routine blood work (complete blood cell count [CBC], serum biochemistry), urinalysis (UA), thoracic radiographs, and abdominal ultrasound do not display major abnormalities in animals with AIP. Some dogs may have increased serum immunoglobulin G (IgG) concentrations.[2]

Electrophysiologic examination should be performed in these patients because some findings are reliable indicators of AIP, especially if the investigation is performed after day 4 of disease.[2] Electromyography (EMG) reveals denervation potentials (fibrillations and positive sharp waves) in 100% of affected dogs (**Fig. 2**). Stimulation of motor nerves elicits compound muscle action potentials (CMAP) of greatly reduced amplitude (75%–100% of dogs) and increased temporal dispersion, but motor nerve conduction (MNC) velocity values remain normal or just mildly decreased (**Fig. 3**). The minimum F-wave latencies are prolonged, the F ratios increased, and the F-wave amplitudes decreased. In severe cases, F waves may even be absent (**Fig. 4**). Sensory nerve conduction (SNC) studies reveal no abnormalities or may show a mild decrease in sensory nerve action potential amplitude without temporal dispersion.[37] All these findings indicate a motor axonopathy affecting the entire length of peripheral nerves but more severe in the proximal portions of motor nerves, ventral nerve roots, or both. In addition, the prolonged F-wave latencies and ratios indicate that there is also demyelination in the ventral nerve roots and proximal portions of motor nerves.

An analysis of lumbar cerebrospinal fluid (CSF) may display albuminocytological dissociation, although there may be a delay in the development of this abnormality.[2] This CSF finding is also true for patients with GBS, in which the CSF protein concentration is usually normal during the first week but increases in more than 90% of patients at the end of the second week of the disease.[14] The increase in protein concentration in lumbar CSF represents the breakdown of the blood-nerve barrier in the subarachnoid portion of the affected ventral nerve roots.[2] It is worth noting that the CSF abnormalities are always observed in lumbar samples and not in cisternal samples and that the CSF cell count usually remains normal.

An enzyme-linked immunosorbent assay (ELISA) using raccoon saliva as antigen showed high sensitivity and specificity in detecting circulating Abs to raccoon saliva in dogs with CHP.[2] For dogs with AIP, the demonstration of anti-GM2 circulating Abs in serum using combinational glycoarrays has shown a diagnostic sensitivity of 60% and specificity of 97%.[28] The demonstration of circulating serum Abs to confirm serologic exposure to different infectious agents, especially *Toxoplasma gondii*, is also recommended in AIP in order to detect the potential triggering factors.[29]

Finally, peripheral nerve biopsy or nerve root biopsy can render information to reach a definitive diagnosis. Histologic findings include leukocytic infiltration of varying composition and intensity (more obvious in the ventral nerve roots and spinal nerves) (**Fig. 5**), segmental demyelination with axon preservation, and concomitant degeneration of axons and myelin.[31] However, peripheral nerve biopsies may not demonstrate any pathologic alteration.[34] A muscle biopsy usually reveals denervation changes, such as atrophy of myofibers and fiber-type grouping if there is reinnervation.[38]

Treatment and Prognosis

There is no specific treatment of this disease. Despite being an immune-mediated disorder, corticosteroid treatment is not effective.[2] Similarly, studies in humans show that steroids are not effective for the treatment of GBS and that prolonged corticosteroid treatment may even slow recovery.[39,40] In humans with GBS, treatment with plasmapheresis or high-dose intravenous (IV) immunoglobulin (IVIg) results in faster recovery rates, shortened times to recover walking without aid, and less frequently required mechanical ventilation. A clinical pilot study in 30 dogs with AIP demonstrated a trend for dogs treated with IVIg toward faster recovery (median 27.5 days) compared with control dogs without IVIg treatment (median 75.5 days).[34] Further prospective studies with a larger number of dogs are needed to confirm the benefits of this treatment modality in dogs.

Currently, the treatment of AIP is limited to supportive care, physical therapy, and proper nutrition. Affected dogs and cats should be kept on soft bedding to avoid

Table 1
Differential features of the most common causes of acute LMN tetraparesis

	Polyradiculoneuritis	Botulism	Tick Paralysis	Acute Fulminating MG
Signalment and history	Any breed or age Cats rarely affected Some: history of raccoon bite Acute, bilateral, progressive ascending tetraparesis-tetraplegia	Any breed or age History of ingestion of carcass/ rubbish May affect several animals Acute, rapidly progressive, flaccid tetraparesis-tetraplegia	Any breed or age Presence of tick bite or female tick attached Travel to endemic area (United States or Australia) Acute LMN tetraparesis-tetraplegia	Canine and feline breed predisposition Regurgitation and profound muscle weakness that develop acutely and progress rapidly to affect respiration
Neurologic signs				
Motor function	Severely reduced-absent	Severely reduced-absent	Decreased, but some motor function might be present	Severe weakness, may be episodic initially
Sensory function	Normal	Normal	Normal	Normal
Autonomic function	Normal	Alterations in HR, mydriasis, constipation, urinary retention, KCS, megaesophagus	Megaesophagus, urinary, CV, and respiratory alterations in Australian form (dilated pupils in advanced cases)	Megaesophagus, increased salivation
Reflexes	Reduced to absent	Reduced to absent	Reduced (withdrawal lost first)	May be preserved
Cranial nerves	Dysphonia-aphonia, facial weakness possible	Decreased gag, facial weakness	Decreased gag (Australian form)	Decreased palpebral, dysphagia, laryngeal weakness
Hyperesthesia	Lumbar hyperesthesia possible	No hyperesthesia	No hyperesthesia	No

Diagnostic tests				
EMG	Fibs and PSWs	Normal	Normal	Normal
MNCV	Normal or slightly decreased; CMAPS of severely reduced amplitude and dispersed	Normal-slightly decreased CMAPS of reduced amplitude, but no dispersion	Normal-slightly reduced, CMAPS may be reduced in size	Normal
F waves	Increased latency, prolonged F ratios, F waves may be absent	Normal	Normal	Normal
Repetitive stimulation	Normal	Small decrease in amplitude at low rates, increase in amplitude at high rate stimulation	Normal	Decremental response at low rate stimulation
CSF analysis	Increased protein concentration (lumbar samples)	Normal	Normal	Normal

Abbreviations: CMAP, compound muscle action potential; CSF, cerebrospinal fluid; CV, cardiovascular; EMG, Electromyography; Fibs, fibrillations; HR, heart rate; KCS, keratoconjunctivitis sicca; MNCV, motor nerve conduction velocity; PSWs, positive sharp waves.

EMG Signals

Interossi EP (Spont)

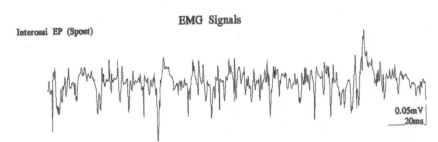

0.05mV
20ms

Fig. 2. Electromyography trace from a dog with AIP showing fibrillations and positive sharp waves.

the development of decubital ulcers; they should be hand fed in sternal position until they are able to reach food and water and should have passive range of motion and massage of all limbs at least 4 times daily to try to maintain muscle mass and delay muscle atrophy.[12] Recumbent animals should be closely monitored with special attention to respiratory function, especially during the progressive phase of the disease (first 4–7 days). If hypoventilation is suspected (increased respiratory effort and respiratory rate), arterial blood gases should be measured and mechanical ventilation initiated if arterial P_{CO_2} is more than 45 mm Hg.[41] Dogs that rapidly become nonambulatory are at a higher risk of developing respiratory paresis-paralysis. The initial emergency approach of an animal with severe, nonambulatory LMN tetraparesis should be the same in all cases regardless the undelying cause (**Fig. 1**) and should be centered on assessing respiration.

Once the clinical signs have stabilized and the animal is able to eat and drink, it can be released from the hospital and go home for continuing nursing care until recovery of enough motor function for ambulation without support. If pulmonary function is not affected, most animals recover over a period of 3 to 6 weeks. However, recovery may take 4 to 6 months in the most severely affected animals.[2]

BOTULISM

This is a rare neuroparalytic disease caused by intoxication with neurotoxins produced by *Clostridium botulinum* (most commonly) but also by *Clostridium baratii* and

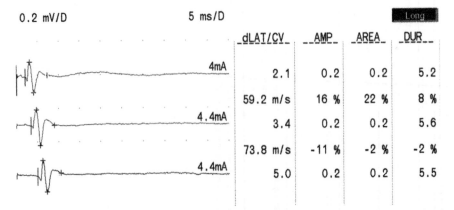

	dLAT/CV	AMP	AREA	DUR
4mA	2.1	0.2	0.2	5.2
	59.2 m/s	16 %	22 %	8 %
4.4mA	3.4	0.2	0.2	5.6
	73.8 m/s	-11 %	-2 %	-2 %
4.4mA	5.0	0.2	0.2	5.5

0.2 mV/D   5 ms/D   Long

Fig. 3. Motor nerve conduction (MNC) study of the tibial nerve of a cat with AIP. Note severely decreased amplitude and area of CMAPs, with just mildly decreased MNC velocity values. dLAT/CV, Latency, condiction velocity; AMP, amplitude; DUR, duration.

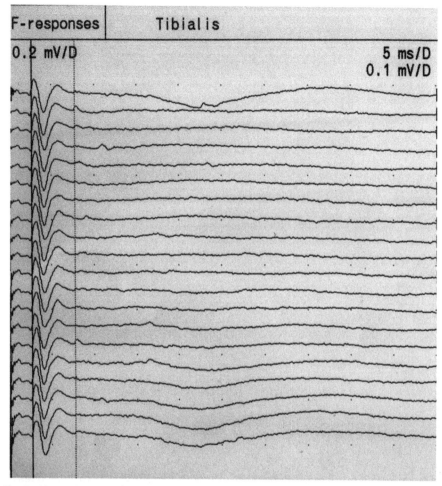

Fig. 4. Absent F waves after stimulation of the tibial nerve in the same cat as in **Fig. 2.** ACh, acetylcholine; BoNT, botulinal neurotoxins.

Clostridium butyricum.[42–44] *C botulinum* is a gram-positive, anaerobic, spore-forming bacterium that is distributed worldwide in soil, marine and freshwater sediments, and the gastrointestinal tracts of mammals and fish.[44,45] *C botulinum* produces all 7 known serotypes of botulinal neurotoxins (BoNT) (A to G), whereas *C baratii* and *C butyricum* produce only one serotype each (F and E, respectively).[46] All BoNT have similar structures and the same pathologic effect, which consists primarily of flaccid paralysis.[42,45] Types A, B, E, and F are associated with human disease. Type D is most prevalent in herbivores. Type C is more prevalent in carnivores and birds.[45] In dogs, the most common toxin associated with clinical illness is BoNT type C (BoNT-C), although 2 cases of type D intoxication were reported from Senegal.[47,48] Natural botulism has only been reported once in a group of 8 cats, and it was also caused by BoNT-C.[49]

   C botulinum forms spores under anaerobic conditions and in environments rich in organic material. Spores are highly resistant to light, heat, desiccation, many chemical agents, and radiation. Toxin production occurs under anaerobic conditions, and both vegetative cells and spores can produce neurotoxin. BoNT are the most potent

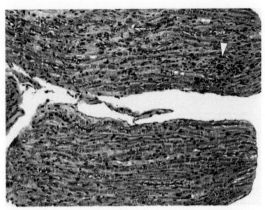

Fig. 5. Longitudinal section of ventral rootlets in a dog showing interstitial and fiber-invasive lymphocytic infiltrates (*arrowhead*) (hematoxylin-eosin). (*Courtesy of* Dr Kaspar Matiasek, Munich, Germany.)

naturally occurring, acutely toxic substances known; they are released only by lysis of the vegetative cell or spore rather than by secretion.[44,45,50]

Pathophysiology

Ingestion of the preformed BoNT causes botulism. The most common source of toxin is uncooked and spoiled food (in dogs, most commonly raw meat) or carrion.[51] The only outbreak reported in cats was caused by ingestion of a pelican carcass.[49] In humans, there are different forms of botulism (infant or intestinal botulism, wound botulism, injection-related botulism, inhalational botulism); but none of these have been described in small animals so far.[45] Following cell lysis of vegetative cells or spores in spoiled food, BoNT are released as progenitor toxins. Once ingested, these are very stable at low pH, which allows them to pass through the stomach and reach the small intestine where the alkaline pH leads to dissociation of the progenitor toxin and release of the BoNT.[52,53] In the small intestine, the toxin is absorbed by endocytosis similar to nutrient proteins, enters the lymphatic system and, from there, goes to the bloodstream. BoNT in the bloodstream rapidly enters tissue fluids and reaches cholinergic nerve terminals.[53] Differences in toxin-binding affinity to nerve terminals explain different species' susceptibility to the effects of BoNT.

Intoxication of the peripheral nervous system (somatic motor and autonomic) involves 4 steps: rapid and specific binding to neuronal surface receptors; internalization of BoNT into endosomal-like compartments; membrane translocation; and finally, enzymatic cleavage of target proteins (Soluble N-ethylmaleimide-sensitive factor activating protein receptor [SNARE] proteins) essential for acetylcholine (ACh) release at the neuromuscular (NM) junction (**Fig. 6**).[44,45] The SNARE proteins are essential for docking and fusion of synaptic vesicles with the presynaptic membrane; thus, by cleavage of these proteins, BoNT prevents synaptic release of ACh at the NM junction, resulting in flaccid LMN paralysis but also in signs of autonomic nervous system dysfunction (sympathetic and parasympathetic). Both the spontaneous release of ACh and its release caused by a nerve action potential are inhibited.[54]

Binding of the BoNT to neuronal surfaces is rapid and irreversible; but during this phase, the toxin is susceptible to inactivation by antitoxin. Once internalized, BoNT is no longer vulnerable to antitoxin.[44,45]

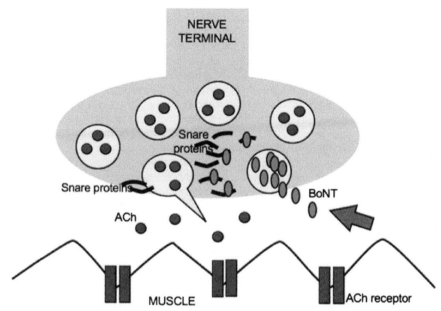

Fig. 6. Mechanism of action of BoNT. Intoxication of the peripheral nervous system (somatic motor and autonomic) involves: rapid and specific binding to neuronal surface receptors, internalization of BoNT into endosomal-like compartments (*arrow*), membrane translocation and, finally, enzymatic cleavage of target proteins (SNARE proteins) essential for acetylcholine (ACh) release at the neuromuscular (NM) junction. SNARE proteins are essential for docking and fusion of synaptic vesicles with the presynaptic membrane, thus by cleavage of these proteins BoNT prevents synaptic release of ACh at the NM junction.

Clinical Signs

Neurologic signs develop within hours up to 6 days after ingestion of contaminated food. Usually, the earlier the signs appear, the more severe are the clinical signs. The severity of the clinical signs depends on the amount of ingested toxin and individual susceptibility.[45,51] Affected dogs develop a progressive, symmetric, ascending flaccid paralysis from the pelvic to the thoracic limbs. Neurologic examination displays flaccid tetraparesis or tetraplegia with severely decreased to absent spinal reflexes but normal mental status and pain perception. Tail wagging is preserved. Cranial nerve dysfunction is evident in many affected dogs, which can show decreased jaw tone, decreased gag reflex with excessive salivation, decreased palpebral reflexes, and aphonia or dysphonia. Severely affected dogs may show decreased abdominal and intercostal muscle tone, maintaining respiration through diaphragmatic movements mainly.[45]

Signs derived of impaired ACh release at autonomic nerve terminals include alterations in heart rate (tachycardia or bradycardia), mydriasis with sluggish pupillary light reflexes, constipation, urinary retention, and keratoconjunctivitis sicca secondary to decreased tear production. Some dogs may also develop megaesophagus and secondary aspiration pneumonia. Death may occur because of respiratory paralysis or from secondary urinary or respiratory infections.[45]

Signs described in cats are very similar to those observed in dogs, except for cranial nerves and signs of autonomic dysfunction, which were not observed in the only feline outbreak reported.[49]

Diagnosis

Suggestive diagnosis of botulism is primarily based on history and clinical presentation. Because of the dietary origin of the toxin, many animals may be affected in the same household or premises, and they all may have a history of exposure to the same spoiled food. However, isolated cases are also possible.

Routine diagnostic tests (CBC, serum biochemistry, UA) do not show any abnormalities. Thoracic radiographs should be performed in all suspected cases to assess for evidence of megaesophagus and subsequent aspiration pneumonia.[43–45]

EMG may show spontaneous electrical activity (fibrillations, positive sharp waves) in any affected muscles after 2 weeks of paralysis but may also be normal.[51,55] MNC and SNC velocity studies are usually within normal reference ranges, but CMAPs are reduced in amplitude without evidence of temporal dispersion. Repetitive nerve stimulation at low frequency rates (3 Hz) may demonstrate a small decrease in amplitude and area of CMAPs. Stimulation at high rates (20–50 Hz) causes a substantial postactivation facilitation in children, which induces an increment in CMAP amplitude and area; but this is present in only 60% of adult human patients. It is thought that this is caused by neurosecretory mechanisms that enhance NM transmission by accumulation of calcium in the nerve terminal, release of ACh, and recruitment of fibers not activated by the first stimulation. However, this postactivation facilitation has not been described in dogs with botulism.[55]

A definitive diagnosis is based on the demonstration of BoNT in blood, feces, vomitus or stomach contents, or in the spoiled food ingested. Samples should be collected early in the disease course and when clinical signs are maximal to be diagnostic. The amounts of sample needed to detect toxin are 10 mL of serum and 50 g of feces, vomitus, stomach contents, or food. Samples should be refrigerated (not frozen) and examined as soon as possible. Samples should also be labeled as biological hazards because people are much more susceptible to botulism toxin than dogs or cats. The most reliable method of identifying BoNT is the mouse inoculation test in which the test sample is inoculated into the peritoneal cavity of 2 groups of mice, one of them protected with antitoxin. Mice are then observed for clinical signs of botulism. The survival of the protected mice and death of unprotected mice confirms diagnosis. However, the test is expensive and involves the use of live animals, thus, is not performed regularly in veterinary medicine.[56] A variety of ELISA, mass spectrophotometry, and polymerase chain reaction–based methods have been developed to measure the enzyme activity of the BoNT by cleavage of artificial substrates; but these are still less sensitive than the mouse inoculation test or are still being evaluated.[45,50,56–58] Because the detection of toxin is difficult, demonstration of a 4-fold increase in BoNT-antibody titer seems to be a reliable diagnostic method in suspected cases. The only limitation of this test is that the final diagnosis is reached when recovery of the disease is well underway or complete.[43]

Treatment and Prognosis

Supportive treatment is essential until patients form new SNARE proteins and functional NM junctions to avoid secondary problems derived from prolonged recumbency. This treatment involves frequent turning and maintaining of affected animals on well-padded, soft, and clean beds to avoid development of pressure sores/ulcers. Urinary bladder management is also important in these patients; manual expression and intermittent or permanent indwelling catheterization is essential to prevent retention cystitis. Artificial tears should also be applied on both eyes frequently (6 times daily at least) in order to protect the corneas from ulcer development. Maintaining daily fluid and nutrition requirements is of utmost importance in these animals, especially those that are recumbent and unable to reach their food or water bowls. Care should be taken when feeding because of the risk of aspiration pneumonia in animals with dysphagia or megaesophagus. In animals with megaesophagus or poor gag reflexes, feeding tubes or parenteral feeding should be considered until they regain the ability to swallow or the megaesophagus resolves (**Fig. 1**).[44] Physical therapy (passive range of motion and massage) is mandatory in these animals to help maintain joint movement and minimize muscle atrophy. In severe cases, arterial blood gases should be checked regularly to monitor respiratory function and mechanical ventilation initiated if necessary (arterial P_{CO_2} >45 mm Hg).[41]

Antibiotics may be necessary in animals with secondary infections (aspiration pneumonia secondary to megaesophagus, urinary infections). In these cases, broad-spectrum antibiotics should be administered; but those that impair NM transmission should be avoided (aminoglycosides, lincomycin, erythromycin, imipenem, ciprofloxacin, penicillamine, polymyxins, and tetracyclines).[12,44] In general, and unless required because of secondary infection, antibiotics should not be used in these animals to avoid alterations in intestinal microflora that could risk overgrowth with C botulinum.[44]

Antitoxin therapy is only effective in people if given early in the course of the disease to limit the severity of clinical signs but not to reverse them. The available human trivalent antitoxin acts against BoNT types A, B, and E; therefore, it is not effective for canine cases, which are all type C.[50]

All affected dogs recover spontaneously in 14 to 24 days, unless secondary complications develop (infections, respiratory failure). Dogs with more rapid onset of clinical signs develop more severe disease, and these are the ones with worse prognosis. In addition, different muscle groups have different susceptibility to the effects of BoNT; therefore, some muscles will be affected last and will recover sooner than others; respiratory, cranial nerves, and thoracic limb muscle function will return first. In the only report of naturally occurring type C botulism in cats, 4 of the 8 affected cats died of respiratory complications, whereas the other 4 cats with milder clinical signs recovered by 5 to 7 days after ingestion of the contaminated food.[49]

Prevention

Heating food to 80°C for 30 minutes or to 100°C for 10 minutes destroys BoNT. Thus, thorough cooking of any food fed to dogs and cats and preventing access to carrion and spoiled food should prevent the disease. Animals do not develop immunity after intoxication because the amount of toxin that produces clinical signs is too low to induce formation of a protective immune response.[59]

In humans, vaccination to elicit protective circulating Abs that bind, neutralize, and clear toxins before they are internalized into cholinergic terminals remains the most effective form of protection against BoNT. Vaccines developed in the past had low potency and immunogenic effects. Efforts are currently focused on the development of recombinant vaccines to elicit superior levels of toxin-neutralizing Abs.[60]

TICK PARALYSIS

Tick paralysis is an NM disorder resulting from envenomation by species of *Ixodes* (Australia) and *Dermacentor* (North America) ticks.[51,61–63] The most important species causing disease in dogs in North America are *Dermacentor andersoni* (the Rocky Mountain wood tick) in the Northwest and *Dermacentor variabilis* (the American dog tick) in the eastern part of the country.[63] In Australia, *Ixodes holocyclus* is the predominant species, although *Ixodes cornuatus* is responsible for some paralysis cases.[62-65] Cats in North America seem to be resistant to the disease, but they are affected in Australia.[62,66] In fact, tick paralysis has been described in several animal species (cattle, sheep, goats, pigs, chickens, dogs, cats) and in people (mainly children).[51,62,63]

The disease has been described primarily in North America and Australia, but cases with apparent tick paralysis have been reported caused by other tick species in Europe.[67] The larger percentage of cases occurs in the Pacific Northwest of the United States, adjacent areas in Southwestern Canada, and across the eastern coast of Australia.[63,66] In Australia, the geographic distribution of *I holocyclus* is determined by the presence of alternative host species (native bandicoots, koalas, and possums) but also by climate and vegetation, with high humidity and low vegetation associated with more tick paralysis cases.[66] In addition, tick paralysis in Australia is a highly seasonal disease, with most cases reported during spring and summer when female tick numbers are highest.[62,66]

Pathophysiology

Tick paralysis is caused by a toxin elaborated in the large salivary glands of feeding females of various species of ticks. The toxin of the Australian ticks (holocylotoxin) is a protein neurotoxin of unidentified chemical structure.[63,67] In any case, the Australian holocylotoxin and the North American *Dermacentor* toxin are secreted into the host through the tick's saliva and act by reducing ACh release from the presynaptic nerve terminal of the NM junction probably by blocking evoked calcium influx from the motor terminal membrane.[68] Thus, the disease is a presynaptic disorder of NM transmission that shares many similarities with botulism. However, the precise cellular mechanisms, which have been delineated for BoNT, remain unknown for tick paralysis toxins.[63] The effects of the Australian holocylotoxin are temperature dependent and more pronounced at higher temperatures. For this reason, high ambient temperatures adversely affect the clinical course of the Australian disease. In addition, holocylotoxin also decreases the release of ACh at autonomic nerve terminals, which results in autonomic imbalance and sympathetic overdrive.[62,68]

Clinical Signs

In North America, a rapidly ascending flaccid paralysis occurs in dogs 5 to 9 days after tick attachment, when the tick is fully engorged. Signs begin usually in the pelvic limbs and progress rapidly to flaccid tetraplegia over 12 to 72 hours. Clinical signs progress more rapidly and are more severe in dogs with heavy infestations. Tendon (stretch) reflexes, such as the patellar reflex, are usually lost before withdrawal reflexes. Cranial nerves are rarely affected, but some animals may show changes in voice, suggesting laryngeal involvement, or facial and masticatory muscle weakness.[51,62] Sensory, urethral, and sphincter functions are unaffected in dogs with American tick paralysis. In severely affected dogs, respiratory paralysis and death may occur if ticks are not removed. However, rapid (hours) improvement is observed after tick removal in most animals.

In Australia, tick paralysis is a far more severe disease. Affected animals (dogs and cats) develop a rapidly ascending, symmetric flaccid paralysis that does not start until 3 days after tick feeding begins, becoming more severe after the fourth day of attachment. In some instances, paralysis may not even start until after the tick has detached.[62] This onset of clinical signs correlates with an increase in salivary gland size in the feeding tick.[69] Although a change in voice is often appreciated early in the disease course, the first consistent sign is pelvic limb ataxia that progresses very quickly (hours) to flaccid tetraplegia. In dogs, other clinical signs associated include bladder dysfunction, variable respiratory and cardiovascular effects, and signs of left-sided congestive heart failure caused by cardiac diastolic dysfunction secondary to sympathetic overdrive. Vomiting might also occur in dogs, sometimes as the first sign of disease, as well as regurgitation secondary to megaesophagus. Dilated and eventually unresponsive pupils may also be observed in advanced cases, and it is a prominent finding in cats.[62] The gag reflex is consistently depressed, and drooling of saliva is seen in dogs that cannot swallow.[62,70] Affected animals show a progressive reduction in respiratory rate and increase in inspiratory effort, which lead to hypoxemia and hypercapnia. The main cause of the respiratory signs seems to be pulmonary edema, but aspiration pneumonia secondary to pharyngeal and laryngeal dysfunction is also a common finding.[71,72] Although signs are most commonly symmetric, recent reports describe asymmetrical focal signs in several dogs and cats, including unilateral facial paralysis, anisocoria, unilateral loss of cutaneous trunci reflex, and Horner syndrome.[70] Removal of the tick does not result in improvement in Australian tick paralysis, with deterioration ensuing despite absence of ticks in the animal's body.[73] Respiratory failure is the main cause of death in animals with Australian tick paralysis, and the only reported fatality rate is 5%.[74]

Diagnosis

The initial diagnosis is made by finding an engorged female tick of the offending species on an animal with the typical clinical signs and by excluding other causes of acute LMN tetraparesis. In some instances, the tick may have already dropped off, so a negative finding does not exclude tick paralysis. In other cases, especially in animals with long hair coats, finding the tick may be difficult; clipping the entire animal may be necessary in order to find the tick. Although a single tick is enough to cause paralysis, if a tick is found, careful search of the whole animal's body should be made looking for more ticks to remove all of them.

In American tick paralysis, rapid improvement (hours to a few days) is observed after tick removal. In Australian tick paralysis, clinical signs often progress after removal of the tick; respiratory paralysis may ensue despite appropriate therapy.[51,62]

Routine diagnostic tests (CBC, serum biochemistry, UA) do not show any abnormalities in animals with American tick paralysis but might show signs of infection if aspiration pneumonia has developed and respiratory acidosis in animals with the Australian form. Thoracic radiographs should be performed in all cases to assess for evidence of megaesophagus and subsequent aspiration pneumonia as well as for pulmonary edema in Australian cases. In these, if respiratory depression is observed, arterial blood gas analyses should be performed to assess oxygenation and ventilation status.[75]

Electrophysiological studies in children with tick paralysis demonstrate a severe reduction in the size of the CMAPs, without evidence of denervation potentials on EMG. Increases in amplitude of the CMAPs might be observed in many patients by cooling the limb tested. Sensory studies and repetitive nerve stimulation are normal, and MNC velocities might be normal or mildly slowed.[73]

Treatment and Prognosis

Removing any ticks attached to patients' bodies results in rapid recovery that may start within hours and continue over several days in North American cases. Ticks should be removed with forceps, applying steady pressure to ensure that the mouthparts are removed from the host. In Australian cases, if the animal is not showing signs of intoxication, removal of the tick may prevent development of the disease.

However, in animals showing neurologic signs, removal of the tick is not enough and the disease is likely to progress.[62,63] Therefore, in most Australian cases, treatment also involves the use of a commercially available tick antitoxin serum (TAS) to neutralize the clinical effects of the holocylotoxin. However, administration of TAS carries the risks of possible adverse systemic reactions. To avoid anaphylactic reactions, an intradermal skin test dose and administration of atropine before TAS have been advocated.[51,76]

Supportive treatment, as described previously for recumbent nonambulatory animals, should be performed. Although rare in North American cases, Australian dogs and cats with tick paralysis may need mechanical ventilation for survival.[71,75]

Tick paralysis in North America is a disease with a good prognosis after the removal of the offending tick. In Australia, tick paralysis is a potentially fatal disease with an estimated mortality rate of 5% despite treatment.[74]

Prevention

After the removal of the ticks, animals should be treated with acaricides and shaved in cases of thick, long hair coats. Regular use of acaricidal solutions or collars does not prevent the disease 100%. As a single tick is enough to cause paralysis, daily search for ticks on the animal's body and manual removal during the spring/summer months is recommended in Australia.

ACQUIRED ACUTE FULMINATING MYASTHENIA GRAVIS

Acquired MG is an immune-mediated disease of the NM junction that has been well described in dogs and cats.[51,61,77,78] In MG, autoantibodies (in most cases IgG) are formed against nicotinic ACh receptors located on the postsynaptic sarcolemmal surface of skeletal muscles. These Abs alter the ACh receptor function by different mechanisms,[51] causing a functional decrease of ACh receptors in the NM junction and, consequently, a decrease in normal NM transmission. Acquired MG has a bimodal age of onset with peaks of incidence at approximately 3 and 10 years of age in dogs and at 2 to 3 and 9 to 10 years of age in cats.[51,79] Dog breeds with the highest risk for acquired MG are Akitas, several terrier breeds, Scottish terriers, German shorthaired pointers, and Chihuahuas. German shepherds, golden retrievers, Labrador retrievers, and dachshunds might be most commonly documented because of the breed popularity.[79,80] Purebred cats, specifically the Abyssinian and related Somali breeds, have the highest relative risk of acquired MG.[81]

Clinical Signs

The clinical manifestation of this decrease in NM transmission is skeletal muscle weakness. Three clinical forms of acquired MG have been described in dogs and cats: focal, generalized, and acute fulminating. The focal and generalized forms present as weakness of isolated muscle groups (focal form) or generalized appendicular muscle weakness (generalized form). Typically, animals demonstrate severe exercise intolerance but regain muscle strength after rest.[51,61,82]

Dogs and cats with acquired acute fulminating MG present with a sudden onset and rapid progression of severe appendicular muscle weakness that does not improve with rest. Affected animals may present nonambulatory in lateral recumbency. Despite severe weakness, spinal reflexes may be preserved in some animals. Skeletal muscle weakness eventually involves the intercostal muscles and/or diaphragm causing severe respiratory distress.[51,77] Sudden onset of megaesophagus with frequent regurgitation of large volumes of fluid and secondary aspiration pneumonia is common in dogs.[83] Signs of weakness of pharyngeal muscles (decreased gag reflex, dysphagia) are also common in dogs,[82] and some animals may have decreased or absent palpebral reflexes.[78,82] The prevalence of this form of MG has been reported to be 16% in dogs[82] and 15% in cats.[77]

Diagnosis

A tentative diagnosis is made based on signalment, history and presenting clinical signs. Dogs and cats with suspected acquired acute fulminating MG should have complete blood work (CBC, serum biochemistry) and UA performed to exclude other systemic causes of generalized NM weakness (endocrinopathies, severe anemia, electrolyte abnormalities, and so forth). In addition, other problems secondary to compromised fluid or nutritional intake might be identified, especially in animals with dysphagia or megaesophagus.[51] Additional endocrine testing, especially of thyroid and adrenal function, should be performed based on findings of the initial blood work.[51,83]

Thoracic radiographs are essential to demonstrate the existence of megaesophagus and aspiration pneumonia, which are common in animals with acute fulminating MG. In addition, thymomas have been associated with acquired MG in humans, dogs, and cats and seem to have the highest incidence in people with the acute fulminating form of MG.[82,83]

An edrophonium chloride challenge test may be performed in dogs (0.1–0.2 mg/kg IV) and cats (0.25–0.5 mg per cat) to support the presumptive diagnosis of acquired MG. A rapid and short-lived (few minutes) increase in muscle strength is expected after the administration of the short-acting anticholinesterase drug. However, some animals with the acute fulminating form may not respond to the test because of insufficient numbers of functional ACh receptors remaining at the NM junction.[83] As an alternative to edrophonium chloride, neostigmine methylsulfate (40 μg/kg intramuscularly or 20 μg/kg IV) may be used to support the presumptive diagnosis of MG.[61]

Electrodiagnostic tests commonly used to support the diagnosis of MG (supramaximal repetitive nerve stimulation, single-fiber EMG) are usually not recommended in these patients because of the risks of general anesthesia in animals with extreme muscle weakness and megaesophagus.

A definitive diagnosis of acquired MG is based on the demonstration of circulating Abs to the ACh receptors. An immunoprecipitation radioimmunoassay that quantifies ACh receptor Abs in serum can be performed in dogs and cats. An ACh receptor antibody titer greater than 0.6 nmol/L in dogs and greater than 0.3 nmol/L in cats is diagnostic of canine and feline MG, respectively.[61]

Treatment and Prognosis

Rapid recognition of the disease is essential for successful treatment because animals with acquired acute fulminating MG require intensive care, which may include respiratory support urgently (**Fig. 1**).

Supportive care and nutritional care are essential and similar to those described for other diseases that cause acute LMN tetraparesis: frequent turning to avoid decubital ulcers, hypostatic lung edema and worsening of possible aspiration pneumonia; fluid therapy to maintain hydration, especially in animals with frequent regurgitation; nutritional support to maintain dietary intake, which should be through enteral administration of food via gastrostomy tube, or parenteral if regurgitation is severe.[61,79] Respiratory support (supplemental oxygen, nebulization and coupage if there is aspiration pneumonia, mechanical ventilation) is frequently required in these animals. Animals with aspiration pneumonia should receive parenteral broad-spectrum antibiotics, ideally based on culture and sensitivity results from tracheal wash samples. Some antibiotics should not be used because of their potential adverse effects on the NM junction (see botulism treatment).

Anticholinesterase therapy should be started as soon as possible; it is the cornerstone of therapy in humans, dogs, and cats. If oral intake is possible or if a gastric tube has been placed, pyridostigmine bromide, a long-acting cholinesterase inhibitor, can be started (0.5–3 mg/kg every 8–12 hours in dogs, 0.25 mg/kg every 8–12 hours in cats) and titrated as needed to improve muscle strength. However, many animals with fulminating MG cannot tolerate oral medications because of frequent regurgitation. In these, parenteral neostigmine can be administered (0.04 mg/kg intramuscularly every 6 hours in dogs). Alternatively, a constant rate IV infusion of pyridostigmine bromide (0.01–0.03 mg/kg/h) can be given to critical animals until oral feeding or an enteral nutrition tube has been placed.[79] Corticosteroids and other immunosuppressive drugs should be initially avoided because of potential worsening of aspiration pneumonia, which is very common in animals with acute fulminating MG. In human patients, expensive short-term therapies, such as IVIg and plasmapheresis (plasma exchange), are used to achieve rapid relief of severe myasthenic symptoms.[84–86] Although successful use of combined plasmapheresis and corticosteroid treatment was reported in a myasthenic dog,[87] IVIg and plasmapheresis are unlikely to be widely used in dogs because of the expense and technical difficulty of performing these therapies.

Thoracotomy and surgical excision of thymic neoplasia in animals with radiographic evidence of thymoma is only advised once the animal is systemically stable and the megaesophagus has resolved. Thymectomy may result in remission of clinical signs of MG, but careful consideration is recommended before performing surgery because of the stress and complications related to anesthesia and thoracotomy in these extremely debilitated patients.

The prognosis for animals with acute fulminating MG is guarded to poor because of the rapid development of respiratory failure and aspiration pneumonia. Most of the reported canine and feline patients died of respiratory failure.[82,83,88]

REFERENCES

1. Chrisman CL. Clinical manifestations of multifocal peripheral nerve and muscle disorders of dogs. Compend Contin Educ Pract Vet 1985;7:355–9.
2. Cuddon PA. Acquired canine peripheral neuropathies. Vet Clin North Am Small Anim Pract 2002;32:207–49.
3. Summers BA, Cummings JF, de Lahunta A. Diseases of the peripheral nervous system. In: Duncan L, McCandless PJ, editors. Veterinary neuropathology. St Louis (MO): Mosby; 1995. p. 402–501.
4. Kingma FJ, Catcott EJ. A paralytic syndrome in coonhounds. Vet Clin N Am 1954;35:115–7.
5. Bors M, Valentine BA, de Lahunta A. Neuromuscular disease in a dog. Cornell Vet 1988;78:339–45.
6. Chetboul V. Cas clinique: Polyradiculoneurite post-vaccinale. Le Point vétérinaire 1989;21:83–5.
7. Harve RS. Acute idiopathic polyradiculoneuritis in a dog (a case report and discussion). Vet Med Small Anim Clin 1979;74:675–9.
8. Northington JW, Brown MJ, Farnbach GC, et al. Acute idiopathic polyneuropathy. A Guillain-Barré-like syndrome in dogs. J Am Vet Med Assoc 1981;179:374–9.
9. Vandevelde M, Oettli P, Fatzer R, et al. Polyradikuloneuritis beim hund: Klinische, histologische and ultrastrukturelle beobachtungen. Schweiz Arch Tierheilkd 1981;123:207–17.

10. Boydell P. Coonhound paralysis in South Yorkshire? Vet Rec 2010;28:351.
11. Rivard G. Case of polyradiculoneuritis (coonhound paralysis) in Quebec. Can Vet J 1977;18:318–20.
12. Olby NJ. Tetraparesis. In: Platt SR, Olby NJ, editors. BSAVA manual of canine and feline neurology. 4th edition. Gloucester (United Kingdom): British Small Animal Veterinary Association; 2013. p. 271–96.
13. Holmes DF, Schultz RD, Cummings JF, et al. Experimental coonhound paralysis: animal model for Guillain-Barré syndrome. Neurology 1979;29:1186–7.
14. Van Doorn PA, Ruts L, Jacobs BC. Clinical features, pathogenesis, and treatment of Guillain-Barrré syndrome. Lancet Neurol 2008;7:939–50.
15. Hadden RD, Karch H, Hartung HP, et al. Preceding infections, immune factors, and outcome in Guillain-Barré syndrome. Neurology 2001;56:758–65.
16. Jacobs DC, Rothbarth PH, van der Meché FG, et al. The spectrum of antecedent infections in Guillain-Barré syndrome: a case-control study. Neurology 1998;51:1110–5.
17. Hughes RA, Cornblath DR. Guillain-Barré syndrome. Lancet 2005;366:1653–66.
18. Haber P, DeStefano F, Angulo FJ, et al. Guillain-Barré syndrome following influenza vaccination. J Am Med Assoc 2004;292:2478–81.
19. Hughes R, Rees J, Smeeton N, et al. Vaccines and Guillain-Barré syndrome. BMJ 1996;312:1475–6.
20. Souayah N, Nasar A, Suri MF, et al. Guillain-Barré syndrome after vaccination in the United States. A report from the CDC/FDA vaccine adverse events reporting system. Vaccine 2007;25:5253–5.
21. Ang CW, de Klerk MA, Endtz HP, et al. Guillain-Barré syndrome and Miller Fisher syndrome-associated Campylobacter jejuni lipopolysaccharides induce anti-GM1 and anti-GQ1b antibodies in rabbits. Infect Immun 2001;69:2462–9.
22. Willison HJ, Yuki N. Peripheral neuropathies and anti-glycolipid antibodies. Brain 2002;125:2591–625.
23. Willison HJ. The immunobiology of Guillain-Barré syndromes. J Peripher Nerv Syst 2005;10:94–112.
24. Halstead SK, O'Hanlon GM, Humphreys PD, et al. Anti-disialoside antibodies kill perisynaptic Schwann cells and damage motor nerve terminals via membrane attack complex in a murine model of neuropathy. Brain 2004;127:2109–23.
25. Rupp A, Morrison I, Barrie JA, et al. Motor nerve terminal destruction and regeneration following anti-ganglioside antibody and complement-mediated injury: an in and ex-vivo imaging study in the mouse. Exp Neurol 2012;233:836–48.
26. Claudie C, Vial C, Bancel J, et al. Antiganglioside antibody profiles in Guillain-Barré syndrome. Ann Biol Clin 2002;60:589–97.
27. Kaida K, Morita D, Kanzaki M, et al. Anti-ganglioside complex antibodies associated with severe disability in GBS. J Neuroimmunol 2007;182:212–8.
28. Rupp A, Galban-Horcajo F, Bianchi E, et al. Anti-GM2 ganglioside antibodies are a biomarker for acute canine polyradiculoneuritis. J Peripher Nerv Syst 2013;18:75–88.
29. Holt N, Murray M, Cuddon PA, et al. Seroprevalence of various infectious agents in dogs with suspected acute canine polyradiculoneuritis. J Vet Intern Med 2012;25:261–6.
30. Cummings JF, Hass DC. Coonhound paralysis. An acute idiopathic polyradiculoneuritis in dogs resembling the Landry-Guillain-Barré syndrome. J Neurol Sci 1967;4:51–81.

31. Cummings JF, de Lahunta A, Holmes DF, et al. Coonhound paralysis. Further clinical studies and electron microscopic observations. Acta Neuropathol 1982;56:167–78.

32. Cummings JF. Canine inflammatory polyneuropathies. In: Kirk RW, Bonagura JD, editors. Current veterinary therapy XI. Philadelphia: WB Saunders; 1992. p. 1034–7.

33. Dewey CW, Cerda-Gonzalez S. Disorders of the peripheral nervous system: mononeuropathies and polyneuropathies. In: Dewey CW, editor. A practical guide to canine and feline neurology. 2nd edition. Ames (IA): Wiley-Blackwell; 2008. p. 427–67.

34. Hirschvogel K, Jurina K, Steinberg TA, et al. Clinical course of acute canine polyradiculoneuritis following treatment with human IV immunoglobulin. J Am Anim Hosp Assoc 2012;48:299–309.

35. Lane JR, de Lahunta A. Polyneuritis in a cat. J Am Anim Hosp Assoc 1984;20:1006–8.

36. Gerritsen RJ, van Ness JJ, van Niel MH, et al. Acute idiopathic polyneuropathy in nine cats. Vet Q 1996;18:63–5.

37. Cuddon PA. Electrophysiologic assessment of acute polyradiculoneuropathy in dogs: comparison with Guillain-Barré syndrome in people. J Vet Intern Med 1998;12:294–303.

38. Dickinson PJ, LeCouteur RA. Muscle and nerve biopsy. Vet Clin North Am Small Anim Pract 2002;32:63–102.

39. Hughes RA, Swan AV, can Koningsveld R, et al. Corticosteroids for Guillain-Barré syndrome. Cochrane Database Syst Rev 2006;(2):CD001446.

40. Hughes RA, Swan AV, van Doorn PA. Intravenous immunoglobulin for Guillain-Barré syndrome. Cochrane Database Syst Rev 2010;(6):CD002063.

41. Sherman J, Olby N, Halling KB. Rehabilitation of the neurological patient. In: Platt SR, Olby NJ, editors. BSAVA Manual of canine and feline neurology. 4th edition. Gloucester (United Kingdom): British Small Animal Veterinary Association; 2013. p. 481–95.

42. Popoff MR. Botulinum neurotoxins: more and more diverse and fascinating toxic proteins. J Infect Dis 2014;209(2):168–9.

43. Bruchim Y, Steinman A, Markovitz M, et al. Toxicological, bacteriological and serological diagnosis of botulism in a dog. Vet Rec 2006;158:768–9.

44. Penderis J. Tetanus and botulism. In: Platt SR, Garosi LS, editors. Small animal neurological emergencies. London: Manson Publishing Ltd; 2012. p. 447–60.

45. Barsanti JA. Botulism. In: Greene CE, editor. Infectious diseases of the dog and cat. 4th edition. St Louis (MO): Elsevier Saunders; 2012. p. 416–22.

46. Simpson LL. Identification of the major steps in botulinum toxin action. Annu Rev Pharmacol Toxicol 2004;44:167–93.

47. Doutre MP. Le botulisme animal de type D au Senegal: premiere observation chez le chien. Rev Elev Med Vet Pays Trop 1982;35:11–4.

48. Doutre MP. Seconde observation de botulisme de type D chez le chien au Senegal. Rev Elev Med Vet Pays Trop 1983;36:131–2.

49. Elad D, Yas-Natan E, Aroch I, et al. Natural *Clostridium botulinum* type C toxicosis in a group of cats. J Clin Microbiol 2004;42:5406–8.

50. Shapiro RL, Hatheway C, Swerlow DL. Botulism in the United States: a clinical and epidemiologic review. Ann Intern Med 1998;129:221–8.

51. Penderis J. Junctionopathies: disorders of the neuromuscular junction. In: Dewey CW, editor. A practical guide to canine and feline neurology. 2nd edition. Ames (IA): Wiley-Blackwell; 2008. p. 517–58.

52. Chaddock JA, Melling J. *Clostridium botulinum* and associated neurotoxins. In: Sussman M, editor. Molecular medical microbiology. San Diego (CA): Academis Press; 2011. p. 1141–52.
53. Rossetto O, Morbiato L, Caccin P, et al. Presynaptic enzymatic neurotoxins. J Neurochem 2006;97:1534–45.
54. Humeau Y, Doussau F, Grant NJ. How botulinum and tetanus neurotoxins block neurotransmitter release. Biochimie 2000;82:427–46.
55. Uriarte A, Thibaud JL, Blot S. Botulism in two urban dogs. Can Vet J 2010;51: 1139–42.
56. Fernandez RA, Ciccarelli AS. Botulism: laboratory methods and epidemiology. Anaerobe 1999;5:165–8.
57. Franciosa G, Fenicia L, Caldiani C. PCR for detection of *Clostridium botulinum* type C in avian and environmental samples. J Clin Microbiol 1996;34: 882–5.
58. Thomas RJ. Detection of *Clostridium botulinum* types C and D toxin by ELISA. Aust Vet J 1991;68:111–3.
59. Coleman ES. Clostridial neurotoxins: tetanus and botulism. Compend Contin Educ Pract Vet 1998;20:1089–98.
60. Webb RP, Smith LA. What next for botulism vaccine development? Expert Rev Vaccines 2013;12:481–92.
61. Shelton GD. Myasthenia gravis and disorders of neuromuscular transmission. Vet Clin North Am Small Anim Pract 2002;32:189–206.
62. Malik R. Tick paralysis in North America and Australia. Vet Clin North Am Small Anim Pract 1991;21:157–71.
63. Edlow JA, McGillicuddy DC. Tick paralysis. Infect Dis Clin North Am 2008;22: 397–413.
64. Beveridge I, Coleman G, Gartrell W, et al. Tick paralysis of dogs in Victoria due to *Ixodes cornuatus*. Aust Vet J 2004;82:642.
65. Jackson J, Beveridge I, Chilton NB, et al. Distribution of the paralysis ticks *Ixodes cornuatus* and *Ixodes holocyclus* in south-eastern Australia. Aust Vet J 2007;85:420–4.
66. Eppleston KR, Kelman M, Ward MP. Distribution, seasonality and risk factors for tick paralysis in Australian dogs and cats. Vet Parasitol 2013;196:460–8.
67. Otranto D, Dantas-Torres F, Tarallo VD, et al. Apparent tick paralysis by *Rhipicephalus sanguineus* (Acari: Ixodidae) in dogs. Vet Parasitol 2012;188: 325–9.
68. Cooper BJ, Spencer I. Temperature-dependent inhibition of evoked acetylcholine release in tick paralysis. Nature 1976;263:693–5.
69. Masina S, Broady KW. Tick paralysis: development of a vaccine. Int J Parasitol 1999;29:535–41.
70. Holland CT. Asymmetrical focal neurological deficits in dogs and cats with naturally occurring tick paralysis (Ixodes holocyclus): 27 cases (1999-2006). Aust Vet J 2008;86:377–84.
71. Webster RA, Haskins S, Mackay B. Management of respiratory failure from tick paralysis. Aust Vet J 2013;91:499–504.
72. Webster RA, Mackie JT, Haskins S. Histopathological changes in the lungs from dogs with tick paralysis: 25 cases (2010-2012). Aust Vet J 2013;91:306–11.
73. Grattan-Smith PJ, Morris JG, Johnston HM, et al. Clinical and neurophysiological features of tick paralysis. Brain 1997;120:1975–87.
74. Atwell RB, Campbell FE, Evans EA. Prospective survey of tick paralysis in dogs. Aust Vet J 2001;79:412–8.

75. Webster RA, Mills PC, Morton JM. Indications, durations and outcomes of mechanical ventilation in dogs and cats with tick paralysis caused by *Ixodes holocyclus*: 61 cases. Aust Vet J 2013;91:233–9.
76. Atwell RB, Campbell FE. Reactions to tick antitoxin serum and the role of atropine in treatment of dogs and cats with tick paralysis caused by *Ixodes holocyclus*: a pilot survey. Aust Vet J 2001;79:394–7.
77. Ducoté JM, Dewey CW. Acquired myasthenia gravis and other disorders of the neuromuscular junction. In: August JR, editor. Consultations in feline internal medicine. 4th edition. Philadelphia: WB Saunders; 2001. p. 374–80.
78. Joseph RJ, Carrillo JM, Lennon VA. Myasthenia gravis in the cat. J Vet Intern Med 1988;2:75–9.
79. Smith Bailey K. Myasthenia gravis. In: Platt SR, Garosi LS, editors. Small animal neurological emergencies. London: Manson Publishing Ltd; 2012. p. 433–45.
80. Shelton GD, Schule A, Kass PH. Risk factors for acquired myasthenia gravis in dogs: 1,154 cases (1991-1995). J Am Vet Med Assoc 1997;211:1428–31.
81. Shelton GD, Ho M, Kass PH. Risk factors for acquired myasthenia gravis in cats: 105 cases (1986-1998). J Am Vet Med Assoc 2000;216:55–7.
82. Dewey CW, Bailey CS, Shelton GD, et al. Clinical forms of acquired myasthenia gravis in dogs: 25 cases (1988-1995). J Vet Intern Med 1997;11:50–7.
83. King LG, Vite CH. Acute fulminating myasthenia gravis in five dogs. J Am Vet Med Assoc 1998;212:830–4.
84. Dewey CW. Acquired myasthenia gravis in dogs – part II. Compend Contin Educ Pract Vet 1998;20:47–59.
85. Van der Meché FG, van Doorn PA. The current place of high-dose immunoglobulins in the treatment of neuromuscular disorders. Muscle Nerve 1997;20:136–47.
86. Keesey J, Buffkin D, Kebo D, et al. Plasma exchange alone as therapy for myasthenia gravis. Ann N Y Acad Sci 1981;377:729–43.
87. Bartges JW, Klausner JS, Bostwick EF, et al. Clinical remission following plasmapheresis and corticosteroid treatment in a dog with acquired myasthenia gravis. J Am Vet Med Assoc 1990;196:1276–8.
88. Ducoté JM, Dewey CW, Coates JR. Clinical forms of acquired myasthenia gravis in cats. Compend Contin Educ Pract Vet 1999;21:440–8.

Inherited Neurologic Disorders in the Dog
The Science Behind the Solutions

Cathryn Mellersh, BSc, PhD

KEYWORDS

- Inherited disorder • DNA testing • Genetic mutation

KEY POINTS

- Inherited neurologic diseases are varied and can be congenital, neonatal, or late onset as well as progressive or stationary.
- Modern genetic technologies are revolutionizing the speed and efficiency with which mutations responsible for inherited neurologic disease are being identified.
- Clinically similar disorders can be caused by different mutations, even within a single breed, and are thus genetically distinct.
- DNA tests can be used by dog breeders to reduce the prevalence of inherited neurologic disorders in specific breeds and help the veterinarian diagnose disease.

BROAD CHARACTERISTICS OF INHERITED DISEASE—WHEN SHOULD A VETERINARIAN SUSPECT A DISEASE IS INHERITED?

There is no definitive or trademark characteristic of an inherited disorder, and the veterinarian should always be open minded about the possibility that a patient may be suffering from an inherited condition. A variety of inherited neurologic diseases has been described in the dog, including examples that are congenital, neonatal, and late onset as well as those that are progressive and stationary, so potentially any neurologic patient could be suffering from an inherited disorder.

It is not possible to tell whether a disease is inherited from a single case; the only indication a disease might be inherited is whether other dogs of the same breed or from the same extended pedigree have also been reported with the same or similar clinical presentation. Mutations that cause inherited disorders arise at random in founder animals and are passed to offspring and subsequent generations if the founder reproduces. If the mutation is recessive, clinically affected animals are only produced when inbreeding has occurred and a dog inherits an identical

Centre for Preventive Medicine, Animal Health Trust, Lanwades Park, Kentford, Newmarket, Suffolk CB8 7UU, UK
E-mail address: cathryn.mellersh@aht.org.uk

Vet Clin Small Anim 44 (2014) 1223–1234
http://dx.doi.org/10.1016/j.cvsm.2014.07.011
0195-5616/14/$ – see front matter
vetsmall.theclinics.com

copy of the mutation from both parents. For this reason, specific inherited diseases are nearly always associated with particular breeds or several closely related breeds.

Sources of Data Regarding Inherited Diseases in Domestic Animals

A literature review might reveal whether a specific disorder has been reported previously. PubMed[1] is a free search engine accessing primarily the MEDLINE database of references and abstracts on life sciences and biomedical topics and is a sensible place to initiate a search for evidence a disease might be inherited.

Another source of evidence that a disorder may be inherited in a domestic species is Online Mendelian Inheritance in Animals (OMIA), which is a catalog/compendium of inherited disorders, other (single-locus) traits, and genes in 214 animal species (other than human and mouse and rats, which have their own resources) authored by Professor Frank Nicholas of the University of Sydney, Australia.[2] OMIA information is stored in a database that contains textual information and references as well as links to relevant PubMed (described above) records at the National Center for Biotechnology Information and to the equivalent database for human inherited disorders, Online Inheritance in Man,[3] and to Ensembl,[4] a software system that produces and maintains automatic annotation on selected eukaryotic genomes.

A database that compiles information specifically about diseases/conditions of pure-bred dogs that are likely to have a genetic component is the Inherited Diseases in Dogs database compiled by Dr David Sargan at Cambridge University.[5]

In addition to online sources of information, an excellent text describing canine and feline disorders that are potentially breed associated is Breed Predispositions to Disease in Dogs and Cats, 2nd Edition by Alex Gough and Alison Thomas,[6] which includes reference to a peer-reviewed publication for each disorder described.

However, not all inherited diseases will have been described in the scientific literature, although considerable anecdotal evidence might still exist to suggest a disease has an inherited component. Breed clubs and breed societies as well as individual breeders are frequently knowledgeable regarding conditions that segregate in their breed, often well before they have been formally recognized by the veterinary profession, so making contact with a breed health coordinator or the equivalent might also yield useful information.

IDENTIFYING THE UNDERLYING CAUSE OF AN INHERITED DISORDER

Once it has been established that a specific disorder is likely to be inherited, by virtue of the fact that it is more prevalent in certain breeds than others, it becomes desirable to identify the mutation(s) or genetic variant(s). Once the causal mutation is known, a DNA test can be developed that breeders can use to guide their breeding decisions and reduce the prevalence of the condition in their breed. The opportunity to minimize the risk of producing clinically affected puppies is particularly desirable when the disorder is challenging to treat effectively or is particularly debilitating—as is frequently the case for diseases of the nervous system.

Over the last decade, the tools available to dissect the genetic basis of canine inherited traits have become increasingly sophisticated since the canine genome was sequenced in its entirety in 2004. The current rapid rate at which disease mutations are identified can be expected to increase further in coming years as next-generation sequencing techniques become increasingly cost effective and therefore within the reach of even the most modestly sized research groups.

Methodology of Mutation Identification

There are 2 main routes to mutation identification; the genomewide investigation approach and the candidate gene approach. During a genomewide investigation, the entire genome is investigated for region(s) likely to harbor the disease-associated mutation(s), using pedigree-based linkage analysis, a genomewide association study (GWAS), or whole genome sequencing. In contrast, during a candidate gene study, only specific genes are investigated. The successful outcome of a genomewide linkage or association study is the identification of a genomic region that is likely to contain the causal mutation being sought. In-depth investigations of the associated region follow, which might involve analysis of candidate genes within the region or a more holistic sequencing approach (known as targeted resequencing, see later discussion). In whole genome sequencing, the entire genome of an affected animal is sequenced and investigated for pathogenic mutations. The different routes to mutation identification are summarized in **Fig. 1** and described later.

Genetic Markers

Both linkage and genomewide association analyses use genetic markers to identify genomic regions associated with disease. Genetic markers are variable or polymorphic regions of DNA that help geneticists navigate their way around the genome and identify regions of DNA that are associated with traits of interest. For genetic markers to be useful, their positions relative to the genome and their positions relative to one another must be known. Microsatellites are one commonly used form of genetic marker that comprise a simple DNA motif repeated in tandem a variable number of times. Often, these repeats consist of the nucleotides, or bases, cytosine and adenosine—so-called CA repeats. The number of repeats present within a given microsatellite may differ between individuals, hence, the term *polymorphism*—the existence of different forms within a population. Single nucleotide polymorphisms (SNPs) are

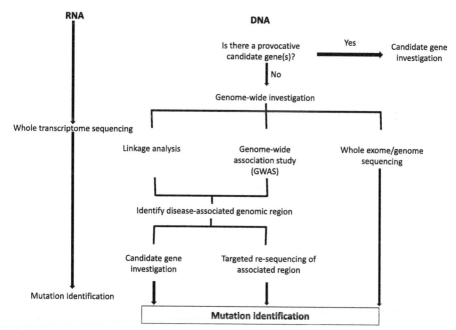

Fig. 1. Schematic illustration of different potential routes to mutation identification.

individual point mutations, or substitutions of a single nucleotide, that do not change the overall length of the DNA sequence in that region. Both SNPs and microsatellites occur frequently and regularly throughout an individual's genome, making them ideal tools for genetic mapping. The alternative forms of a gene or genetic marker that occupy the same locus on a chromosome are known as alleles.

Genetic Linkage Analysis

Markers, genes, or mutations that are located on the same chromosome as one another tend to be inherited together, whereas markers on different chromosomes are inherited independently. The closer 2 markers are to each other the less likely they are to be separated by genetic recombination, the process that occurs during meiosis when chromosome pairs align and physical breakage and exchange of genetic materials between the homologous chromosomes can occur. Recombination results in a combination of genes/markers different from that of either parent. By analyzing large numbers of genetic markers from all over the genome (a genomewide scan) in dogs from pedigrees segregating an inherited condition, researchers can identify markers that are being co-inherited with the disease. Because the location of genetic markers within the genome is known, the position of the disease-causing mutation can also be inferred. The above process is known as pedigree linkage analysis and requires the analysis of DNA from both affected and unaffected related members of an extended family. The precision with which a mutation can be located depends on several factors, including the numbers of animals in the study, the numbers of genetic markers analyzed, and the fortuitous occurrence of recombination in critical dogs within the pedigree.

Example

In practice, it is often difficult to collect DNA samples from sufficient family members for a successful linkage analysis unless a research colony is available. However, the technique was used very successfully in 1999 by Lin and colleagues[7] to identify a mutation in the *hypocretin (orexin) receptor 2* gene (*Hcrtr2*) that was responsible for a well-established canine model of narcolepsy.

Genomewide Association Studies

An alternative approach to linkage analysis is to use a GWAS, also known as association mapping, whereby unrelated affected and unaffected individuals (cases and controls) are drawn from the population, and the frequency with which certain alleles are present in each of these groups is tested for association with a disease. Similar to linkage analysis experiments, the successful outcome of an association study is the identification of a region of the genome containing a mutation that is responsible for the disease under investigation. Because modern breeds of dog have been developed relatively recently, often from a small number of founders, individuals of the same breed exhibit low levels of intrabreed variation and usually share long regions of chromosomes (haplotype blocks) that are identical by descent. This extensive linkage disequilibrium is in contrast to that in humans and means that far fewer, less densely spaced markers are sufficient to map genomic regions associated with traits in the dog. The disadvantage of long linkage disequilibrium is that although it is relatively easy to map disease regions, the regions are long, relative to corresponding regions that are mapped in more genetically diverse species. But once a broad region of interest has been identified, the geneticist can take advantage of the high levels of interbreed variation. Different breeds are genetically isolated from one another, meaning the genetic profiles of different breeds are distinctive. Traits shared by different breeds can be linked to large genomic regions using a single breed, and then the associated region can be refined and reduced by identifying the minimum haplotype that is shared across breeds segregating the same trait. Although each breed studied will carry the gene of interest on a large haplotype block, each breed's haplotype will be different, having arisen from an independent set of recombination events; the overlapping region that is common to all breeds contains the gene being sought.

Example

An example of the successful use of a GWAS is that of Forman and colleagues[8] who used this method to successfully identify the mutation for spinocerebellar ataxia (SCA) in the Parson Russell terrier (PRT). SCA in the PRT is a disease of progressive incoordination of gait, and loss of balance and pedigree analysis indicated an autosomal recessive mode of inheritance. Clinical signs usually become apparent between 6 and 12 months of age with affected dogs presenting with symmetric SCA particularly in the pelvic limbs. The degree of truncal ataxia, pelvic limb hypermetria, and impaired balance is progressive, particularly during the initial months of disease. A certain degree of stabilization and intermittent worsening may occur. At the later stages of the disease, ambulation often becomes difficult, with owners usually electing to euthanatize affected dogs on welfare grounds. Using a GWAS approach followed by targeted resequencing (see later discussion), a SNP in the *CAPN1* gene, encoding the calcium-dependent cysteine protease calpain1 (mu-calpain), was identified for which all affected dogs were homozygous. The SNP is a missense mutation causing a cysteine to tyrosine substitution at residue 115 of the CAPN1 protein. Cysteine 115 forms a key part of a catalytic triad of amino acids that are crucial to the enzymatic activity of cysteine proteases. The *CAPN1* gene shows high levels of expression in the brain and nervous system, and roles for the protein in both neuronal necrosis and maintenance have been suggested. Given the association with SCA in the PRT, the functional implications and high level of conservation observed across species, CAPN1 represents a novel potential cause of ataxia in humans.[8]

Targeted Resequencing

Targeted resequencing is the term used to describe the process of sequencing a small subset of the genome, such as a particular chromosome or a chromosomal region of interest. The technique is commonly used once a GWAS has implicated a particular genomic region to be associated with a disease under investigation (see previous discussion). The associated region is typically resequenced in some cases and controls and their sequences compared to identify any variants that are predicted to be pathogenic. The term *resequencing* is used because the method is used to identify genomic variations of a DNA sample, or small cohort of samples, in relation to a common reference sequence. A detailed description of targeted resequencing methodology is outside the scope of this review, but briefly, after fragmenting the genome, fragments from the desired region are captured by hybridizing the sample to complementary biotinylated probes, which can then be separated from the rest of the genome using streptavidin-labeled magnetic beads, followed by a wash step to remove unbound, nontargeted fragments. The resulting DNA is then used to prepare a standard library for sequencing.

Example

The method was used to successfully identify the mutation responsible for episodic falling (EF) in the Cavalier King Charles spaniel.[9] In this study, a GWAS and targeted resequencing of DNA from just 5 dogs were used to simultaneously map and identify mutations for 2 distinct inherited disorders that both affect the Cavalier King Charles Spaniel. The authors investigated EF, a paroxysmal exertion-induced dyskinesia, alongside the phenotypically distinct condition, congenital keratoconjunctivitis sicca and ichthyosiform dermatosis, commonly known as *dry eye curly coat syndrome*. EF is characterised by episodes of exercise-induced muscular hypertonicity and abnormal posturing, usually occurring after exercise or periods of excitement. The causal mutation for EF was identified as an approximately 16-kilobase (kb) deletion encompassing the first 3 exons of the brevican gene (BCAN). Brevican is one of the central nervous system–specific members of the hyaluronan-binding chondroitin sulfate proteoglycan family. Brevican is important in the organization of the nodes of Ranvier in myelinated large-diameter axons, and disruption of this region results in a delay in axonal conduction.[9]

Candidate Gene Analysis

Candidate gene analysis is the term used when a gene or subset of genes, as opposed to the entire genome, are investigated for their potential association with a disease under investigation. Candidate genes can be identified at the start of a study based on a priori knowledge of the gene's biological function, an association with a similar disease in a different species, or at completion of a successful GWAS when a gene may be identified as a positional as well as a functional candidate.

Example

A good example of a study in which a disease-associated mutation was identified in a gene that was both a functional and positional candidate was that of Zeng and colleagues[10] who used this approach to identify the mutation for Bandera's Neonatal Ataxia (BNAt) in the Coton de Tulear breed of dog. Dogs affected with this condition, which is named after one of the first puppies to be clinically evaluated, are usually identified as soon as their littermates develop coordinated movements. They exhibit titubation of the head and intention tremors. Most are unable to walk but can scoot in sternal recumbency as a means of purposeful locomotion. Spinal reflexes remain intact, but righting reflexes are delayed, and proprioceptive positioning is severely decreased or absent. Affected puppies are visual but lack a menace response and exhibit fine vertical ocular tremors at rest and saccadic dysmetria together with an upbeat nystagmus during dorsal positioning.[11] Zeng and coworkers[10] undertook a GWAS with 12 cases and 12 controls that identified a 713-kb region on canine chromosome 1 that was significantly associated with the disease. The region contained 4 genes, one of which was the metabotropic glutamate receptor 1 gene (*GRM1*) that was considered to be the most likely candidate to contain the BNAt-causing mutation because naturally occurring and experimentally induced *Grm1* deficiencies produced disease phenotypes in mice that resembled that of the BNAt-affected canine puppies. Resequencing *GRM1* from affected dogs identified a 62-base pair (bp) insertion in exon 8 that was concluded to be the cause of BNAt.[10]

Whole Genome Sequencing

Another route to mutation identification is to compare the sequence of an affected individual's entire genome with those of unaffected individuals. This is known as *whole genome sequencing* and is undertaken in the absence of prior association mapping that can narrow the hunt for the mutation to a small fraction of the genome and a subset of genes. Whole genome sequencing poses a considerable challenge, from a computational and bioinformatics perspective, because of the vast number of variants that are typically detected between the genomes of different individuals, even when those individuals are members of the same breed of dog. A refinement of whole genome sequencing is to sequence just the coding exons of all genes, a technique known as *whole exome sequencing*. This method is less computationally challenging than whole genome sequencing, because the exome is typically less than 5% the size of the whole genome, but relies on the hypothesis that most mutations associated with disease lie in the coding regions of genes. The method will not lead to the successful identification of causal mutations that lie outside coding exons.

Example

Whole genome sequencing has recently been used successfully for the first time in the dog to identify the mutation responsible for a form of inherited SCA associated with myokymia, seizures, or both known to affect Jack Russell terriers, Parson Russell terriers, and Russell terriers (collectively referred to as Russell group terriers).[12] The authors of this study sequenced the entire genome of a single Russell group terrier with SCA and myokymia and compared it with the whole genome sequences from 81 other canids that were normal or had other diseases. A mutation in the gene coding for the inwardly rectifying potassium channel Kir4.1 (*KCNJ10*) was identified that changed an amino acid and was predicted to be pathogenic. All dogs that were homozygous for this mutation had SCA with varying combinations of myokymia and seizures.[12] This form of ataxia is different and genetically distinct from the form described above that is caused by the *CPN1* mutation,[8] although both forms are characterized by similar and overlapping clinical signs and affect the same breeds.

Whole Transcriptome Sequencing

All of the methods described above use genomic DNA as the substrate for mutation identification. An alternative to sequencing genomic DNA is so-called mRNA sequencing from a tissue that is central to the trait. Because mature mRNA is effectively an RNA copy of the exome, mRNA sequencing can be considered a form of targeted resequencing, allowing nature to do the target capture rather than the in vitro methods that are required for exome sequencing.

Example

Sequencing of mRNA has, to date, only been used once to identify a disease-associated mutation in the dog. Forman and colleagues[13] used the method to identify the mutation responsible for neonatal cerebellar cortical degeneration (NCCD) in the beagle. NCCD-affected beagles are unable to ambulate normally from the onset of walking, and the main pathologic findings include Purkinje cell loss with swollen dendritic processes. In this landmark investigation, mRNA sequence from the cerebellum of a single NCCD case was generated, and the sequence of 27 genes known to cause ataxia in humans was analyzed. The causal mutation, located in the β-III spectrin gene (*SPTB2*), was an 8-bp coding deletion that is predicted to cause both an aberrant run of 27 extra amino acids and premature termination of mRNA (**Fig. 2**). The mutation segregated perfectly as an autosomal recessive in the small family tested, was found in the heterozygous state in other unaffected but at-risk dogs and was absent in 37 other breeds. As expected, cerebellar tissue from the affected dog showed a near total loss of β-III spectrin mRNA and protein when compared with a control dog. Spectrins are a family of cytoskeletal proteins, with tetrameric structures comprising 2 α and 2 β subunits, with diversity and specialization of function. β-III spectrin is primarily expressed in the nervous system and the highest levels of expression are found in Purkinje cell soma and dendrites.[14]

A

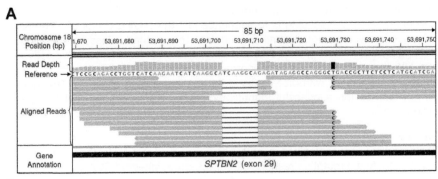

B

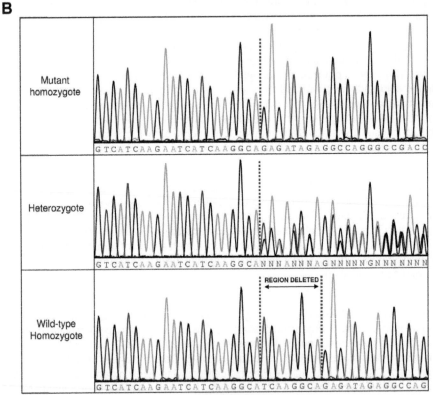

Fig. 2. Sequencing data show mutation responsible for NCCD in the beagle. (*A*) RNA sequencing reads from the mRNA-seq experiment aligned across the deletion and visualized in the software Integrative Genomics Viewer (IGV).[24] Reads are represented by gray bars, with the deletion indicated with a black horizontal line in reads. A single, benign nucleotide polymorphism (c.5580 T > C) is also located 18 bp downstream of the deleted sequence in the NCCD case and is highlighted in blue. (*B*) Sanger sequencing to confirm the 8-bp deletion in the case, the sire of the case (obligate heterozygote), and a wild-type individual (sibling). The 8-bp sequence upstream of the deletion is identical to the deleted sequence.

DNA TESTING

Once a mutation has been identified, using one or a combination of the methods outlined previously, a DNA test can be developed and offered to the public. Worldwide there are now many facilities offering canine DNA tests.[15] The process of DNA testing is simple and involves the submission of a sample of a dog's DNA to an appropriate testing laboratory. The DNA can often be submitted as a cheek swab that an owner can take themselves, although some tests or laboratories may require a blood sample. The testing laboratory analyses the DNA for the presence or absence of the relevant mutation and will report back, usually within a few weeks, with the result (the dog's genotype). The results will inform the veterinarian or owner whether the dog being tested has zero, 1, or 2 copies of the mutation for which the dog is being tested.

DNA Tests for Disease-Associated Mutations—What Do the Test Results Mean?

It is worth considering what the results of a DNA test mean to the owner, the veterinarian, and the dog. The primary consumer of DNA tests is the dog breeder, and the benefits of DNA tests to breeders wishing to reduce the prevalence of disease have been widely discussed.[16–19] As increasing pressure is put on breeders to improve the genetic health of the dogs they produce, the judicious use of DNA tests in this endeavor has never been more topical. It is important for both the breeder and the veterinarian to remember that clinically similar conditions can be caused by different mutations, and although clinically affected dogs of the same breed will usually share the same causal mutation, it is possible for genetically distinct forms of the same disease to segregate within the same breed. A good example of this is illustrated by the 2 clinically similar but genetically distinct forms of ataxia that affect Jack and Parson Russell terriers that were described previously. It is important for owners and veterinarians to appreciate that most DNA tests only assay for a single, specific mutation and not for any other mutations that cause clinically similar conditions. A clear DNA test result is not, therefore, an absolute guarantee that a dog will never have a clinically similar disease to that being for which it is being tested, although dogs that are clear of specific mutations can be considered at low risk of disease development.

Basic Genetics

Most of the DNA tests currently available are for mutations responsible for simple or single gene diseases and include all of the disorders described previously. This means that the disease is a result of a single mutation; no other genes or environmental factors are involved. For these diseases, the results of DNA tests are easy to interpret, and an individual dog's risk of developing the condition can be estimated with a high level of certainty from the DNA test results. Many simple inherited conditions have a recessive mode of inheritance. Recessive diseases are the result of mutations that cause the loss of function of a biologically important gene as opposed to dominant conditions, which usually result from mutations that cause an inappropriate gain of function of a gene. Every dog has 2 copies of each gene, one inherited from the dam and one from the sire, and carriers that have inherited a single copy of the normal gene from one parent and a single copy of a mutant gene from the other parent usually have sufficient functional protein to remain clinically healthy. It is only when a dog inherits a faulty gene from both parents that it becomes clinically affected. Consequently, if a mutation is recessive, then dogs with zero or 1 copy of the mutation will remain clinically free of the disease, although heterozygous carriers will pass the mutation onto around half of their offspring. Dogs with 2 copies of the mutation (homozygotes) will almost certainly have the disease during their lifetime, although they might be clinically clear at the time of testing. If a mutation is dominant, dogs with 1 or 2 copies of the mutation will get the condition (unless there is evidence of incomplete penetrance), whereas dogs that are clear of the mutation will remain healthy.

Some diseases are more complex, and result from mutations in multiple genes or the interaction between genes and the environment. Individual mutations might increase a dog's risk of getting the associated condition but cannot predict with certainty whether a dog will become clinically affected.

Using DNA Test Results to Reduce the Prevalence of Disease

DNA tests can play a critically important role in the control and eventual elimination of inherited diseases. Recessive diseases are notoriously difficult for the dog breeder to eliminate because of the existence of clinically healthy carriers within the population that can only be detected retrospectively, once they have produced affected offspring or one of their parents has been diagnosed as affected. The problem is confounded for late-onset conditions in which affected animals may be innocently bred before they are diagnosed, and this problem is applicable to dominant and recessive diseases.

The availability of a DNA test is often the only way in which a recessive condition or a late-onset dominant condition can be reliably eliminated from a breed. Breeders should have their breeding stock tested before mating and make sensible breeding choices, based on the genotype of their dog, that minimize the risk of producing affected offspring. Disease mutations can be common within specific breeds, and once a DNA test becomes available, the instinct of many breeders is to only breed from clear dogs. This practice will obviously eliminate the disease mutation from the breed rapidly but may do so at the expense of genetic diversity if large numbers of dogs are instantly removed from the gene pool. High levels of inbreeding and loss of genetic variation are well documented to have detrimental effects on the health and fertility of animals. For common recessive mutations, it is therefore advisable for breeders to continue breeding with carriers, at least for the first-generation after DNA test development. Provided all carriers are paired with DNA-tested, clear mates, only clear and carrier puppies will be born; no clinically affected dogs will be produced, and breeders can select a clear dog to breed on from the resulting litters. **Table 1** details the outcomes of mating dogs with different genotypes (with respect to a recessive mutation) and whether they can result in clinically affected offspring.

Table 1
Outcomes of mating dogs with different autosomal recessive genotypes

Combination of Dogs	Outcome	Possibility of Clinically Affected Offspring?
Clear × Clear	All puppies will be clear	No
Clear × Carrier	50% of puppies will be clear 50% of puppies will be carriers	No
Clear × Affected	All puppies will be carriers	No
Carrier × Carrier	25% of puppies will be clear 25% of puppies will be affected 50% of puppies will be carriers	Yes
Carrier × Affected	50% of puppies will be affected 50% of puppies will be carriers	Yes
Affected × Affected	All puppies will be affected	Yes

For dominant mutations, the situation is different. All offspring that inherit a disease-associated dominant mutation will have clinical signs at some stage during their lives, so breeding with animals that carry such mutations is harder to justify.

Using DNA Test Results to Aid Differential Diagnosis

Another, often overlooked, role of the DNA test is to help the veterinarian diagnose disease. There can be considerable overlap between the clinical signs of genetically different disorders, and DNA tests, where they exist, can come to the rescue. For example, several neurologic syndromes have been described in Cavalier King Charles spaniels, including occipital hypoplasia/syringomyelia, episodic collapse, epilepsy, and vestibular disorders, and clinical signs of these disorders can overlap.[20] In 2012, the mutation responsible for one of these conditions, EF, was identified (described previously), and now a DNA test is available for veterinarians to use to assist their investigations for those patients whose clinical signs are consistent with EF.[9] Similarly, L-2-hydroxyglutaric aciduria is a neurometabolic disorder that produces a variety of clinical neurologic deficits, including psychomotor retardation, seizures, and ataxia, and can thus be misdiagnosed as epilepsy. However, since 2007, when the molecular defect responsible for this condition in Staffordshire bull terriers was characterized, veterinarians can determine whether a dog is carrying 2 copies of the causal mutation and therefore whether it is in fact affected with L-2-hydroxyglutaric aciduria or another condition.[21]

Although a useful aid to differential diagnosis, the results of DNA testing should rarely be used in isolation by the veterinarian. One additional factor is the typical age of onset of specific diseases; inherited disorders typically have a characteristic age of onset, and this should always be considered alongside the DNA test results. One disease in which this is particularly pertinent is degenerative myelopathy (DM), for which a DNA test based on a mutation in a gene called *SOD1* is available to multiple breeds.[22] The age of onset of DM is variable, ranging from 6 to 15 years of age or even older, and some dogs that are homozygous for the DM mutation may die before any DM signs develop. Therefore, a young dog that is homozygous for the DM mutation and showing clinical signs consistent with DM, may be suffering from an entirely different condition.

Some inherited disorders require an environmental trigger or exposure in addition to carrying a risk mutation. An example is the condition known as exercise-induced collapse (EIC) in Labrador retrievers. EIC is an autosomal recessive syndrome caused by a mutation in the *DNM1* gene, which causes a defect in nerve communication during intense exercise.[23] Dogs that are homozygous for the mutation will collapse, but only after intense exercise, so alternative diagnoses should be considered for dogs that have not exercised before collapse, regardless of their DNA test result for the *DNM1* mutation.

DNA tests represent a valuable tool with which to reach a differential diagnosis but, as with all test results, should be considered as part of the complete clinical history for a patient and not in isolation.

Resources listing currently available DNA tests:

http://www.akcchf.org/canine-health/health-testing/

http://research.vet.upenn.edu/DNAGeneticsTestingLaboratorySearch/tabid/7620/Default.aspx

http://www.thekennelclub.org.uk/media/14688/dnatestsworldwide.pdf

REFERENCES

1. Available at: http://www.ncbi.nlm.nih.gov/pubmed/. Accessed July 2014.
2. Available at: http://omia.angis.org.au/home/. Accessed July 2014.

3. Available at: http://www.omim.org/. Accessed July 2014.

4. Available at: http://www.ensembl.org/index.html. Accessed July 2014.

5. Available at: http://www.vet.cam.ac.uk/idid/. Accessed July 2014.

6. Gough A, Thomas A. Breed predispositions to disease in dogs and cats. 2nd edition. Blackwell Publishing; 2010. p. 330.

7. Lin L, Faraco J, Li R, et al. The sleep disorder canine narcolepsy is caused by a mutation in the hypocretin (orexin) receptor 2 gene. Cell 1999;98(3):365–76.

8. Forman OP, De Risio L, Mellersh CS. Missense mutation in CAPN1 is associated with spinocerebellar ataxia in the parson russell terrier dog breed. PLoS One 2013;8(5):e64627.

9. Forman OP, Penderis J, Hartley C, et al. Parallel mapping and simultaneous sequencing reveals deletions in BCAN and FAM83H associated with discrete inherited disorders in a domestic dog breed. PLoS Genet 2012;8(1):e1002462.

10. Zeng R, Farias FH, Johnson GS, et al. A truncated retrotransposon disrupts the GRM1 coding sequence in Coton de Tulear dogs with Bandera's neonatal ataxia. J Vet Intern Med 2011;25(2):267–72.

11. Coates JR, O'Brien DP, Kline KL, et al. Neonatal cerebellar ataxia in Coton de Tulear dogs. J Vet Intern Med 2002;16(6):680–9.

12. Gilliam D, O'Brien DP, Coates JR, et al. A homozygous KCNJ10 mutation in Jack Russell Terriers and related breeds with spinocerebellar ataxia with myokymia, seizures or both. J Vet Intern Med 2014;28(3):871–7.

13. Forman OP, De Risio L, Stewart J, et al. Genome-wide mRNA sequencing of a single canine cerebellar cortical degeneration case leads to the identification of a disease associated SPTBN2 mutation. BMC Genet 2012;13(1):55.

14. Sakaguchi G, Orita S, Naito A, et al. A novel brain-specific isoform of beta spectrin: isolation and its interaction with Munc13. Biochem Biophys Res Commun 1998;248(3):846–51.

15. Available at: http://www.offa.org/dna_alltest.html. Accessed July 2014.

16. Mellersh C. DNA testing man's best friend. Vet Rec 2011;168(1):10–2.

17. Mellersh C, Sargan D. DNA testing in companion animals - what is it and why do it? Practice 2011;33(9):442–53.

18. Mellersh C. DNA testing and domestic dogs. Mamm Genome 2012;23(1–2):109–23.

19. Mellersh C. DNA testing: diagnosing and preventing inherited disorders in dogs. Vet Rec 2013;172(10):264–5.

20. Rusbridge C. Neurological diseases of the Cavalier King Charles spaniel. J Small Anim Pract 2005;46(6):265–72.

21. Penderis J, Calvin J, Abramson C, et al. L-2-hydroxyglutaric aciduria: characterisation of the molecular defect in a spontaneous canine model. J Med Genet 2007;44(5):334–40.

22. Awano T, Johnson GS, Wade CM, et al. Genome-wide association analysis reveals a SOD1 mutation in canine degenerative myelopathy that resembles amyotrophic lateral sclerosis. Proc Natl Acad Sci U S A 2009;106(8):2794–9.

23. Patterson EE, Minor KM, Tchernatynskaia AV, et al. A canine DNM1 mutation is highly associated with the syndrome of exercise-induced collapse. Nat Genet 2008;40(10):1235–9.

24. Robinson JT, Thorvaldsdottir H, Winckler W, et al. Integrative genomics viewer. Nat Biotechnol 2009;29(1):24–6.

Neuronavigation in Small Animals

Development, Techniques, and Applications

Fred Wininger, VMD, MS[a,b,*]

KEYWORDS

- Stereotaxy • Localization • Brain • Central nervous system • Biopsy • Intracranial
- Tumor

KEY POINTS

- Localization of lesions for minimally invasive biopsy of the brain is challenging.
- Modern techniques for navigation within the central nervous system rely predominantly on frameless systems and depend on cross-sectional imaging by CT or MRI.
- Rigidly affixed external markers define relationships between landmarks within and outside the cranial vault and are used to plan surgical trajectories.
- Surgical instruments can be labeled so as to provide real-time feedback on positioning within sites of minimal surgical access.
- Modern neuronavigation techniques have huge potential to revolutionize diagnosis, and therefore treatment, of intracranial lesions and will likely play a role in the development of minimally invasive techniques for spinal stabilization.

THE NEED FOR NEURONAVIGATION

The central nervous system is characterized by an intricate anatomy that necessitates precise localization methods to acquire representative biopsy material (**Figs. 1–5**). The brain is opaque; some regions are convoluted into gyri and sulci, and it is enclosed by the boney opaque calvarium that is inconsistently spatially matched with the content and has few identifiable prominences. Furthermore, it is segmented into specific white matter tracts and nuclei, all difficult to identify grossly, but most with independent essential functions. Localization within this uniquely complex structure is further complicated by pulsatile deformation of shape associated with blood flow and permitted by the surrounding cerebrospinal fluid. These obstacles, coupled with its poor handling quality and a lack of forgiveness to manipulation, make it perhaps the most difficult structure to surgically navigate in the entire body.[1]

[a] Department of Neurology/Neurosurgery, Veterinary Specialty Services, 1021 Howard George Drive, Manchester, MO 63021, USA; [b] University of Missouri-College of Veterinary Medicine, Veterinary Medicine and Surgery, 900 E Campus Drive Columbia, MO 65211, USA
* Veterinary Specialty Services, 1021 Howard George Drive, Ballwin, MO 63021.
E-mail address: fredwininger@gmail.com

Vet Clin Small Anim 44 (2014) 1235–1248
http://dx.doi.org/10.1016/j.cvsm.2014.07.015
0195-5616/14/$ – see front matter © 2014 Elsevier Inc. All rights reserved.

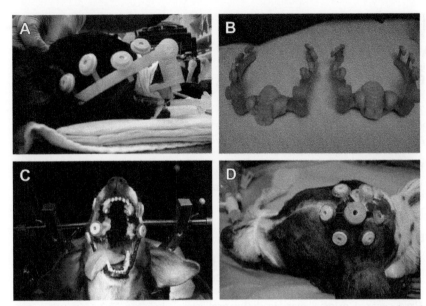

Fig. 1. Examples of artificial fiducial arrays. (*A, B*) Temporary bite arrays are easily fitted to patients, are minimally invasive, and can be removed between procedures. (*C*) More rigid dental arrays may improve accuracy but require a single anesthetic event. (*D*) Implantable arrays are more invasive but otherwise provide greater accuracy and confidence of neuronavigation. The illustrated array can be removed and the calvarial plug covered by the skin.

Localization aids for neurosurgery have been an essential part of successful intervention since its functional anatomy has been defined. This concept is considered essential in veterinary neurology: localization based on clinical presentation and physical examination findings is the crux of the discipline. The identification of "eloquent cortical regions" by Paul Broca and Carl Wernike, in which lesions would have serious consequences for the patient, is arguably the initiator of neuronavigation. Although dogs do not have eloquent cortex per se, the dog and cat homunculus is mostly known and surgical manipulation of specific supratentorial structures can cause important clinical consequences.[2,3] Because domestic animals' primary motor functions are thought to be largely extrapyramidal, compromise of basal nuclear and other subcortical structures may be of relatively greater importance.[4]

Development of Neuronavigation Devices

Initial neuronavigation techniques relied on the "terrestrial globe model" developed in humans, who have a spherical head of stereotypical size and proportions. Kocher and Kronlein's "Craniometer" and Zernov's "Encephalometer" used these proportions along with external craniofacial landmarks to target internal brain structures for symptomatic resection.[5] Because imaging other than radiography was not available at that time, intervention was based largely on the symptoms of the patient and functional neuro-anatomic atlases. Techniques relying on specific correlation of extracranial and intracranial structures are not applicable to many animal models because of craniofacial variability and nonuniformity of brain proportions.

The earliest image-based neuronavigation techniques were termed "stereotaxy," a term derived from the latin *stereos* = (geometric) solid and *taxis* = positioning

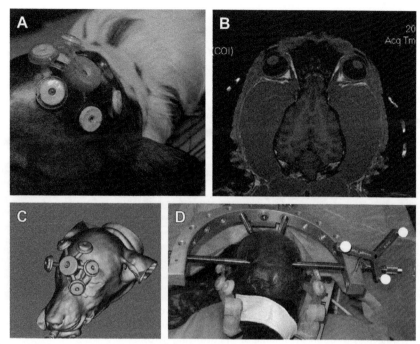

Fig. 2. Steps in neuronavigation (*A*) The patient is fitted with an artificial fiducial array (here a skull implant). (*B*) The image data set, a high-resolution T1-weighted 3D study, is acquired. In this example, a dental block fiducial array is used; the hyperintense paramagnetic markers are seen surrounding the head. (*C*) The image is reconstructed in 3D space. The fiducial centers are labeled and the target identified, which creates the "image space." (*D*) The subject tracker, with reflective balls, is affixed to the head of the patient using skull pins.

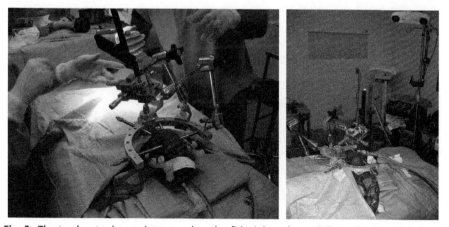

Fig. 3. The tracker tool or pointer touches the fiducial markers while in the line of sight of the infrared camera and links the image space with the anatomic space. The tracking tool is stabilized in an articulating arm to allow manipulation to reach target and complete the procedure.

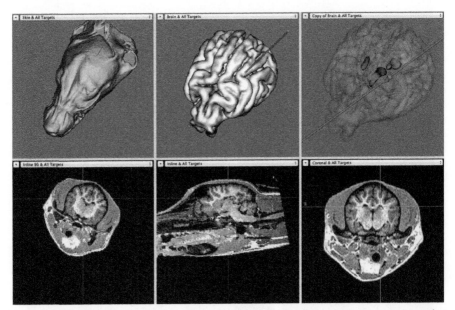

Fig. 4. 3D data sets allow for surface reconstructions of skin, bone, brain, or any tissue that can be identified as a region of interest. Here a lateral ventricular target has been selected with a trajectory through the middle of the overlying gyrus.

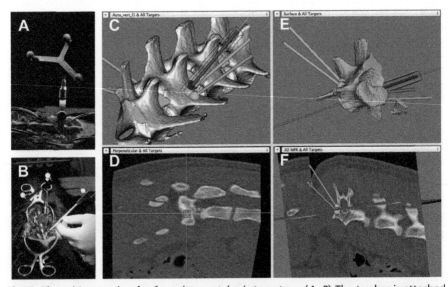

Fig. 5. The subject tracker for frameless vertebral stereotaxy. (*A, B*) The tracker is attached via clamps to any bony protuberance. Other iterations can be directly drilled into individual segments. (*C–F*) Planning is similar to intracranial application but requires each vertebrae to be treated as an individual unit with their own natural fiducial landmarks. ([*A, B*] *Courtesy of* Nicholas Archambault, DVM, University of Missouri.)

or placement. Stereotaxy is based on a 3-plane x-axis, y-axis, and z-axis Cartesian coordinate system, and the earliest systems required a frame to be rigidly affixed to the skull. Distances from a central point origin in these axes correspond to positions in the dorsal, transverse, and sagittal plane. The frames often have defined and consistent points of stabilization; in humans, fixation points vary from modular bite plates to implantable skull pins. In animals, ear bars placed into the external acoustic meatus, an upper dental arcade rest for the incisors and ventral orbital clamps, are most common. Frame-based systems can apply the numerical values of the coordinate system to predefined anatomic atlases, which are readily available for rodents and primates. Radiography and ventriculography can be used to identify mineralized internal reference points (eg, a calcified pineal body) to set an intracranial origin point and further increase the accuracy of the coordinate system.

Tomographic modalities applying cross-sectional imaging such as CT and MRI revolutionized neuronavigation because of the superior spatial and contrast-resolving properties. Because of the superior soft tissue contrast, normal and pathologic anatomy for an individual patient could now be assessed. Advancing thin cross-sectional imaging with computers capable of compiling data in 3-dimensional (3D) space allowed frameless systems to be developed because the Cartesian coordinate system could now be rotated into convenient positions.

Framed systems are generally cumbersome and difficult to accurately and reproducibly affix to the skull. For best results, patients must be within a frame while the imaging procedure is performed. Many systems require the frame to remain affixed between imaging and surgical procedures, necessitating surgery within the imaging gantry or incurring difficulties during patient transport. Framed systems often limit surgical exposure and prevent optimal patient positioning, particularly for skull-base and ventral procedures. Because frameless systems can overcome these obstacles, they have largely supplanted frame-based systems.

Frameless systems

Frameless systems can be classified as arm-based or pointer-based. Arm-based systems operate through a "proprioceptive theory." An articulating arm is affixed rigidly to the head using clamps and the system identifies location by calculating its own position in space relative to a fixed point, through measurements of angles of each joint and crank arm length, similar to a biological arm sensory system. Arm-based systems still struggle with many of the steric obstacles of frame-based systems, such as limited trajectories and inaccessible surgical sites. However, they do not require an optic external tracking system, which allows the operator to be closer to the surgical field without blocking the line of sight. Pointer systems operate on a principle similar to global positioning systems and use either optical or electromagnetic assessments. Twin sources (cameras) calculate distance through measurement of sphere diameter and distance from each other. Most recent studies show accuracy of less than 0.5 mm in even the deepest of human brain locations, on par with framed systems. For this reason, they have largely replaced framed systems in human medicine.[6]

STRUGGLES IN VETERINARY STEREOTAXY

Many limitations have prevented the application of neuronavigation systems to clinical veterinary medicine, of which anatomic variability is the greatest. The human skull is more or less spherical and relatively thin (5–13 mm) and has small overlying sinuses, thin muscles of mastication, and little variability in size or shape.[7] The dog skull is highly variable in general size, shape, and thickness (sometimes >10 mm), making frame placement difficult. This conformation presents challenges when creating focal craniotomy defects, because the external skull surface is often oblique to the brain-calvarium interface. The large diploic cavity and sinuses also complicate focal hole-drilling if compared with similar techniques in the relatively homogenous human skull. Furthermore, the large muscles of mastication make application of a frame and single burr hole approaches difficult (although enclosed biopsy channels that cut, pene-trate, and separate muscle provide a partial solution).

The varying sizes of the dog head have also prevented the development of a stan-dardized atlas of neuroanatomy. In the rodent and primate, imaging is often not neces-sary as a prerequisite, particularly if using framed techniques, because the variability in brain and brain-skull ratios is so limited that surgery can be performed based on general species anatomy.[8]

POINTER-BASED FRAMELESS NEURONAVIGATION TECHNIQUE

The frameless pointer techniques create a virtual reality between anatomic space (ie, the reality of the patient head in the operating room) and "image space," which is the 3D reconstruction of the tomographic data set. In this image space, the different structures of the brain and pathologic lesions can be identified and preoperative planning completed. Successful fusion of anatomic and image spaces makes neuro-navigation possible.

Frameless stereotactic systems consist of a series of components that must be linked together: (1) tomographic image data set; (2) identifiable fiducial markers than can be localized in both data set and intraoperatively; (3) computer capable of rendering the data set into 3D space; (4) a subject tracker (usually affixed to the skull) that "registers" (ie, aligns) the patient with the 3D model; (5) an instrument tracker to register interventional tools with the anatomic space. The specific details of each of these are considered below.

Tomographic Data Set

Various methods of cross-sectional imaging can be used for neuronavigation techniques.

Ultrasound was the initial modality of choice because it allowed for reasonable tissue contrast, the ability to identify the biopsy device, flexibility for real-time manip-ulation, and portability (ie, it could be used in the operating suite).[9] However, its limitations of shallow depth of field, bleeding/gas susceptibility, and penetration char-acteristic of sound waves preclude its use in minimally invasive neuronavigation without large craniotomies. CT revolutionized brain imaging with the ability to provide cross-sectional intracranial imaging. CT has excellent spatial resolution and fair contrast resolution. The downsides to the modality are that it requires "in- and out-of-the-room technology," meaning that the practitioner makes adjustments to the procedure but must leave the surgical suite if reimaging is required because of the ionizing radiation, which may also be a safety concern to the patient because multiple image sets may be required.

MRI is the current gold standard for intracranial imaging and provides several advantages over CT, including exponentially improved soft tissue contrast resolution facilitating identification of small anatomic targets and avoidance of collateral damage to essential nuclei. Multiple pulse sequences allow for directed contrast resolution to improve conspicuity of tissues of interest, particularly when paramagnetic contrast is used. Aside from the standard anatomic imaging, the data sets can be fused with other functional studies, such as diffusion, perfusion, spectroscopy, angiography, and BOLD imaging. Like CT, thin slices allow for multiplanar reconstructions; however, MR has no associated ionizing radiation and vessel imaging does not require administration of contrast agent. MR is not so amenable to framed systems that require intraprocedure imaging because of susceptibility artifacts to metallic substances and safety concerns within the 5-G line. Within this fringe field, ferromagnetic instruments attracted toward the MR gantry can become dangerous projectiles. Creating surgical instruments without ferrous components is technically challenging and expensive.[10] Because frameless neuronavigation surgery occurs outside the imaging area, this is not a rate-limiter.

When acquiring the data set, the smallest volume isotropic voxels should be selected without compromising signal-to-noise ratio. "Isotropic voxels" are cubes of imaging data acquired in one plane that can be reconstructed into any planar (including oblique) views for image guidance. Smaller voxels generally provide higher resolution, but if too small, they can be information-deficient and create grainy or "signal-starved" images. On CT, voxels are acquired at 5 mm in the author's facility. On MRI, T1-weighted gradient-based sequences are commonly used and have different names depending on vendor (eg, MPRage [Siemens Medical Solutions USA, Inc, Malvern, PA], fast spoiled gradient echo FSPGR [GE Global Diagnostic Imaging, Pewaukee, WI]). The sequences can be acquired postcontrast and are generally submillimeter voxels with acquisition times between 10 and 20 minutes on a 1.5-T MRI. Increased acquisition times allow for more averaging and higher resolution but longer anesthesia times. More recently, T2-weighted 3D sequencing, such as SPACE (Siemens) or CUBE (GE), have become available and provide the clinical benefit of showing fluid-based lesions, such as edema, which are not visible on T1-weighted 3D imaging.

Identifiable Fiducial Markers

Fiducial markers are the landmarks by which image space and anatomic space are melded. As such, they must be easily identified on the image data sets and in the operating room. Furthermore, these markers must be finite in both regions, because accuracy of the system is directly related to the precise identification in both spaces. These fiducial markers are rigidly associated with the skull, and any variability of the fiducials between the 2 spaces will lead to failed registration. The closer the fiducial system is to the target tissue, the higher the accuracy. Generally, 3 fiducial points in the varying planes are needed for adequate registration, but it is recommended to have multiple fiducial markers available. Markers that appear usable in image space may be inaccessible in the operating room if, for example, they are blocked by the head clamp or too close to the borders of the aseptic field.

Fiducial markers can be either natural visible landmarks, such as bony protuberances or teeth, or artificially implanted arrays. The advantage of natural landmarks is that they do not require an implantation procedure before imaging. Also, if surgery was not anticipated before imaging and an artificial array was not placed, neuronavigation is still possible. However, natural landmarks tend to be less defined in both image and anatomic space and may require more extensive surgical dissection to identify them. Furthermore, if destroyed during the craniotomy, registration cannot be reperformed if needed. These natural landmarks are more amenable to CT than MRI data sets because of the superior mineral resolution.

Artificial landmarks are generally small pinpoint discs that can be registered in both image and anatomic spaces. They are constructed of materials visible to the specific modality: radiopaque mineral for CT and paramagnetic material for MR. These arrays cannot contain any ferromagnetic substances that would cause a susceptibility artifact on MRI and so they are generally made from MR-safe plastics such as PEEK and the fiducial markers colabeled with copper sulfate and iodinated contrast. In general, any artificial fiducial array should be removable after imaging and be replaceable in the identical orientation for surgery.

Artificial dental landmarks are commonly used in both human and veterinary medicine. Dental bite blocks are minimally invasive and can be quickly formed before imaging or in the gantry once a lesion is identified. They are distant to the intracranial space, which decreases accuracy but is advantageous in not interfering with the surgical approach. Nevertheless, there is potential for significant user error, particularly because of movement, which considerably decreases procedural accuracy. An alternative technique is to drill superficial small-bore holes in the teeth that are then painted with paramagnetic solution. However, this more invasive technique must be performed before imaging and requires intraoperative access to the oral cavity potentially compromising aseptic technique.

An alternative technique is to use implantable fiducial arrays, which can be placed anywhere on the skull. These implantable fiducial arrays often comprise an implantable cranial plug that can be sutured under the skin and a fitted screw attached to fiducial markers. They are associated with the greatest accuracy because of their proximity to the target and repeatable space orientation without motion, but they do necessitate a short preimaging surgery.

Imaging of frameless neuronavigation procedures can be performed well before surgery, so long as there is no physical change in the cranial structure or proportions in the interim period; this would exclude growing patients or those with lesions that change in shape and size, so altering the proximity of the target structure to the fiducial system.

Creation of Image Space

Once loaded, the image data set can be converted into 2-dimensional and 3D reconstructions. Regions of interest can be identified and reformatted into volume renderings that will be later used for surgical guidance. These anatomic images can be used with functional imaging or other anatomic data sets. The fiducial landmarks are identified and labeled for later registration with anatomic space. Specific targets for surgery are also labeled. Predetermined trajectories may be created to reach these targets while preserving vital structures. Intraoperative trajectories can later be prescribed and are useful when a planned trajectory is not possible because of surgical field limitations.

The Subject Tracker

Tracker systems

The frameless neuronavigation of the tracking systems allows for real-time communication between image and anatomic spaces and, currently, is mostly optical or electromagnetic. Optical sensors use dual infrared cameras that focus on 3 specifically oriented reflective balls. Based on the diameters of the balls, the camera determines the distance of the tracker from itself. These systems are accurate and economical, but require an uninterrupted line of sight for adequate performance; if the surgeon breaks the beam between camera and surgical field, the system is rendered useless. Electromagnetic systems provide the advantage of not requiring line of site access, but require a generator, which can be cumbersome, expensive, and less accurate.[11]

The tracking system identifies 2 groups of points, the subject tracker and the pointer/tracker tool. The subject tracker is equivalent to the origin point of the virtual space in the coordinate system. It is from this point that the computer correlates the registered fiducials, merging image, and anatomic space. It is generally affixed to the skull via a C-clamp or partial "halo." This halo can be affixed to the operating table by an articulating arm, enabling the surgeon to manipulate the entire head and system into the most ergonomic position. The halo also serves as a platform for placement of other manipulators/surgical tools.

The Image Tracker

The tracking tool, or pointer, is also connected to 3 reflective balls monitored by an infrared camera. Once the subject tracker is affixed to the skull, the pointer is used to register the fiducial markers in anatomic space with those in image space. At this point, the camera/computer can identify any point in image space with those in anatomic space based on its position from the subject tracker. Although registration is performed with the pointer, the tracking tool can be calibrated with any surgical tool, including biopsy needles, syringes for injection, ultrasonic aspirator, or probe. During surgery, the computer provides real-time feedback on target and trajectory with multiplanar images to monitor the potential path to surgical target. Once this path is set and the tracking tool is locked in place, the depth to target is displayed. Accurate depth in surgery can be attained by neuronavigation and corroborated using calipers.

Summary of Frameless Stereotactic Technique

1. Affixing artificial fiducials before imaging (unless using natural fiducials)
2. Acquisition of image data set
   a. CT versus MRI
3. Creation of 3D image space
4. Assignment of fiducial localizers in image space
5. Target designation in image space
6. Surgical approach and affixing of the subject tracker
7. Assignment of fiducial markers in anatomic space
8. Target approach in surgical space

SOURCES OF ERROR

Neuronavigation errors can vary in severity from minor inaccuracy to complete procedure failure but can generally be classified into 2 groups according to previously published criteria.[12]

Type I errors include a change of position between image acquisition and the procedure.

Brain deformation/shift is a common error when the subject's anatomy differs between imaging and surgery, which inevitably occurs when the skull and/or dura are opened. In humans, deformation can be as great as 5.6 mm from durotomy alone[13] and may be even larger in a patient with altered intracranial dynamics. Once the parenchyma is manipulated or a structural lesion is removed, the initial image space and neuronavigation may be rendered useless. Other preprocessing errors that lead to inaccuracy can be image distortion (echo planar imaging being the most susceptible), inaccurate tumor definition, or poorly resolved image data sets.

Type II errors include problems in creation of the virtual reality of image and anatomic space fusion.

Wang[12] describes these errors as either transformation errors because of neuronavigation imperfection (type IIA) or errors based on surgeon error (type IIB). Type IIA errors reflect inherent inaccuracy of the tracking system; optical systems have a reported root-mean-square error of 0.25 mm, whereas in electromagnetic systems it is ~1 mm. Any damage to the tracking devices can also cause this form of error because the spheres are specifically spaced and alteration in intersphere distance or angulation will lead to localization error. Placement of the fiducials distant from the target will also increase this form of error.

Type IIB error is performance error, essentially caused by inaccurate identification of fiducials in either the image space during surgical planning or anatomic space during registration. In addition, poor replacement or movement of the fiducial array between imaging and surgery will lead to mal-registration. Intraoperative movement of the subject tracker or C-clamp can also cause severe navigation error.[14]

VETERINARY APPLICATIONS

Framed stereotaxy has been used in animals nearly as long as it has been used in humans, initially in research and later in clinical veterinary medicine. The first applications used center-of-the-arc techniques and had a relatively high level of accuracy. However, initial framed systems were bulky, provided limited surgical access and limited trajectories, required multiple imaging samples, so-called out-of-the room technology,[15–19] and were based largely on CT imaging. Later, real-time CT veterinary navigation devices have been described that obviate multiple scans between procedures.[20] Many of these systems are still in use today.

Kopf (David Kopf Instruments, Tujunga, California) framed systems are a mainstay of stereotaxy in rodent research and the company also produces systems for large animals (dogs, cats, and primates). Newer iterations of the system have an imaging frame that can be used during the imaging procedure, and derived localization values can be used in the actual surgical frame, making the system MR safe and usable in a designated surgical suite. Accuracy studies of this system show an overall mean error in needle placement in a dorsoventral trajectory of 0.9 ± 0.9 mm for dogs and 1.0 ± 1.1 mm for cats. Because of greater obliquity error, the system is considered accurate for lesions 3.3 mm in depth.[21]

In the past several years, veterinary-specific frameless systems have been introduced into multiple practices. A CT-specific frameless system using a bite plate was recently described as having an accuracy ranging between 2.0 and 3.9 mm for deep intracranial biopsies.[22] The commercially available veterinary-specific Brainsight vet system (Rogue Research, Montreal, Quebec) is compatible with CT but is primarily designed for MR data sets. An evaluation of this system showed a mean needle placement error for all target sites of 1.79 ± 0.87 mm. The upper bound of error for this stereotactic system was 3.31 mm for deeper subcortical structures.[23]

Neuronavigation has many applications in the veterinary clinical arena and several have been evaluated at this point. Perhaps the primary utility of these systems is to biopsy intra-axial tissue for definitive diagnosis of MR identified lesions.[24,25] Freehand biopsy techniques using a frameless neuronavigation technique to sample encephalitic cases through a 4-mm burr hole had a definitive diagnostic rate of 82% with a less specific diagnosis of encephalitis of 94% (although such figures also depend on the nature of the sampled population). The morbidity of this technique neared 29% but most clinical consequences were transient.[26] Sixteen-gauge side-cutting needles have been shown to provide samples adequate for diagnostic interpretation greater than 96% when aspirated to less than 2.0 cc of negative pressure.

The texture of intracranial masses can present certain obstacles, because extra-axial masses or highly mineralized tissue is more difficult to penetrate than the softer underlying neuroparenchyma.[27] Although not specifically used with neuronavigation, a cryogenic-based biopsy device has recently been described for use in the dog brain.[28]

This tool uses a carbon dioxide cartridge to freeze the tissue before biopsy, and the technique was not associated with any morbidity and had high diagnostic yield.

Neuronavigation has been also used for guidance of tumor resection in open craniotomies, for both identification and completeness of excision. However, once the procedure is initiated, much of the image space data become inaccurate because of brain shift and deformation. The need for modern neuronavigation systems for tumor approaches may be in question with the increased frequency of intraoperative MR capabilities.[29] Modern surgical suites can monitor neurosurgical procedures in real time, obviating many of the errors associated with neuronavigation, which are reliant on preprocedural imaging. Intraoperative MR is highly expensive, because of both the imaging equipment and the need for MR safe/compatible surgical equipment, which may limit this approach in veterinary medicine.

OTHER USES FOR NEURONAVIGATION

In addition to removing tissue, neuronavigation can be used to place therapeutic substances or implants. In the author's program, neuronavigation is most commonly used for the injection of gene therapy to intraventricular or intraparenchymal targets.[30] Similarly, the technique may be used for placement of ventricular shunting devices in animals without significantly dilated ventricles. This and endoscopic techniques (ventriculoscopy) lend themselves to guidance by neuronavigation techniques.[31] Deep brain stimulators are used with increased frequency in human medicine to treat epileptiform and movement disorders. A technique for placement of these electrodes into dogs has been evaluated in which the electrodes were successfully placed in 3 of 4 dogs with a mean accuracy of 4.6 ± 1.5 mm.[32]

Neuronavigation techniques are not restricted to the brain and have application to the vertebral column as well. Specific spinal cord neurolocalization is likely not feasible based on the mobility of the cord itself relative to its adjacent vertebral segments, but the utility for the neuronavigation instead lies in the placement of vertebral implants that gain adequate bone purchase without compromising the vertebral canal and its contents. A major consideration for spinal neuronavigation is that each vertebral unit is separate and must be registered individually. The techniques generally use CT imaging with natural fiducial markers that are exposed in the anatomic space.[33-35] These techniques are currently under investigation in the veterinary field, and preliminary pilot data have quantitatively shown the ability to place bicorticate implants in ideal bone purchase corridors without spinal column compromise.[36]

Transphenoidal hypophysectomy (TSH) is frequently described in the human and veterinary literature but one of the primary limitations of this technique is the lack of consistent external anatomic landmarks that can indicate the safe surgical corridor to the hypophyseal sella. Previous guided approaches include CT assessment of the distance from the hamular processes, nasopharyngeal catheters, or staged surgery with pilot hole–based CT localization. An alternate technique is the use of frameless neuronavigation for surgical corridor guidance. In addition to high accuracy and reduced surgical time, the neuronavigation system permits the use of oblique trajectories and therefore easier surgical access with less restriction from the mandible. In a recent review of 208 pituitary adenoma cases, Eboli and colleagues[37] reported integration of intraoperative CT data with preoperative MR data into an electromagnetic-based navigational system and demonstrated 100% concordance between bony landmarks in the imaging data set with the intraoperative probe location, leading to successful procedural navigation. A cadaveric study for validation of frameless neuronavigation in dog TSH showed an accuracy median of 0.89 mm with all approaches successfully within the hypophyseal sellae.[38] A secondary value of the frameless systems is a more agile form of patient positioning for this technique, permitting head angle changes during the procedure. TSH is often performed in the human medical field with the assistance of endoscopic magnification and illumination.

Veterinary neurologists are using neuronavigation for multiple applications more frequently, but its utility in the clinical arena is still somewhat unknown. Although the diagnostic specificity of MR is estimated to be high,[39] a tissue sample is usually required for definitive diagnosis, and certainly for determining tumor grade and malignancy. Although extra-axial masses can be sampled by these techniques, the advantage of possible complete excisions through open surgical approaches means that the primary attraction of neuronavigation in this context is for intra-axial sampling. However, it could be argued that with the currently limited neoplastic and encephalitic treatments (that are often similar), the value of tissue diagnosis may lie more in prognosis than therapy. On the other hand, novel intervention cannot be developed without accurate pretherapeutic diagnoses. It is likely that, as the ease and accuracy of these techniques improve, their value will become clearer.

REFERENCES

1. Ishii M, Gallia GL. Application of technology for minimally invasive neurosurgery. Neurosurg Clin N Am 2010;21:585–94.
2. Bagley RS. Recognition and localization of intracranial disease. Vet Clin North Am Small Anim Pract 1996;26:667–709.
3. King AS. Physiological and clinical anatomy of the domestic mammals: central nervous system, vol. 1. Oxford, UK: Wiley-Blackwell; 1999.
4. DeLahunta AG. Veterinary neuroanatomy and clinical neurology. St Louis (MO): Saunders Elsevier; 2009.
5. Grunert P. From the idea to its realization: the evolution of minimally invasive techniques in neurosurgery. Minim Invasive Surg 2013;2013:171369.
6. Owen CM, Linskey ME. Frame-based stereotaxy in a frameless era: current capabilities, relative role, and the positive- and negative predictive values of blood through the needle. J Neurooncol 2009;93:139–49.
7. Hwang SC, Im SB, Kim BT, et al. Safe entry point for twist-drill craniostomy of a chronic subdural hematoma. J Neurosurg 2009;110:1265–70.
8. Greitz T, Bohm C, Holte S, et al. A computerized brain atlas: construction, anatomical content, and some applications. J Comput Assist Tomogr 1991;15:26–38.
9. Weiss CR, Nour SG, Lewin JS. MR-guided biopsy: a review of current techniques and applications. J Magn Reson Imaging 2008;27:311–25.
10. Darakchiev BJ, Tew JM, Bohinski RJ, et al. Adaptation of a standard low-field (0.3-T) system to the operating room: focus on pituitary adenomas. Neurosurg Clin N Am 2005;16:155–64.
11. Zaaroor M, Bejerano Y, Weinfeld Z, et al. Novel magnetic technology for intraoperative intracranial frameless navigation: in vivo and in vitro results. Neurosurgery 2001;48:1100–7.
12. Wang MN, Song ZJ. Classification and analysis of the errors in neuronavigation. Neurosurgery 2011;68:1131–43.
13. Kuhnt D, Bauer MH, Nimsky C. Brain shift compensation and neurosurgical image fusion using intraoperative MRI: current status and future challenges. Crit Rev Biomed Eng 2012;40:175–85.
14. Widmann G, Schullian P, Ortler M, et al. Frameless stereotactic targeting devices: technical features, targeting errors and clinical results. Int J Med Robot 2012;8:1–16.

15. Moissonnier P, Blot S, Devauchelle P, et al. Stereotactic CT-guided brain biopsy in the dog. J Small Anim Pract 2002;43:115–23.
16. Moissonnier P, Bordeau W, Delisle F, et al. Accuracy testing of a new stereotactic CT-guided brain biopsy device in the dog. Res Vet Sci 2000;68:243–7.
17. Giroux A, Jones JC, Bøhn JH, et al. A new device for stereotactic CT-guided biopsy of the canine brain: design, construction, and needle placement accuracy. Vet Radiol Ultrasound 2002;43:229–36.
18. Koblik PD, LeCouteur RA, Higgins RJ, et al. CT-guided brain biopsy using a modified Pelorus Mark III stereotactic system: experience with 50 dogs. Vet Radiol Ultrasound 1999;40:434–40.
19. Coffey RJ, Lunsford LD. Animal research stereotactic instrument modified for computed tomographic guidance. Appl Neurophysiol 1987;50:81–6.
20. Flegel T, Podell M, March PA, et al. Use of a disposable real-time CT stereotactic navigator device for minimally invasive dog brain biopsy through a mini-burr hole. AJNR Am J Neuroradiol 2002;23:1160–3.
21. Troxel MT, Vite CH. CT-guided stereotactic brain biopsy using the Kopf stereotactic system. Vet Radiol Ultrasound 2008;49:438–43.
22. Taylor AR, Cohen ND, Fletcher S, et al. Application and machine accuracy of a new frameless computed tomography-guided stereotactic brain biopsy system in dogs. Vet Radiol Ultrasound 2013;54:332–42.
23. Chen AV, Wininger FA, Frey S, et al. Description and validation of a magnetic resonance imaging-guided stereotactic brain biopsy device in the dog. Vet Radiol Ultrasound 2012;53:150–6.
24. Kubben PL, ter Meulen KJ, Schijns OE, et al. Intraoperative MRI-guided resection of glioblastoma multiforme: a systematic review. Lancet Oncol 2011;12: 1062–70.
25. Orringer DA, Golby A, Jolesz F. Neuronavigation in the surgical management of brain tumors: current and future trends. Expert Rev Med Devices 2012;9: 491–500.
26. Flegel T, Oevermann A, Oechtering G, et al. Diagnostic yield and adverse effects of MRI-guided free-hand brain biopsies through a mini-burr hole in dogs with encephalitis. J Vet Intern Med 2012;26:969–76.
27. Schneider AR, Chen AV, Haldorson GJ. (2010, June). Evaluation of a 14 and 16 Gauge Side-Cutting Biopsy Needle and Four Different Aspiration Pressures Used to Obtain Brain Tissue in Dogs. ACVIM Forum, Anaheim, CA.
28. Marino DJ, Loughlin CA. (2012, June). The Sanarus Cassi IITM Freeze Core Biopsy System for Brain Tumor Biopsy: A Prospective Comparison with Surgical Tissue Biopsy Sections. ACVIM Forum, New Orleans, LA.
29. Black P, Jolesz FA, Medani K. From vision to reality: the origins of intraoperative MR imaging. Acta Neurochir Suppl 2011;109:3–7.
30. Katz ML, Coates JR, Sibigtroth CM, et al. Enzyme replacement therapy attenuates disease progression in a canine model of late-infantile neuronal ceroid lipofuscinosis (CLN2 disease). Journal of Neuroscience Research 2014. http://dx. doi.org/10.1002/jnr.23423.
31. Krombach GA, Rohde V, Haage P, et al. Virtual endoscopy combined with intraoperative neuronavigation for planning of endoscopic surgery in patients with occlusive hydrocephalus and intracranial cysts. Neuroradiology 2002;44: 279–85.
32. Long S, Frey S, Freestone DR, et al. Placement of deep brain electrodes in the dog using the brainsight frameless stereotactic system: a pilot feasibility study. J Vet Intern Med 2014;28:189–97.

33. Moses ZB, Mayer RR, Strickland BA, et al. Neuronavigation in minimally invasive spine surgery. Neurosurg Focus 2013;35:E12.

34. Shin BJ, James AR, Njoku IU, et al. Pedicle screw navigation: a systematic review and meta-analysis of perforation risk for computer-navigated versus freehand insertion. J Neurosurg Spine 2012;17:113–22.

35. Tjardes T, Shafizadeh S, Rixen D, et al. Image-guided spine surgery: state of the art and future directions. Eur Spine J 2010;19:25–45.

36. Wininger FA, Archambault N, Frey S. (2013, August). MR frameless stereotactic Vertebral Pin Placement in dogs. Veterinary neurosurgical society annual meeting, Portland OR.

37. Eboli P, Shafa B, Mayberg M. Intraoperative computed tomography registration and electromagnetic neuronavigation for transsphenoidal pituitary surgery: accuracy and time effectiveness. J Neurosurg 2011;114:329–35.

38. Wininger FA, Bentley M, Coates JR, Frey S (2011, August). MR-Based frameless Stereotactic System for Surgical Approach in Trasnphenoidal Hyposphysectomy. Veterinary neurosurgical society annual meeting, Portland, ME.

39. Young BD, Fosgate GT, Holmes SP, et al. Evaluation of standard magnetic resonance characteristics used to differentiate neoplastic, inflammatory, and vascular brain lesions in dogs. Vet Radiol Ultrasound 2014;55v:399–406.

Index

Note: Page numbers of article titles are in **boldface** type.

A

Acquired acute fulminating myasthenia gravis, 1216–1218
    clinical signs of, 1216–1217
    diagnosis of, 1217
    introduction, 1216
    prognosis of, 1217–1218
    treatment of, 1217–1218
Acute idiopathic polyradiculoneuritis (AIP), 1202–1208
    clinical signs of, 1203–1204
    diagnosis of, 1204–1205
    introduction, 1202–1203
    pathophysiology of, 1203
    prognosis of, 1205–1208
    treatment of, 1205–1208
Acute lower motor neuron (LMN) tetraparesis, **1201–1222**. *See also specific types, e.g., Botulism*
    acquired acute fulminating myasthenia gravis, 1216–1218
    AIP, 1202–1208
    botulism, 1208–1213
    introduction, 1201–1202
    tick paralysis, 1213–1216
Acute repetitive seizures (ARS)
    defined, 1104
Acute spinal cord injury (SCI), **1131–1156**. *See also* Spinal cord injury (SCI), acute
Adoptive immunotherapy
    in brain tumor management
        in dogs and cats, 1028–1029
Age
    as factor in prognosis after SCI, 1147
Aging
    in canine brain, **1113–1129**
        clinical implications of, 1121–1122
        introduction, 1113–1114
        lysosomal storage diseases, 1118–1119
        neurobiology of, 1114–1119
            brain atrophy, 1114–1115
            selective neuron loss, 1115
            senile plaques, 1115–1116
            vascular disorders, CAA, 1116–1117
        oxidative damage and mitochondrial dysfunction, 1118
        tau neuropathology of, 1117
    in feline brain, **1113–1129**

Vet Clin Small Anim 44 (2014) 1249–1263
http://dx.doi.org/10.1016/S0195-5616(14)00150-8
0195-5616/14/$ – see front matter © 2014 Elsevier Inc. All rights reserved.

Aging (*continued*)
     clinical implications of, 1121–1122
     introduction, 1113–1114
     neurobiology of, 1119–1121
        Aβ, 1119–1120
        neuron loss and atrophy, 1119
        neuronal loss in NPC disease, 1120–1121
        tau phosphorylation, 1120
AIP. *See* Acute idiopathic polyradiculoneuritis (AIP)
Altered states of consciousness
   in small animals, **1039–1058**. *See also* Consciousness, altered states of
ARS. *See* Acute repetitive seizures (ARS)
Ataxia(s)
   hereditary
      canine, **1075–1089**. *See also* Hereditary ataxia(s), canine

B

Bacteria
   in infectious CNS disease
      testing for, 1194–1195
Biomarker(s)
   for neural injury and infection in small animals, **1187–1199**. *See also* Neural injury,
      biomarkers for
   in prognosis after SCI, 1148
Blood pressure
   abnormalities in
      after SCI
        in dogs, 1137
Border Terriers
   epileptoid cramping in, 1098
Botulism, 1208–1213
   clinical signs of, 1211
   diagnosis of, 1212
   introduction, 1208–1210
   pathophysiology of, 1210
   prevention of, 1213
   prognosis of, 1212–1213
   treatment of, 1212–1213
Boxers
   paroxysmal dyskinesia in, 1099
Brain
   aging of
      in canine and feline brain, **1113–1129**. *See also* Aging, in canine brain; Aging,
        in feline brain
Brain biopsy
   in MUO evaluation, 1171
Brain tumors
   treatment of
      in dogs and cats, **1013–1038**. *See also specific methods, e.g.,* Stereotactic
        radiosurgery

CED, 1020–1026. *See also* Convection-enhanced delivery (CED)
    current options, 1014–1015
    immunotherapy, 1026–1031. *See also* Immunotherapy
    introduction, 1013–1015
    stereotactic radiosurgery, 1015–1020

C

CAA. *See* Cerebrovascular amyloid angiopathy (CAA)
Candidate gene analysis
    in identifying underlying cause of inherited neurologic disorders in dogs, 1228
Canine multiple system degeneration (CMSD), 1085–1086
Carbon dioxide
    oxygen and
        in altered states of consciousness management, 1052–1054
Cat(s)
    brain of
        aging effects on, **1113–1129**. *See also* Aging, in feline brain
    brain tumors in
        treatment of, **1013–1038**. *See also* Brain tumors, treatment of, in dogs and cats
    experimental models with SCI
        cell transplantation in, 1144–1145
    intervertebral disk disease in
        as factor in prognosis after SCI, 1147–1148
    SE in
        treatment of, 1107
Cavalier King Charles spaniels
    episodic falling in, 1093–1095
CED. *See* Convection-enhanced delivery (CED)
Cell transplantation
    in acute SCI management
        evidence for, 1142–1144
    in clinical cases with SCI, 1145
    in experimental models of SCI
        canine, 1144
        feline, 1144–1145
Central nervous system (CNS) disease
    immune-mediated
        neuroinflammation and, 1159–1161
    infectious
        testing for, 1193–1196
            introduction, 1193
            microbial agent–related, 1194–1196
            PCR–based techniques, 1193–1194
                limitations of, 1194
    noninfectious inflammatory
        categorization of, 1158
Central nervous system (CNS) neoplasia
    glucocorticoids for, 1065
Cerebellar cortical degeneration
    canine, 1080–1083

Cerebellar (*continued*)
    mapped diseases, 1083
    RAB24, 1083
    SEL1 mutation, 1082
    SPTBN2, 1083
Cerebrospinal fluid (CSF) analysis
  in MUO evaluation, 1171
Cerebrospinal fluid (CSF) production
  reduction in
    corticosteroid use and
      in small animal neurology, 1062
Cerebrovascular amyloid angiopathy (CAA)
  in canine brain
    aging and, 1117–1118
Chinooks
  PNKD in, 1095
Cleaved tau
  for neural injury and infection in small animals, 1191
Cluster seizures
  defined, 1104
  treatment of, 1109
CMSD. *See* Canine multiple system degeneration (CMSD)
CNS. *See* Central nervous system (CNS)
Consciousness
  altered states of
    in small animals, **1039–1058**
      coma scales in
        future uses, 1056
      described, 1040–1041
      diagnostic approach to, 1049–1052
        electrodiagnostic evaluation, 1051–1052
        laboratory and ancillary investigations, 1049
        neuroimaging, 1049–1051
      immediate emergency treatment for, 1052–1055
        diuretics, 1055
        fluid therapy, 1054–1055
        general care, 1052
        oxygen and carbon dioxide management, 1052–1054
      introduction, 1039–1040
      neurologic evaluation of, 1043–1049
      prognosis of, 1056
  impaired
    in small animals, 1040–1041. *See also* Consciousness, altered states of,
    in small animals
  neuro-anatomical basis of, 1041–1042
Convection-enhanced delivery (CED)
  in brain tumor management
    in dogs and cats, 1020–1026
      infusion techniques, 1024–1026
      introduction, 1020–1021

procedure, 1021–1022
technical factors governing insulate distributions in brain, 1022–1024
Corticosteroid(s)
in small animal neurology, **1059–1074**
detrimental effects of, 1068–1069
glucocorticoids for specific conditions, 1063–1068. *See also* Glucocorticoid(s),
in small animal neurology
introduction, 1059–1060
mechanisms of activity, 1060–1063
activity via nongenomic effects, 1061
activity via nuclear effects, 1060–1061
immune system effects, 1062–1063
metabolic effects, 1061–1062
blood pressure effects, 1062
CSF production reduction, 1062
gluconeogenic effects, 1061
therapeutic effects of glucocorticoids, 1061
CSF. *See* Cerebrospinal fluid (CSF)
Cutaneous trunci muscle reflex
as factor in prognosis after SCI, 1147
CyberKnife stereotactic radiosurgery
in brain tumor management
in dogs and cats, 1017–1018
Cytokine immunomodulation
in brain tumor management
in dogs and cats, 1027

D

Diarrhea
corticosteriod therapy and, 1068
Diuretics
in altered states of consciousness management, 1055
DNA testing
in inherited neurologic disorders in dogs, 1231–1233
Dog(s)
blood pressure abnormalities in
after SCI, 1137
brain of
aging effects on, **1113–1129**. *See also* Aging, in canine brain
brain tumors in
treatment of, **1013–1038**. *See also* Brain tumors, treatment of, in dogs and cats
experimental models with SCI
cell transplantation in, 1144
hereditary ataxia in, **1075–1089**. *See also* Hereditary ataxia(s), canine
inherited neurologic disorders in, **1223–1234**. *See also* Neurologic disorders,
inherited, canine
paroxysmal movement disorders in, **1091–1102**. *See also* Movement disorders,
paroxysmal, canine
SE in, 1107–1109

Dyskinesia(s)
    paroxysmal. *See* Paroxysmal dyskinesia
    phenobarbital-induced, 1100

E

Encephalitis
    necrotizing
        signalment, neurologic signs, and histopathologic features of, 1166–1168
Epileptoid cramping
    in Border Terriers, 1098
Episodic ataxia
    canine, 1086
Episodic head tremor syndrome
    canine, 1098–1099

F

Fluid therapy
    in altered states of consciousness management
        in small animals, 1054–1055
Focal seizure
    defined, 1104
Fosphenytoin
    for SE in dogs, 1109
Fungus(i)
    in infectious CNS disease
        testing for, 1196

G

Gamma Knife stereotactic radiosurgery
    in brain tumor management
        in dogs and cats, 1016–1017
Generalized seizure
    defined, 1103
Genetic linkage analysis
    in identifying underlying cause of inherited neurologic disorders in dogs, 1226
Genetic markers
    in identifying underlying cause of inherited neurologic disorders in dogs, 1225–1226
Genetic testing
    in MUO evaluation, 1172
Genome-wide association studies (GWAS)
    in identifying underlying cause of inherited neurologic disorders in dogs, 1226–1227
GFAP. *See* Glial fibrillary acidic protein (GFAP)
Glasgow Coma Scale
    modified
        in neurologic evaluation of impaired consciousness, 1043–1049
Glial fibrillary acidic protein (GFAP)
    for neural injury and infection in small animals, 1190–1191
Glucocorticoid(s)
    in small animal neurology

for CNS neoplasia, 1065
contraindications to, 1067–1068
for corticosteroid-responsive meningitis, 1063
for immune-mediated disease, 1063
for immune-mediated myositis, 1064–1065
for infectious disease, 1066
for MUO, 1064
for myasthenia gravis, 1065–1066
for pain control, 1066–1067
for polyradiculoneuritis, 1065–1066
therapeutic effects of, 1061
Granulomatous meningoencephalomyelitis
signalment, neurologic signs, and histopathologic features of, 1163–1166
Growth factors
for neural injury and infection in small animals, 1192
Gut ulceration
corticosteriod therapy and, 1068
GWAS. See Genome-wide association studies (GWAS)

H

Hereditary ataxia(s)
canine, **1075–1089**
cerebellar cortical degeneration, 1080–1083
classification of, 1076–1077
clinical approach to, 1077–1080
CMSD, 1085–1086
episodic, 1086
introduction, 1075
spinocerebellar degeneration, 1083–1085
without neurodegeneration, 1085

I

Immune-mediated CNS disease
glucocorticoids for, 1063
neuroinflammation and, 1159–1161
Immune system
corticosteroid use effects on
in small animals, 1062–1063
Immunosuppression
corticosteriod therapy and, 1068
Immunotherapy
in brain tumor management
in dogs and cats, 1026–1031
active immunotherapy, 1029–1030
adoptive immunotherapy, 1028–1029
cytokine immunomodulation, 1027
future directions in, 1030–1031
history/rationale, 1027
introduction, 1026

Immunotherapy (*continued*)
      monoclonal antibodies, 1027–1028
      passive immunotherapy, 1027–1029
      strategies, 1027–1030
Infectious disease(s)
  CNS
      testing for, 1193–1196. *See also* Central nervous system (CNS) disease, infectious,
          testing for
    glucocorticoids for, 1066
    testing for
      in MUO evaluation, 1171–1172
Inflammatory disease(s)
  noninfectious
    of CNS
      categorization of, 1158
Inherited neurologic disorders
  in dogs, **1223–1234**. *See also* Neurologic disorders, inherited, canine
Intervertebral disk disease
  in cats
    as factor in prognosis after SCI, 1147–1148

L

Leukoencephalitis
  necrotizing
    signalment, neurologic signs, and histopathologic features of, 1168
Levetiracetam
  for SE in dogs, 1107–1109
Linear accelerator stereotactic radiosurgery
  in brain tumor management
    in dogs and cats, 1016
LMN. *See* Lower motor neuron (LMN)
Lower motor neuron (LMN)
  vs. UMN
    in clinical evaluation of patient following severe SCI, 1134
Lower motor neuron (LMN) tetraparesis
  acute, **1201–1222**. *See also* Acute lower motor neuron (LMN) tetraparesis
Lysosomal storage diseases
  canine
    aging effects on, 1118–1119

M

Magnetic resonance imaging (MRI)
  in prognosis after SCI, 1148
Matrix metalloproteinases (MMPs)
  for neural injury and infection in small animals, 1192
MBP. *See* Myelin basic protein (MBP)
Meningitis
  corticosteroid-responsive
    glucocorticoids for, 1063

Meningoencephalitis
    necrotizing
        signalment, neurologic signs, and histopathologic features of, 1167–1168
Meningoencephalomyelitis
    granulomatous
        signalment, neurologic signs, and histopathologic features of, 1163–1166
Meningoencephalomyelitis of unknown origin (MUO), **1157–1185**
    diagnostic evaluation of, 1168–1172
        brain biopsy in, 1171
        cross-sectional imaging in, 1169–1170
        CSF analysis in, 1171
        infectious disease testing in, 1171–1172
    glucocorticoids for, 1064
    granulomatous meningoencephalomyelitis, 1163–1166
    histopathologic features of, 1161–1163
    introduction, 1157–1159
    necrotizing encephalitis, 1166–1168
    neuroinflammation in, 1161–1163
    neurologic signs of, 1161–1163
    prognosis of, 1175–1176
    signalment of, 1163–1168
    treatment of, 1172–1175
Metabolism
    corticosteroid use effects on
        in small animals, 1061–1062
Microbial agents
    in infectious CNS disease
        testing for, 1194–1196
            bacteria, 1194–1195
            fungus, 1196
            protozoa, 1195
            rickettsia, 1196
            viruses, 1195
MMPs. See Matrix metalloproteinases (MMPs)
Monoclonal antibodies
    in brain tumor management
        in dogs and cats, 1027–1028
Movement disorders
    paroxysmal
        canine, **1091–1102**
            inherited diseases, 1093–1099
                epileptoid cramping in Border Terriers, 1098
                episodic falling in Cavalier King Charles spaniels, 1093–1095
                episodic head tremor syndrome, 1098–1099
                PNKD in Chinooks, 1095
                Scottie cramp in Scottish Terriers, 1095–1098
            introduction, 1091–1093
            involuntary, 1100
            paroxysmal dyskinesia, 1099–1100
                in boxers, 1099
            phenobarbital-induced dyskinesia, 1100

Movement (*continued*)
      phenobarbital-responsive paroxysmal dyskinesia, 1099–1100
      sporadic reports, 1099–1100
MUO. *See* Meningoencephalomyelitis of unknown origin (MUO)
Muscle wasting
  corticosteriod therapy and, 1068–1069
Mutation identification
  in identifying underlying cause of inherited neurologic disorders in dogs, 1225
Myasthenia gravis
  acquired acute fulminating, 1216–1218. *See also* Acquired acute fulminating
    myasthenia gravis
  glucocorticoids for, 1065–1066
Myelin basic protein (MBP)
  for neural injury and infection in small animals, 1190
Myositis
  immune-mediated
    glucocorticoids for, 1064–1065

N

Necrotizing encephalitis
  signalment, neurologic signs, and histopathologic features of, 1166–1168
Necrotizing leukoencephalitis
  signalment, neurologic signs, and histopathologic features of, 1168
Necrotizing meningoencephalitis
  signalment, neurologic signs, and histopathologic features of, 1167–1168
Neoplasia(s)
  CNS
    glucocorticoids for, 1065
Neural injury
  biomarkers for, **1187–1199**
    cleaved tau, 1191
    in diagnostic testing, 1188
    GFAP, 1190–1191
    growth factors, 1192
    introduction, 1187–1188
    limitations of, 1188–1192
    MBP, 1190
    MMPs, 1192
    NSE, 1190
Neurodegeneration
  ataxias without, 1085
Neurofilament heavy chain (NF-H)
  phosphorylated
    for neural injury and infection in small animals, 1191–1192
Neuroinflammation
  histopathology of, 1161
  in immune-mediated CNS disease, 1159–1161
  in MUO, 1161–1163
  overview of, 1159–1163

Neurologic disorders
   inherited
      canine, **1223–1234**
         characteristics of, 1223–1224
         DNA testing for, 1231–1233
         identifying underlying cause of, 1224–1230
            candidate gene analysis, 1228
            genetic linkage analysis, 1226
            genetic markers, 1225–1226
            GWAS, 1226–1227
            mutation identification, 1225
            target resequencing, 1227–1228
            whole genome sequencing, 1228–1229
            whole transcriptome sequencing, 1229–1230
         sources of data regarding, 1224
Neuron-specific enolase (NSE)
   for neural injury and infection in small animals, 1190
Neuronavigation, **1235–1248**
   devices for
      development of, 1236–1239
   frameless systems, 1239
   need for, 1235–1236
   pointer-based frameless technique, 1240–1243. *See also* Pointer-based frameless
      neuronavigation technique
   sources of error with, 1243–1244
   uses of, 1244–1246
   veterinary applications, 1244–1245
   veterinary stereotaxy–related struggles and, 1239–1240
NF-H. *See* Neurofilament heavy chain (NF-H)
Niemann-Pick type C (NPC) disease
   feline
      neuronal loss in
         aging and, 1120–1121
Noninfectious inflammatory disease
   of CNS
      categorization of, 1158
NPC disease. *See* Niemann-Pick type C (NPC) disease
NSE. *See* Neuron-specific enolase (NSE)

O

Oxygen and carbon dioxide
   in altered states of consciousness management, 1052–1054

P

Pain control
   glucocorticoids for, 1066–1067
Pain sensation
   detectable
      as factor in prognosis after SCI, 1147

Paroxysmal dyskinesia
   in boxers, 1099
   phenobarbital-responsive
      canine, 1099–1100
Paroxysmal movement disorders
   canine, **1091–1102**. See also Movement disorders, paroxysmal, canine
Paroxysmal nonkinesigenic dyskinesia (PNKD)
   in Chinooks, 1095
PCR. See Polymerase chain reaction (PCR)
Phenobarbital-induced dyskinesia
   canine, 1100
Phenobarbital-responsive paroxysmal dyskinesia
   canine, 1099–1100
Phosphorylated neurofilament heavy chain (NF-H)
   for neural injury and infection in small animals, 1191–1192
PNKD. See Paroxysmal nonkinesigenic dyskinesia (PNKD)
Pointer-based frameless neuronavigation technique, 1240–1243
   described, 1240
   identifiable fiducial markers, 1241–1242
   image space creation, 1242
   image tracker, 1243
   subject tracker, 1242–1243
   tomographic data set, 1240–1241
Polymerase chain reaction (PCR)–based techniques
   in infectious CNS disease testing, 1193–1194
      limitations of, 1194
Polyradiculoneuritis
   glucocorticoids for, 1065–1066
Protozoa
   in infectious CNS disease
      testing for, 1195

R

Radiosurgery
   stereotactic
      in brain tumor management
         in dogs and cats, 1015–1020. See also Stereotactic radiosurgery, in
         brain tumor management, in dogs and cats
Refractory status epilepticus (RSE)
   defined, 1104
   super
      defined, 1104
Rehabilitation
   after SCI
      role for, 1146
Respiratory dysfunction
   SCI and, 1137–1138
Rickettsia
   in infectious CNS disease
      testing for, 1196
RSE. See Refractory status epilepticus (RSE)

S

Schiff-Sherrington syndrome
  clinical evaluation of patient following severe SCI and, 1134–1135
SCI. *See* Spinal cord injury (SCI)
Scottie cramp
  in Scottish Terriers, 1095–1098
Scottish Terriers
  Scottie cramp in, 1095–1098
SE. *See* Status epilepticus (SE)
Seizure(s)
  acute repetitive
    defined, 1104
  cluster
    defined, 1104
    treatment of, 1109
  focal
    defined, 1104
  generalized
    defined, 1103
  terminology related to, 1103–1104
Sensory dysfunction
  SCI and, 1135–1136
Spinal cord function
  assessment of
    ancillary methods in, 1138–1142
      clinical scoring, 1138
      electrophysiologic measures, 1141–1142
      kinematics, 1139
      MRI advances, 1139–1140
Spinal cord injury (SCI)
  acute, **1131–1156**
    introduction, 1131–1132
    treatment of
      cell transplantation in
        evidence for, 1142–1144
        in experimental canine models, 1144
        in experimental feline models, 1144–1145
      new pharmacologic interventions in, 1142
      standard of care with urinary retention management, 1145–1146
  blood pressure abnormalities following
    in dogs, 1137
  causes of, 1132–1133
  clinical cases with
    cell transplantation in, 1145
  early rehabilitation after
    role for, 1146
  experimental canine models of
    cell transplantation in, 1144
  prognosis following, 1147–1148
  respiratory dysfunction following, 1137–1138

Spinal (*continued*)
  sensory dysfunction following, 1135–1136
  severe
    clinical evaluation of patient following, 1133–1138
      normal locomotion, 1133
      sequential appearance of neurologic deficits after spinal cord damage,
        1133–1134
      spinal shock and Schiff-Sherrington syndrome, 1134–1135
      UMN *vs.* LMN, 1134
    standards of care for, 1142–1146
    treatment of, 1142–1146
    urinary dysfunction following, 1136–1137
Spinal shock
  clinical evaluation of patient following severe SCI and, 1134–1135
Spinocerebellar degeneration
  canine, 1083–1085
SRSE. *See* Super refractory status epilepticus (SRSE)
Status epilepticus (SE), **1103–1112**
  convulsive
    defined, 1104
  defined, 1103
  introduction, 1104–1105
  nonconvulsive
    defined, 1104
  refractory
    defined, 1104
    super
      defined, 1104
  treatment of, 1105–1109
    current and historical drug therapy in, 1106–1107
      in cats, 1107
      in dogs, 1107
      in humans, 1106–1107
    fosphenytoin in, 1109
    future possibilities in, 1110
    general considerations in, 1105–1106
    general standard of practice, 1107
    initial
      single-agent *vs.* combined therapy for, 1109
    levetiracetam in, 1108–1109
Stereotactic radiosurgery
  in brain tumor management
    in dogs and cats, 1015–1020
      CyberKnife stereotactic radiosurgery, 1017–1018
      described, 1019–1020
      Gamma Knife stereotactic radiosurgery, 1016–1017
      introduction/history, 1015
      linear accelerator stereotactic radiosurgery, 1016
      radiobiological considerations, 1018–1019
      technical aspects, 1015–1018

Super refractory status epilepticus (SRSE)
 defined, 1104

T

Target resequencing
 in identifying underlying cause of inherited neurologic disorders in dogs,
  1227–1228
Tetraparesis
 acute LMN, **1201–1222**. See also Acute lower motor neuron (LMN) tetraparesis
Tick paralysis, 1213–1216
 clinical signs of, 1214–1215
 diagnosis of, 1215
 introduction, 1213–1214
 pathophysiology of, 1214
 prevention of, 1216
 prognosis of, 1215–1216
 treatment of, 1215–1216
Transplantation
 cell. See Cell transplantation
Tumor(s)
 brain. See Brain tumors

U

UMN. See Upper motor neuron (UMN)
Upper motor neuron (UMN)
 vs. LMN
  in clinical evaluation of patient following severe SCI, 1134
Urinary dysfunction
 SCI and, 1136–1137

V

Vascular disorders
 in canine brain
  aging and, 1116–1117
Veterinary sternotomy
 struggles related to
  neuronavigation and, 1239–1240
Virus(es)
 in infectious CNS disease
  testing for, 1195
Vomiting
 corticosteriod therapy and, 1068

W

Whole genome sequencing, 1228–1229
Whole transcriptome sequencing
 in identifying underlying cause of inherited neurologic disorders in dogs,
  1229–1230

United States Postal Service

Statement of Ownership, Management, and Circulation
(All Periodicals Publications Except Requestor Publications)

1. Publication Title	2. Publication Number	3. Filing Date
Veterinary Clinics of North America: Small Animal Practice	0 0 3 - 1 5 0	9/14/14

4. Issue Frequency	5. Number of Issues Published Annually	6. Annual Subscription Price
Jan, Mar, May, Jul, Sep, Nov	6	$310.00

7. Complete Mailing Address of Known Office of Publication *(Not printer)* *(Street, city, county, state, and ZIP+4®)*

Elsevier Inc.
360 Park Avenue South
New York, NY 10010-1710

Contact Person: Stephen R. Bushing
Telephone (Include area code): 215-239-3688

8. Complete Mailing Address of Headquarters or General Business Office of Publisher *(Not printer)*

Elsevier Inc., 360 Park Avenue South, New York, NY 10010-1710

9. Full Names and Complete Mailing Addresses of Publisher, Editor, and Managing Editor *(Do not leave blank)*

Publisher *(Name and complete mailing address)*

Linda Belfus, Elsevier, Inc., 1600 John F. Kennedy Blvd. Suite 1800, Philadelphia, PA 19103-2899

Editor *(Name and complete mailing address)*

Patrick Manley, Elsevier, Inc., 1600 John F. Kennedy Blvd. Suite 1800, Philadelphia, PA 19103-2899

Managing Editor *(Name and complete mailing address)*

Adrianne Brigido, Elsevier, Inc., 1600 John F. Kennedy Blvd. Suite 1800, Philadelphia, PA 19103-2899

10. Owner *(Do not leave blank. If the publication is owned by a corporation, give the name and address of the corporation immediately followed by the names and addresses of all stockholders owning or holding 1 percent or more of the total amount of stock. If not owned by a corporation, give the names and addresses of the individual owners. If owned by a partnership or other unincorporated firm, give its name and address as well as those of each individual owner. If the publication is published by a nonprofit organization, give its name and address.)*

Full Name	Complete Mailing Address
Wholly owned subsidiary of	1600 John F. Kennedy Blvd, Ste. 1800
Reed/Elsevier, US holdings	Philadelphia, PA 19103-2899

11. Known Bondholders, Mortgagees, and Other Security Holders Owning or Holding 1 Percent or More of Total Amount of Bonds, Mortgages, or Other Securities. If none, check box ☐ None

Full Name	Complete Mailing Address
N/A	

12. Tax Status *(For completion by nonprofit organizations authorized to mail at nonprofit rates) (Check one)*
The purpose, function, and nonprofit status of this organization and the exempt status for federal income tax purposes:
☒ Has Not Changed During Preceding 12 Months
☐ Has Changed During Preceding 12 Months *(Publisher must submit explanation of change with this statement)*

PS Form 3526, August 2012 (Page 1 of 3 (Instructions Page 3)) PSN 7530-01-000-9931 **PRIVACY NOTICE:** See our Privacy policy in www.usps.com

---

13. Publication Title	14. Issue Date for Circulation Data Below
Veterinary Clinics of North America: Small Animal Practice	July 2014

15. Extent and Nature of Circulation		Average No. Copies Each Issue During Preceding 12 Months	No. Copies of Single Issue Published Nearest to Filing Date
a. Total Number of Copies *(Net press run)*		1,489	1,688
b. Paid Circulation (By Mail and Outside the Mail)	(1) Mailed Outside-County Paid Subscriptions Stated on PS Form 3541. *(Include paid distribution above nominal rate, advertiser's proof copies, and exchange copies)*	951	1,066
	(2) Mailed In-County Paid Subscriptions Stated on PS Form 3541 *(Include paid distribution above nominal rate, advertiser's proof copies, and exchange copies)*		
	(3) Paid Distribution Outside the Mails Including Sales Through Dealers and Carriers, Street Vendors, Counter Sales, and Other Paid Distribution Outside USPS®	192	212
	(4) Paid Distribution by Other Classes Mailed Through the USPS (e.g. First-Class Mail®)		
c. Total Paid Distribution *(Sum of 15b (1), (2), (3), and (4))*	▲	1,143	1,278
d. Free or Nominal Rate Distribution (By Mail and Outside the Mail)	(1) Free or Nominal Rate Outside-County Copies Included on PS Form 3541	103	110
	(2) Free or Nominal Rate In-County Copies Included on PS Form 3541		
	(3) Free or Nominal Rate Copies Mailed at Other Classes Through the USPS (e.g. First-Class Mail)		
	(4) Free or Nominal Rate Distribution Outside the Mail (Carriers or other means)		
e. Total Free or Nominal Rate Distribution *(Sum of 15d (1), (2), (3) and (4))*	▲	103	110
f. Total Distribution *(Sum of 15c and 15e)*	▲	1,246	1,388
g. Copies not Distributed *(See instructions to publishers #4 (page #3))*	▲	243	300
h. Total *(Sum of 15f and g)*	▲	1,489	1,688
i. Percent Paid *(15c divided by 15f times 100)*	▲	91.73%	92.07%

16. Total circulation includes electronic copies. Report circulation on PS Form 3526-X worksheet.

17. Publication of Statement of Ownership
If the publication is a general publication, publication of this statement is required. Will be printed in the <u>November 2014</u> issue of this publication.

18. Signature and Title of Editor, Publisher, Business Manager, or Owner

[signature] Stephen R. Bushing – Inventory Distribution Coordinator

Date: September 14, 2014

I certify that all information furnished on this form is true and complete. I understand that anyone who furnishes false or misleading information on this form or who omits material or information requested on the form may be subject to criminal sanctions (including fines and imprisonment) and/or civil sanctions (including civil penalties).

PS Form 3526, August 2012 (Page 2 of 3)

Moving?

Make sure your subscription moves with you!

To notify us of your new address, find your **Clinics Account Number** (located on your mailing label above your name), and contact customer service at:

Email: journalscustomerservice-usa@elsevier.com

800-654-2452 (subscribers in the U.S. & Canada)
314-447-8871 (subscribers outside of the U.S. & Canada)

Fax number: 314-447-8029

Elsevier Health Sciences Division
Subscription Customer Service
3251 Riverport Lane
Maryland Heights, MO 63043

*To ensure uninterrupted delivery of your subscription, please notify us at least 4 weeks in advance of move.